"In *The Lions of Winter: Survival and Sacrifice on Mount Washington*, author Ty Gagne masterfully weaves a gripping narrative of heroism, endurance, and heartbreak in one of the harshest environments on Earth. Set amidst the unforgiving winter wilderness of Mount Washington, Gagne tells the true story of a daring search and rescue mission to find two missing climbers who have fallen prey to extreme weather conditions. Through vivid storytelling, Gagne brings to life the extreme challenges faced by the rescuers—subzero temperatures, blizzard conditions, and treacherous terrain—as they risk everything to save those in peril. The book is both a tribute to the bravery and selflessness of these heroes who put their lives on the line to save others and a powerful meditation on the delicate balance between humanity and nature's most formidable forces. A must-read for anyone captivated by the raw, untamed beauty of the White Mountains and the extraordinary people who brave its dangers."

—Tiffany Eddy, CEO of Tiffany Eddy Media and former anchor/reporter for WMUR-TV

"In *The Lions of Winter*, Ty Gagne tells a compelling story of camaraderie and loss in the harsh winter mountains of New Hampshire, weaving intricate chain-reaction timelines and stark alpine landscapes with themes of fellowship, self-sacrifice, survival, providence, and redemption. Along the way, *Lions* offers profound insights into the corporeal struggles of the rescuers who risk all to find lost souls and the rescued struggling to survive unimaginable conditions."

—Mike & Stomp, "Sounds Like a Search and Rescue" podcast

The Lions of Winter
Survival and Sacrifice on Mount Washington

Copyright © Ty Gagne 2024

ISBN: 979-8-9899998-3-5

Printed in Canada by Friesens Corporation,
 Altona, Manitoba

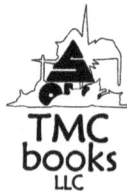

TMC
books
LLC

731 Tasker Hill Rd.
Conway, NH 03818
USA
www.tmcbooks.com

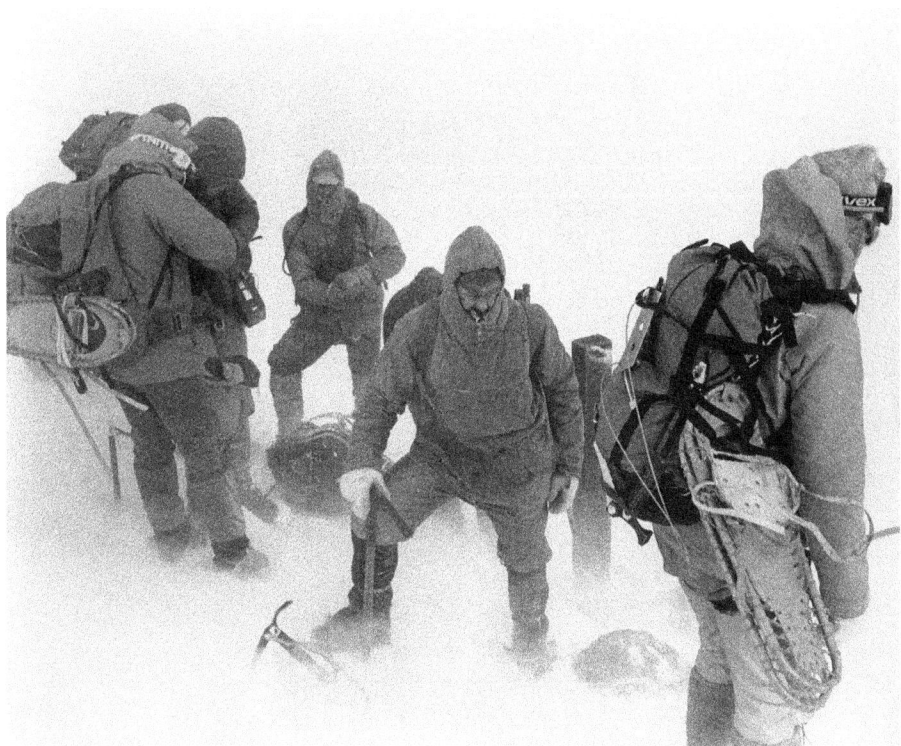

The Lions of Winter

Survival and Sacrifice on Mount Washington

Ty Gagne

FOR

Mom, who encouraged me to see the beauty of each stone.
And Dad, who instilled in me the belief that none of them
should be left unturned.
I love you both.

And

Ron Reynolds; my friend, teacher, and climbing mentor, who
showed me that some of the most enriching and meaningful
learning experiences are found in high places.

"Ty Gagne is a very fine writer. Struck by the number of lives that changed forever in this tragedy of two lost climbers and those who endangered themselves to help them, he has compiled an exceptionally full recounting of this historic rescue mission. The amount of detail Gagne has gathered is truly admirable, and his work honors everyone involved."

—Alison Osius, senior editor at *Outside*, former editor of *Climbing* and *Rock and Ice* magazines, and author of *Second Ascent: The Story of Hugh Herr*

"It has been over 40 years since a volunteer rescuer was killed while searching for two lost climbers in the White Mountains. In gripping detail, Ty Gagne examines the tragedy, describing how the young climbers got lost, the risks taken by the rescuers, and the discovery of the climbers just as hope faded for their safe recovery. He writes about the changes brought about by the incident and its effect on those involved. Gagne skillfully weaves together interviews and historical records to place the reader directly at the scene, and the result is a book that is impossible to put down. It is sure to be the definitive account of an event that has haunted the climbing community for decades."

—Barbara Tetreault, longtime North Country reporter and managing editor

"Ty Gagne is a fearless storyteller. Fearless because, in the revealing of this tale and others, he walks directly into the most harrowing of human experiences. Two young men who believe they are going to die, another who has no idea that his life will end that day. A family who has no warning of the agony about to hit, and others that will feel unimaginable relief. How do people survive? How do rescuers continue to push through their own fear and exhaustion? How do these people manage such loss? Using the mountains as his canvas, Gagne explores the compartments humans somehow create in our minds and our bodies, compartments that allow us to seek the beauty of life's unpredictable adventures amidst the ever-victorious power of nature."

—Lynn Lyons, LICSW, anxiety expert, author, and host of the "Flusterclux" podcast

"A captivating read of life, love, and selflessness in the White Mountains of New Hampshire. The tragic loss of Albert Dow's life in an avalanche in 1982 on Mount Washington during a search for two lost climbers illustrates the indelible impact of his sacrifice, his character, and his memory. Gagne pulls together the puzzle pieces of facts, weather, survival, passion, and fate in this timeless tale. The page-turning journey honors the many people who make up the bedrock of the outdoor community and the members of the Mountain Rescue Service who are the real-life action heroes of the Granite State."

—Dan Egan, extreme ski pioneer, host of the "603Podcast," and author of *Thirty Years in a White Haze*

"On virtually any given day, the majestic White Mountains of New Hampshire can turn sheer joy to despair and contentment into survival. The line between them can be disturbingly thin. The sacrifices of those who keep us on this side of the line are stories that need to be known. In *The Lions of Winter*, Ty Gagne achieves this in a compelling and emotional retelling of a real-life event that forever changed the course of search and rescue in the Whites. I will be making it required reading for anyone who comes out with me."

—Commissioner Taylor Caswell, New Hampshire Department of Business and Economic Affairs

"This is a captivating read about the bravery and skill of rescuers in the White Mountains of New Hampshire. It will interest anyone who would like to understand how challenging such rescues can be and the incredible sacrifices made by the heroic volunteers and their families. It is refreshing to learn of the willingness of so many selfless people to help others in times of distress and need. Gagne's masterful storytelling captures the action and emotion in great detail, keeping you turning the pages."

—Patrik Frisk, former president of Timberland

"Ty Gagne has written a gripping and vivid account of two teenage climbers lost on Mount Washington in 1982 and the heroic yet tragic rescue mission that followed. Through extensive research and interviews with many who were involved, Gagne brings this harrowing ordeal to life in dramatic detail. As the director of a documentary on this subject, I found *The Lions of Winter* completely absorbing and filled with new and astonishing details. The book is outstanding. I could not put it down."

—Matthew Orr, director of *Augmented*

"For most New Englanders, including myself, Mount Washington is shrouded in legend, beauty, and danger. *The Lions of Winter* highlights one of the most trying tales the mountain has seen in recent history. Ty Gagne offers a unique look into both sides of a complex rescue attempt that impacted the community in more ways than those could have imagined. For anyone not familiar with the region, Gagne's detailed research paints a vivid image of a harsh landscape that has defined the lives of so many around it. The relationship between rescuers and victims leaves readers asking themselves questions about risk, sacrifice, and the true cost of exploration."

—Nick Martini, director of *109 Below* and founder of Stept Studios

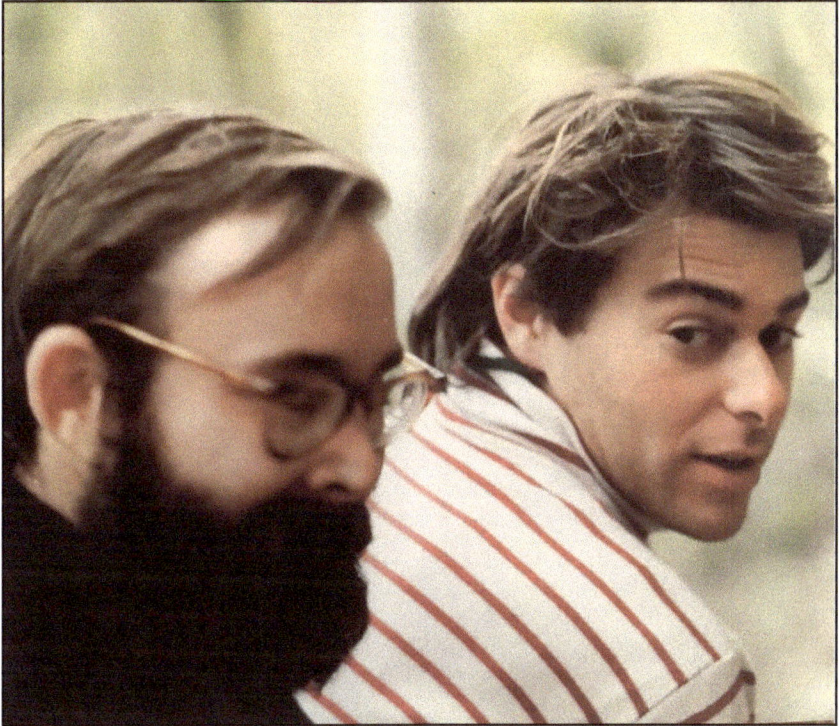

This book is dedicated to Albert Dow III (right) and Michael Hartrich
of Mountain Rescue Service, true friends and steadfast teammates, who
demonstrated that within the beauty of selflessness lies the gift of sacrifice.

It is an iron rule of history that what looks inevitable in hindsight was far from obvious at the time.

—Yuval Noah Harari, *Sapiens: A Brief History of Humankind*

Contents

Author's Note

*One of the great contradictions of climbing writing is that the bigger
and deeper the experience the more difficult they tend to be
to write about.*

—Marc-André Leclerc, world-renowned alpinist killed in an
avalanche in 2018

When Albert Dow III was killed in an avalanche on New Hampshire's Mount Washington on Jan. 25, 1982, while searching for two young ice climbers, I was in the eighth grade. Although I lived in the same state and was just a 90-minute drive away, I was oblivious to the tragedy and subsequent heartbreak that swept through the Mount Washington Valley and beyond.

As an awkward and uninformed teenager, my concerns at the time drifted between the very local and more distant matters. Would I start in the upcoming middle-school basketball game? No, I would not. At the next dance, could I summon enough intestinal fortitude to approach a girl? Sadly, I remained seated during Led Zeppelin's eight-minute epic "Stairway to Heaven." Would President Ronald Reagan protect us from nuclear war with the Soviet Union? Thankfully, mutually assured destruction was averted.

I first learned of Albert Dow in the mid-1990s during a winter trip on Mount Adams with my climbing partner and mentor Ron Reynolds. Ron was my middle-school industrial arts teacher who introduced me to rock climbing during my sixth-grade year. I obviously couldn't dance or excel athletically, and I was deathly afraid of heights at the time, but somehow Ron thought rock climbing would be a good outlet for me. Decades after that first terrifying rappel, we were still connected by the strong bond of friendship.

Ron had been a longtime member of the North Conway-based all-volunteer Mountain Rescue Service, the same team Albert was on when he was killed. Although they hadn't been on any callouts together, Ron had climbed with Albert at one of the many crags found throughout the Mount Washington Valley.

Our snow-climbing route that winter day would take us up the steep headwall of King Ravine on the western side of Mount Adams. It is well-known avalanche terrain, and during our long slog into the base of the ravine we talked about the risks involved in what we were about to do. To drive the point home, Ron shared with me how Albert and teammate Michael Hartrich had been caught in an avalanche on Mount Washington's Lion Head during a search. The slide had occurred in a glade of birch trees on what was considered to be innocuous terrain. At the time of the avalanche, it seemed unimaginable to anyone with knowledge of that terrain that it could happen there. Ron and I enjoyed hard-packed névé snow as we ascended the headwall unroped using crampons and a mountaineering axe. The greatest risk we assumed that day was a "long sliding fall," a more frequent cause of injury and death in the Presidential Range than avalanches.

I briefly recalled Ron's mention of Albert Dow in February 1999 when I climbed the Winter Route on Lion Head with Rick, a work colleague, and my brother-in-law Tom. After summitting Mount Washington, we realized that our descent back to Lion Head would be over ice-coated terrain and that a fall by any one of us could be catastrophic. We opted for the better part of valor and made an unplanned descent down the Mount Washington Auto Road. Upon reaching Route 16, I was forced to hitchhike for my first and last time in order to get back to my vehicle at Pinkham Notch Visitor Center.

Later that evening on WMUR-TV, I learned that shortly after we started our descent of the Auto Road, a hiker was seriously injured while glissading and wearing crampons in the ice-covered southeast snowfields that we'd been on hours earlier. The incident required a technical rescue by 20 rescuers, including Mount Washington Observatory summit staff, the Appalachian Mountain Club, the U.S. Forest Service, and Mountain Rescue Service, which would conclude at 2:30 a.m. the following morning.

The events of that day on Mount Washington returned the story of Dow's fate to the back of my mind, where it remained dormant until almost two decades later, when I began writing stories of tragedy and survival in the White Mountains. Those efforts included conversations with dozens of past and present members of the New Hampshire search and rescue community. In almost every discussion, there was one name that consistently emerged: Albert Dow. With each interaction and other information gleaned during my research, it became clear that Dow's tragedy was a watershed moment for New Hampshire's backcountry search and rescue operations and has had significant influence on the way they are managed today.

As I moved closer and closer to this story and the desire to write it, I had serious reservations about doing so because I and many others consider the tragedy on Lion Head to be literally and figuratively on sacred ground. I knew I'd be opening some old and still painful emotional wounds. As I shared time with those closest to Albert and this tragedy, there were moments of deep sorrow and also immense joy as friends, family, and teammates reflected on his life. For that I am truly grateful to Albert's sisters, Susan Dow-Johnson and Caryl Dow, past and present members of the New Hampshire search and rescue community representing several agencies and organizations, and countless others who contributed to my work. I spoke with as many people as I could who were directly involved in the 1982 mission, including the young climbers for whom rescuers were searching, Hugh Herr and Jeff Batzer. I am grateful to both for their willingness to share their stories in hopes that others may learn from their multi-day ordeal.

Since 1982, a small number of those involved have passed away, and a small number have chosen not to participate. My heart goes out to the families of those who are no longer here to share their experiences, and I understand and respect the wishes of those who declined my request to talk. I'd also be remiss if I didn't acknowledge the work of writer Alison Osius, who early on wrote so eloquently of the search for Hugh and Jeff, and the loss of Albert Dow, in her excellent biography of Herr, *Second Ascent: The Story of Hugh Herr*, which was published in 1991 and is no longer in print.

The pain of Dow's sudden death at age 28 is still evident on the faces and in the words of his family and search and rescue teammates. It remains a traumatic event for those who were directly involved, and the passage of time has affected recall and perception. When thinking back on these types of events, people who were standing shoulder to shoulder might remember seeing, hearing, and experiencing completely different things. With that in mind, I have done my best to share these memories as authentically as they were shared with me. I take full responsibility for any errors, misrepresentations, or omissions.

Why did I decide to write about a search and rescue mission that happened more than 40 years ago? Besides wanting to raise awareness of avalanche hazard on Mount Washington and the surrounding peaks and the consequences our actions can have on those who venture into the backcountry to help us, I was inspired to write the story following a conversation I had with Albert Dow's close friend and teammate Michael Hartrich at the Pope Memorial Library in North Conway, N.H. Hartrich was mere steps away from Albert that day on Lion Head and was also buried in the avalanche that took Albert's life, but survived without serious injury.

Sitting at a high-top table amid shelves of books and beautifully restored wood trimmings, Hartrich looked down at the hot cup of tea cradled in both hands and offered his thoughts on the value of Albert's story being brought back into the light:

> No one much talks about Albert, and I think most of the climbing community have been kind of silent and have this undercurrent of sorrow about it. It's sad, really, because you figured he'd be somebody you'd know long enough—you'd know his kids, you'd see him around, you'd still do things together once in a while. And then he's completely gone.

I felt the time had come to revive the story of Albert Dow in an effort to pay tribute to the man, his selflessness, and the important legacy he left behind in the White Mountain search and rescue community. It is in many ways a timeless story, and I am honored to tell it.

INTRODUCTION

A CHRISTMAS MEMORY

*Anyone can have a friend, but the one that would
walk in a storm to find you is all you will ever need.*
—Shannon L. Alder, author and life coach

**Marjorie and Albert Dow Jr.'s home
Tuftonboro Corner, N.H.
Saturday, Dec. 26, 1981
Morning**

Albert Dow III was feeling joyful during this holiday time with his family. A day after Christmas, the festive aura remained strong at his childhood home. On Christmas Eve he'd made the 45-minute drive southwest from the apartment in Brownfield, Maine, that he shared with his partner, Joan Wrigley, who was out of state celebrating Christmas with her own family. It was the last holiday the couple would spend apart, since they planned to announce their engagement on Valentine's Day. But later that day during the family visit, 28-year-old Albert planned to share the news with his mother Marjorie in a private conversation.

During this holiday season, the Dow home might easily have been mistaken for a winter feature in *Yankee Magazine*. Inside, a large, fully dressed balsam fir anchored the first-floor living room. Albert's father, Albert Jr., was known for cutting off the lower branches and plugging them into holes that he drilled in sparse sections of the tree. Homemade garlands threaded their way through stair banisters, and pine boughs were decorously placed in bowls, around candle holders, and along the fireplace's mantle.

Outside, the front of the house frequently drew the admiring eyes of passersby. The front door was framed by more garland, and two giant wreaths adorned the doors of the large attached barn. A carriage lamp atop a pole was wrapped in colorful lights. When snowflakes fell, the effect was of a quintessential holiday greeting card.

At varying intervals that morning, family members awoke and shuffled in the direction of the kitchen, the home's traditional mustering point. As they drifted toward the muffled sound of conversation and the wafting aroma of freshly brewed coffee, the floorboards of the center-chimney New England colonial creaked and groaned in response. It was impossible to move undetected as the entire structure protested winter's bite, which had so easily penetrated the antique house. But for Marjorie and Albert Jr., these sounds signaled happiness. Their loved ones were home, an increasingly rare occurrence as the family grew in age and number.

Marjorie moved effortlessly between countertop and stove, as daughters Susan Dow-Johnson, 29, and Caryl Dow, 23, stood ready to help. It was well known in this picturesque New Hampshire village, one of four encompassing the town of Tuftonboro, that Marjorie was an excellent and fiercely independent cook. It had been years since her daughters had given up on expressing their frustration and resigned themselves to the role of spectators.

Just off the kitchen Albert Jr. was in casual conversation with their son-in-law Charles, Susan's husband. Both were careful to avoid any involvement in the kitchen's dynamics, letting Marjorie and her daughters work things out among themselves. For Albert, his wife's total confidence in the kitchen was a far cry from the early days of their marriage. He often shared the story of how, on one morning not long after their nuptials, he walked into the kitchen and found his wife weeping. "I don't know how to cook," she told him. Albert had navigated that situation with a perfect blend of compassion and encouragement, and from that moment on Marjorie pursued the art of cooking with passionate abandon.

As years passed, the couple entertained frequently. "My mother often sought out new recipes, and even if Dad didn't like every one, he never wanted to deflate her effort," recalls Caryl. "She loved hostessing for sure. It was their fun."

Four-year-old Amy, wide awake and oblivious to the chill, toddled back and forth between mother Susan and Uncle Albert. Quick to remind everyone that she was on the cusp of her fifth birthday, Amy sought brief respite at her mother's side in order to catch her breath from fits of laughter. Dressed in pajama bottoms and his beloved navy blue, reindeer-patterned sweater that an aunt had knitted for him, her Uncle Albert was in full-on Kermit the Frog mode, imitating the famed Muppet with the precision of an expert impressionist. He would often call his niece, who lived in Pennsylvania, and spend their entire conversation in character. There was a strong bond between them, and Amy was clearly delighted to experience her uncle's humor in person.

While the group awaited breakfast, conversation turned to young Albert's membership in the all-volunteer North Conway-based Mountain Rescue Service (MRS). Less than two weeks earlier, Albert had been with MRS on Mount Washington and its iconic Auto Road in severe weather, searching for a missing Thiokol snow tractor operator from the Poland Spring, Maine-based WMTW television station, which at that time broadcast the weather from the summit. The search, still fresh in the minds of those in and around the Mount Washington Valley, had garnered significant attention throughout New England.

Since its inception in 1972, MRS generally operated under the radar, which was right where it wanted to be. But for the Dow family, it felt as though backcountry callouts were becoming more and more frequent during Albert's three years with the team, and they were worried for his safety. Joe Lentini, a friend and fellow MRS teammate of Albert's, says today that callouts were indeed on the rise during that time. "Rescues seemed to be more frequent back then, and there are two reasons for that. [Climbing] gear wasn't as advanced, and the winters were colder. When people get hypothermic, they make mistakes."

Despite his family's wariness, Albert felt at ease sharing his recent experience on the Mount Washington Auto Road. He was clearly passionate about the work and the meaning it held for him. But with his niece hanging on his every word, he was careful not to instill a sense of fear in her. "He was a great storyteller," Susan said of her younger brother. "He noticed details, and I can remember him describing how incredibly cold it was on that particular mission."

———————————

Mount Washington Observatory Surface Weather Observations (9:00 to 10:00 a.m.): Temperature 9°F; winds out of the northwest averaging 22 mph; visibility 0 miles; fog/snow/freezing drizzle; windchill -11°F.

Mount Washington Auto Road
Sargent's Purchase, N.H.
Wednesday, Dec. 16, 1981
9:30 a.m.

The search and rescue story Albert Dow shared with his family that day was both harrowing and inspiring, especially when combined with details recorded in official incident reports and the Mount Washington Observatory News Bulletin.

Phil Labbe was an hour behind schedule. It was Wednesday, which meant shift change for both the Observatory and WMTW-TV summit crews, who were charting the weather. Labbe's job was to get a warm, well-rested television crew and their supplies up the mountain via the TV station's Thiokol snow tractor to replace the team who'd been on the summit during the previous week. He'd been held up in Gorham waiting for a stockpile of groceries that was delayed due to snow-covered roads. When he finally arrived at Glen House at the base of Mount Washington, he loaded the Thiokol, made sure his four passengers were ready, and headed for the summit. Winds were barely discernible, and visibility was poor but manageable for the slow crawl up the 7.6-mile road to the Sherman Adams Building at the high point of the 60-acre Mount Washington State Park.

At 65 years old, having previously served on the summit as part of the U.S. Air Force's Aeronautical Icing Research Laboratory and then for WMTW-TV as a mechanical engineer, Labbe was in his 32nd winter on the mountain and was intimately familiar with the terrain and route. "He could walk that road blindfolded," said an unidentified veteran of Mount Washington to United Press International on Dec. 16, 1981. "He's a part of the mountain."

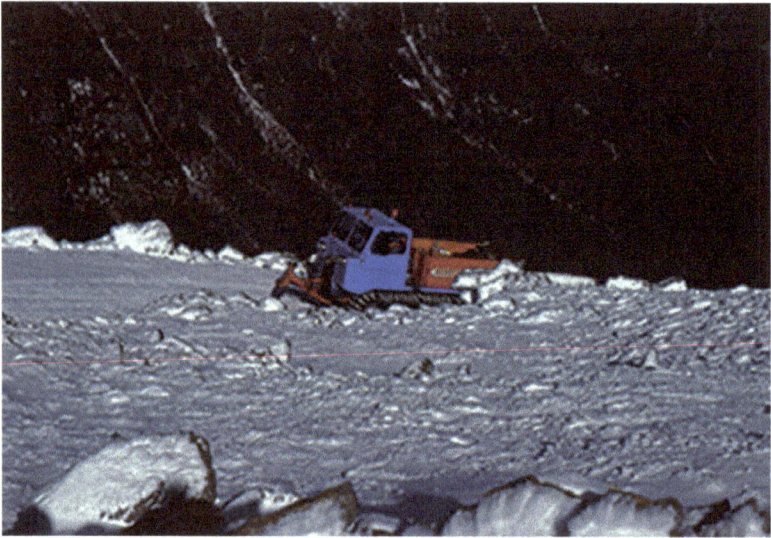

The 1980s-era Mount Washington Observatory Thiokol slogging up the Auto Road.

Not long after Labbe began his climb from the base to the 6,288-foot summit, an Observatory Thiokol snow tractor operated by Ken Rancourt and carrying two passengers headed up the mountain as well.

As is often the case at the "Home of the World's Worst Weather," the higher the two machines climbed, the worse the conditions became. By 11:00 a.m. the temperature had dropped to 8°F on the summit, and winds were averaging 78 mph, putting the windchill near -24°F. High winds were conspiring with the freshly fallen snow to create whiteout conditions. In minutes, visibility went from poor to almost nil. Labbe was just above the seven-mile post when he decided it was too dangerous to proceed any farther and turned the Thiokol around to descend.

Two miles lower, Ken Rancourt was at a full stop because his Thiokol had triggered a small avalanche. Decades later, Rancourt reflects on the precarious situation he and his passengers found themselves in. "That kind of avalanche happens when you cut out enough snow to form a level bed to drive on," he explains today. "It's not uncommon but still scary, and it's also frustrating because it negates all the work you've had to do to reach higher on the road. Avalanches mostly happen at mile five, where we were that day, but they could also occur on a smaller scale at the four-mile mark. It all depends on wind direction."

Meanwhile, as Labbe's Thiokol limped across Cow Pasture, he took a wrong turn and lost sight of the snow-covered roadway. "What happens over time is you do so many trips that you get used to it being bad," Rancourt says. "Then it goes up one more notch, and it's not just bad, it's impossible. That's when you get in trouble."

Dressed in a full-body, hooded snowmobile suit and wearing a winter hat and gloves, Labbe set the emergency brake and climbed out of the snow tractor. He was instantly pinned against the machine by winds gusting at over 100 mph and a windchill of -27°F. Careful not to tear his suit on the vehicle's sharp tracks, he worked his way carefully across the cleats and dropped to the ground. He was concerned he might drive the Thiokol off the edge and hoped that by not having to peer through the cab window he'd regain his bearings and reconnect with the elusive Auto Road.

But the wind gusts and bitter cold proved too much for Labbe. "I started down the road behind the machine and slipped on some ice," he told Martha Petrowski of *The Berlin Reporter* for her Dec. 29, 1981 article. "The winds were so strong I was literally twisted around and lost my sense of direction. I hunted for the machine but just couldn't find it." Far above the safety of treeline, completely disoriented and fully exposed to the extreme weather, he was soon unable to find the Thiokol he had just left.

Inside the machine, his four passengers waited anxiously as the minutes ticked by. With no sign of their driver, they began gunning the Thiokol's engine and flashing its headlights in hopes that Labbe would catch a glimpse of the machine. Oblivious to these audio-visual signals, Labbe spent the next 15 minutes moving in short bursts over the terrain so as not to get even farther away from his intended target. He was getting colder, this winter day was short, and he knew that to remain in that environment any longer could prove fatal, so he began to descend the mountain.

Rob Kirsch, a former Mount Washington Observatory weather intern and summer crew member and current member of the Observatory's Board of Trustees, penned an article on this incident for the Observatory's News Bulletin titled "The Longest Day." Describing Labbe's behavior, he wrote, "Keeping the wind at his back in an attempt to maintain at least a minimal sense of direction, he struck out at an angle that he believed would bring him to the road."

With still no sign of their driver, the WMTW crew radioed Rancourt in the Observatory's Thiokol and alerted him to the fact that Labbe was missing on the mountain. At 11:52 a.m., Rancourt radioed the news to Dave Warren, the huts manager for the Appalachian Mountain Club (AMC), located at Pinkham Notch Camp, known today as the Visitor Center. Warren immediately notified Mountain Rescue Service and Lt. Bill Hastings of New Hampshire Fish and Game, the agency with jurisdiction over search and rescue missions in that area of the Presidential Range.

With the two Thiokols often used during search and rescue missions incapacitated high on the mountain, additional resources were needed to find Labbe. So Thiokols owned by the National Forest Service and Wildcat Mountain, both in close proximity, were transported by flatbed trucks to the base of the mountain, where search teams from MRS and the AMC were already assembling. By 2:00 p.m., rescue crews were headed up the Auto Road by Thiokol and on foot. Winds on the summit were sustained at over 100 mph. It had been three hours since Labbe had been lost. "At one point there were four Thiokols on the Auto Road looking for Phil," recalls Rancourt. "From the Forest Service, Wildcat Mountain, the Observatory, and WMTW. It was pretty impressive."

Standing idle and feeling helpless, Rancourt decided to turn the Observatory Thiokol around and descend to the bottom of the winter cutoff, hoping Labbe might emerge there. Located between the 4½- and six-mile markers, the cutoff was a winter shortcut for snow tractors ascending and descending the mountain. Two miles above Rancourt, ice buildup on the carburetor of the WMTW Thiokol had caused it to stall, which eliminated the TV crew's main heat source. Anticipating a brutally cold night ahead and to prevent the high winds from permeating the cab, they hastily stuffed clothing, paper towels, and anything pliable they could find into every nook and cranny.

Labbe was in a fight for his life and unknowingly crossed the Auto Road at Cow Pasture. "The mountain wanted me bad, but I wasn't going to give up without a fight," he told Martha Petrowski. He feared that he was well below the road itself and continued to avoid descending too directly. "Through a combination of experience, common sense, and instinct, [Labbe] appears to have held a course relatively close to that of the road," Kirsch wrote. "His progress was slow and painful, and the constant pummeling of the wind forced him to spend much of his time on all fours. Several times he took refuge behind rocks, attempting to rest and evaluate his situation. On each occasion he roused himself, knowing that his survival depended on continued descent."

Wind gusts on the mountain had increased to 125 mph. Remarkably, the stranded WMTW crew members were able to get the machine restarted. Using the wind as a guide, the designated driver headed in what they collectively believed to be the right direction. With the sun dropping to the west and daylight fading, two crew members took turns walking out in front of the Thiokol to ensure it stayed on the Auto Road.

At 3:30 p.m., a second WMTW Thiokol with a six-person capacity but packed with eight geared-up rescuers from MRS and the AMC, including Albert Dow, was almost halfway up the Auto Road in the vicinity of the cutoff. The windblown snowdrifts were so high across the road that the team exited into winds over 100 mph and windchills below -30°F. They attacked the drifts with shovels while the Thiokol, operated by WMTW Chief Engineer Parker Vincent, plowed its way forward.

Joe Lentini, who was part of the rescue team riding in the Thiokol, remembers conditions as if it were yesterday. "We got up there, and the winds were gusting to 140 mph on the summit. I don't know how high up we got because it was whiteout conditions; it was goddamn crazy. We took ropes and strung them on either side of the Thiokol, and there were four of us on either side at different intervals as we searched. We were attached to the Thiokol by rope, so we could clip on or off, and we wouldn't get lost. Gusts would hit us in the high 80s and 90s and would just level us. Our Thiokol driver, Parker Vincent, was terrified for Phil. They had been working together for decades."

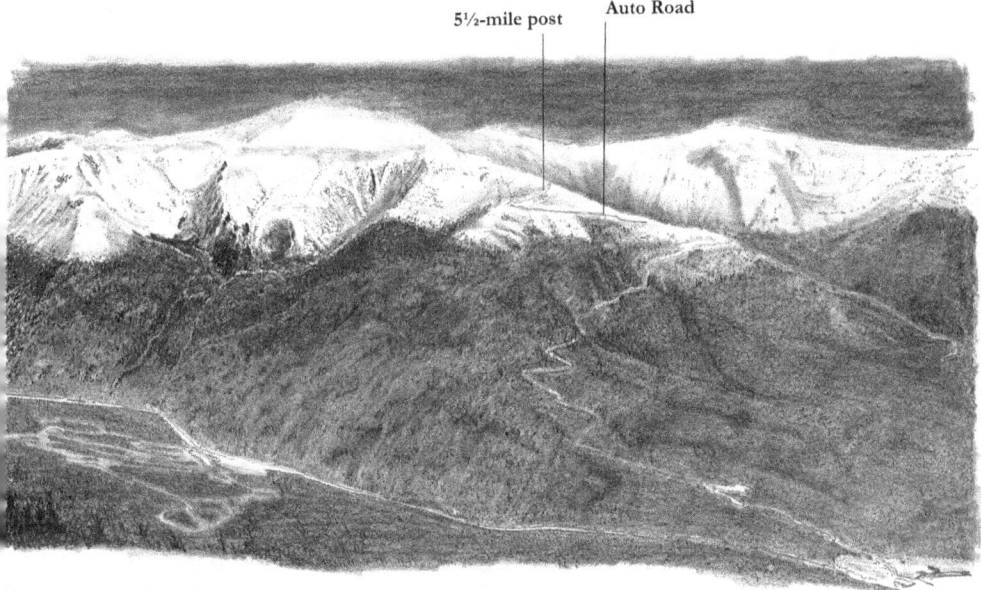

5½-mile post   Auto Road

Above them, Labbe continued moving across the terrain on all fours. Upon reaching the 5½-mile post, he recognized a pole that was used as a marker. "For the first time I knew where I was," he told Petrowski. "It was such a good feeling to recognize something."

Rancourt's descent in the Observatory Thiokol was painstakingly slow. Over the course of two hours, he descended only three-quarters of a mile. It was after 4:00 p.m., and Frank Hubley, a Motorola radio technician who was headed to the summit with Rancourt to do repairs, was shoveling drifts in front of their Thiokol as Rancourt plowed ahead. Through the blowing snow, Hubley saw something that would change the dire mood of that day. Rob Kirsch wrote: "Seeing a form looming from behind the machine, Frank dropped his shovel and raced to meet it. After more than 4½ hours in the elements, Labbe had stumbled upon the road and caught up with those trying to find him. He was immediately put inside the heated Thiokol cab, where the process of de-icing his face and head commenced."

Rancourt remembers the moment the needle found the haystack. "Phil approached my Thiokol, and he was in pretty sad shape," he recalls. "His face and wrists were frostbitten, and he'd lost a glove."

Minutes after Labbe was located, the WMTW Thiokol carrying the rescue team arrived. "I remember that we stopped when we got to the other snowcat," says Alec Behr, an MRS team member and close friend of Albert Dow. "When I got out of our machine, it was a complete whiteout because the winds were so strong. If I had walked a hundred and fifty feet from the snowcat, I wouldn't have known where it was."

During the descent to the waiting ambulance, Labbe was treated for frostbite, dehydration, and exhaustion by Dr. Robert Jaffee, an AMC volunteer who was in the second WMTW Thiokol. With a train of machines headed down the mountain, picking up rescuers who had been ascending on foot, the road was cleared by 7:00 p.m. Just 45 minutes earlier, the Observatory had recorded its peak gust of the day at 142 mph.

During the search mission, eight different radio channels were used by multiple agencies to communicate with each other. Thirty-six people contributed to the effort, including two individuals who sat with Phil Labbe's wife while rescuers searched the mountain for her husband.

Often after the unexpected happens, organizations will debrief the incident and implement changes in policy, training, equipment, and process. That is exactly what happened in this case. "After Phil's incident, we started carrying 50-foot-long ropes with carabiners on them," says Ken Rancourt. "In really poor visibility, you could latch yourself to the window frame of the Thiokol and then you'd be tied to the machine. The person out front could go left to right to gauge where the road was."

Rancourt, who is now a member of the Mount Washington Observatory Board of Trustees, says the practice is still utilized today, "but only under very rare circumstances, that is, when the snowcat operator has gone beyond the natural weather limitations of dense blowing snow, fog, and high winds."

Philip Labbe survived the incident and died on July 8, 2010, at age 94.

Despite this story's happy ending, it only served to heighten the Dow family's worries about Albert's practice of going out on rescue missions in extreme conditions. Marjorie Dow was the one to broach the subject with her son when he finished recounting his role in the rescue. "Why would you go out to look for him?" she asked. It was less a question than a statement from a concerned parent: "I wish you wouldn't do this, Albert, go out in such cold."

"We had a call and he needed help, Mom," Albert's sisters recall him replying. "If I was lost on the side of a mountain and needed help, I wouldn't want to be ignored."

That comment became a chilling memory for the Dow family. In less than a month—and with haunting irony—Albert's selflessness and his commitment to helping others in trouble would lead to his own tragic fate.

Albert Jr. would die on Jan. 19, 2006, at age 82, and Marjorie on Nov. 20, 2017, at 89. They lived for decades with their grief, but they and the rest of the Dow family took some measure of comfort knowing that young Albert's tragic story would forever change the future of search and rescue operations in the White Mountains, making them safer for those who followed him.

I
EXUBERANCE

I contemplate young mountaineers hung with ropes
and ice-axes, and think that they alone have understood
how to live life.
—Vita Sackville-West in a letter to Virginia Woolf

Garden State Parkway
Cape May, N.J.
Friday, Jan. 22, 1982
3:00 a.m.

Jeff Batzer and Hugh Herr are lost. They departed Herr's home in Holtwood, Pa., seven hours earlier, intending to drive 500 unimpeded miles north to Pinkham Notch, N.H. Instead, they have found themselves some 125 miles off course at the southern-most point of New Jersey. Frustrated by this costly navigational error, they reorient themselves and point Batzer's Datsun pickup truck north on the Garden State Parkway. Batzer, who lives 40 minutes north of Herr in Manheim Township, Pa., still recalls his dismay: "That was just ridiculous. It was one of the most horrible things I'd ever done driving," he says. "Three and a half hours of going south instead of north."

Now headed in the right direction, they hope that by the time they arrive at Pinkham Notch there will still be enough daylight remaining to do some reconnaissance of Huntington Ravine on Mount Washington, where they plan to climb the following day.

After working all day Thursday as a tool and die apprentice at Precision Machine Company, the 20-year-old Batzer had hurried home, where he lived with his parents Richard and Joan, to make last-minute preparations for his weekend trip. In between laps back and forth from his bedroom to his truck, Batzer talked excitedly with his father, who was expressing worry about his son's trip and the forecast he'd read calling for bad weather. "I remember Dad being concerned, but it was mild," Batzer recalls. "Here you have your 20-year-old son heading out on an adventure. What are you going to do?"

In fact, Batzer realized only later that his father was feeling more than mild anxiety. "In talking with my brother, I learned that my dad had all he could do to let me go that day," says Batzer. "I was climbing almost every day at the time, but there was something about that trip that really scared him."

Batzer, the middle child of three, was no stranger to adventure in the backcountry. His parents exposed all three boys to the wild outdoors from a young age. "We were always big campers and did a lot of hunting, hiking, and fishing together," says Batzer. "I could use a map and compass and start a fire. My parents instilled in us a 'watch your back and be aware of your surroundings' mentality."

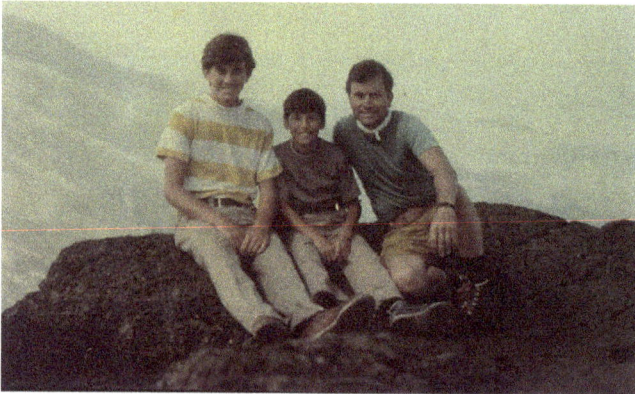

Jeff Batzer (middle) is flanked by brother Rich (left) and father Richard after summiting Mount Washington in 1973.

As Batzer grew up, his already deep connection to the outdoors evolved into a fascination with vertical cliffs and high-mountain peaks. "At 10 years old, I was intrigued by rock climbing and mountaineering," he said. "I loved reading features in *National Geographic* about Mount Everest."

In the summer of 1978, at age 16, Batzer graduated from scrambles on all fours up rocky slopes to more vertical climbs. "From the moment I first touched rock, I was all out," he recalls. In a 1982 interview with Phil Kukielski of the *Providence Journal*'s *Sunday Journal Magazine*, Joan Batzer would say of her son, "Climbing gave him something to say. ... He's always been the little guy between the two big fellows. He had to prove he could be as strong and endure more. This was one thing that really drove Jeff on."

On that Thursday afternoon before their weekend trip, Hugh Herr had left Penn Manor High School and headed straight home, where he lived with parents John and Martha. Though only 17 years old and a junior in high school, Herr did not encounter any worry from his parents about his impending hike on Mount Washington. The Herrs had always given Hugh and his four older siblings a lot of latitude and instilled in each of them a strong sense of self-reliance and discipline. "Every summer as a family we'd go on these road trips across America," recalls Herr. "It was generally an outdoor adventure involving fishing, camping, and hiking."

Herr started rock climbing when he was just six years old, and by the time he was eight it had become, in his own words, "an all-consuming passion." The more time he spent in the backcountry, the more accustomed he became to exploring the terrain alone. "Mountain adventures transitioned from hiking to climbing, and from glacier walking to rock climbing," he says, adding, "I was very schooled in avalanche avoidance and all aspects of technical rock and ice climbing, and I did a lot of glacier work out West."

Herr's precocious climbing talent has been well documented over the years. In her 2012 book *Up: A Mother and Daughter's Peakbagging Adventure*, Patricia Ellis Herr describes former husband Hugh's amazing progression: "He had his first crampons at age 7, and by age 8 he had hiked 11,624-foot Mount Temple in the Canadian Rockies and attempted 14,411-foot Mount Rainier with his father and two older brothers. The weather forced them to turn back, but Hugh returned to the peak when he was 11 and reached the summit."

In *Second Ascent: The Story of Hugh Herr* (1991), Alison Osius writes that as Herr grew older, his climbing routes grew more technical: "At age 13, he and [older brother] Hans had climbed the Exum Ridge of 13,766-foot Grand Teton in Wyoming."

Herr himself recognized the rare attributes he possessed early on. "I was a very unusual teenager," he says. "I was very analytical and calculating. I had an interest in Zen, mind control, meditation, and what they now call 'the zone' in athleticism." Osius adds that "Hugh was tantalized by concepts of the mental control needed to perform in a risk-taking, problem-solving situation."

For Herr, entering "the zone" led to profound mindfulness. "On some of my ascents, there'd be 30-foot sections that I'd have absolutely no memory of," he says. "I was really deeply in the zone. I'd practice meditation and visualization and imagine my body in exact movements. I was and remain afraid of heights, but I'm able to condition my mind. If we were to go climbing right now, I'd be terrified, but if we climbed for a month, I'd say, 'Oh yeah, these ropes, they work.'"

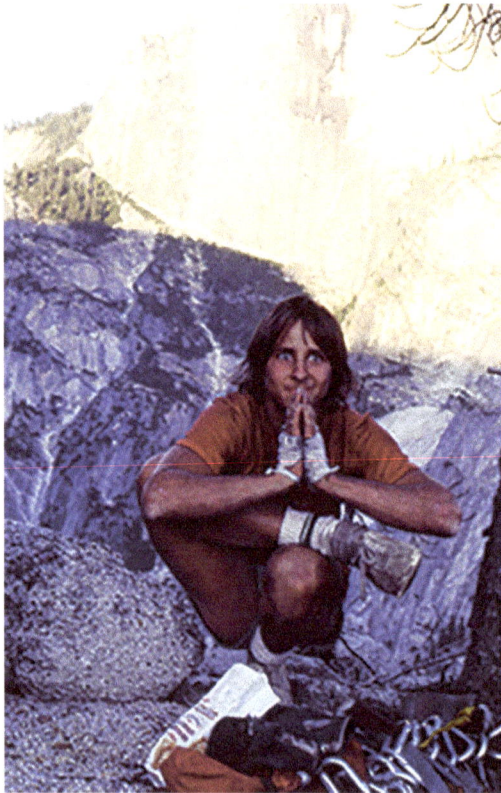

Hugh Herr, age 16, finds a moment of Zen in Yosemite after ascending Astroman, a 2,000-foot climb. Half Dome is in the background.

Herr's approach and style were heavily influenced by other climbers of that era, especially Henry Barber. Now in his 70s, Barber has always been a fierce advocate for clean, minimalistic climbing. This style requires using techniques and gear that avoid damaging the rock. At the time, Barber was laser focused on his craft and how far he could take it, but he was oblivious to the effect he was having on the greater climbing community. "Honestly, I never really knew what my influence was on anybody," he says. "I think it was about my style and ethics. I was climbing pure, ground up, on-sight, with only nuts and a swami belt. It's not what I did as much as how I did it."

"Barber was world class, and Hugh was kind of in the same category," says Batzer. "I was 20, he was 17 and I was well aware that Hugh was already one of the best climbers in the country."

Herr knew of Barber's groundbreaking ascents, and Barber began hearing of the young Herr as well. "He was up-and-coming in the Gunks [short for the Shawangunks, located near New Paltz, N.Y.]," says Barber. "There's a couple of climbs he did that were very noteworthy and at the upper end of the scale. I knew he was doing these things."

Herr, also nicknamed "Boy Wonder" because of his status as a child prodigy of the sport, climbed Bugaboo Spire (10,512 ft.) and Snowpatch Spire (10,118 ft.), part of the Bugaboo Mountain Range in British Columbia, at age 15. In the summer of 1981, he was completing highly challenging routes in Yosemite and the Gunks. "I was very, very advanced," he says today. "By 17, I was a top climber in the United States."

Batzer met Herr in 1979, when he was 17 and Herr was 14, while both were bouldering at a popular climbing spot in Lancaster County, Pa. Bouldering is a form of climbing that is done without ropes or harnesses on smaller rock features. Depending on the height or difficulty of the challenge, the climber may be spotted by someone at ground level and/or use a "crash pad" to prevent or minimize the risk of injury in the event of a fall.

Shortly after that first meeting, the two started climbing together. "There was chemistry between us," says Batzer. "Hugh had a greater appetite for risk, but he was always very sensitive to me. He was very careful with me because I think he realized I was still kind of a rookie even after two years. I was still cutting my teeth."

Despite their different comfort levels with risk-taking, Batzer says he and Herr were compatible climbing partners. "I was never somebody who really enjoyed the risk part, but I'd definitely be described as an adrenaline junkie," he says. "I climbed scared, and I tended to be overly careful at times. To counteract that, I pushed myself into difficult situations on hard climbs. I looked at myself as a technical climber, and I really wanted to achieve ice- and rock-climbing excellence."

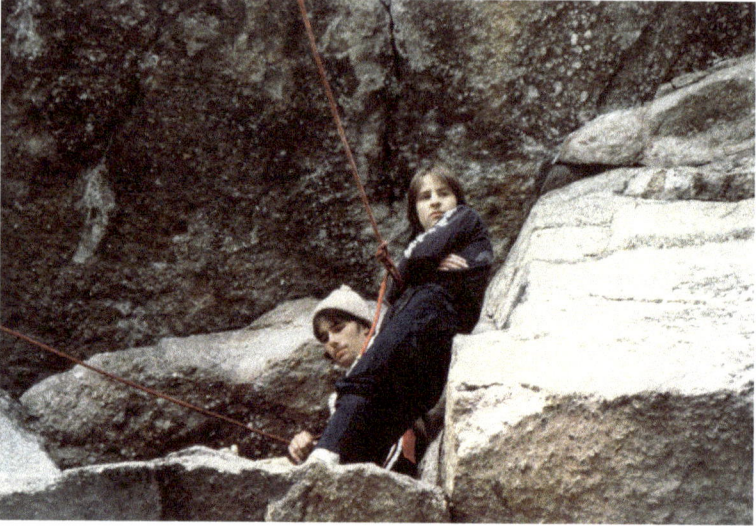

Jeff Batzer (left) and Hugh Herr beneath the Kansas City Route in the Shawangunks in New York in 1981. "Hugh got Kansas City that day, but I did not," recalls Batzer. "Although I tried!"

Herr viewed the hazards of climbing as an inherent part of the sport and a challenge to be embraced. "I would take risks, but I believe they were manageable," he says today. At age 16, he was drawn to soloing. "The subculture of mountaineering and climbing was about purity and ethics," he says. "By that I mean a minimalist approach. If you climb the mountain without any assistance, that's the most pure. Henry Barber was my idol. I had other idols who wouldn't even use chalk; they would climb barefoot. I was part of that tradition, which my father thought was absolute nonsense. He was deeply upset by that culture."

Alison Osius writes that it wasn't only Herr's father who was upset with his "pure," ropeless ascents. His older brother Tony objected as well. "[Tony's] little brother, the kid he taught to climb, was pushing it too far and could get killed. He felt that Hugh was too young to contemplate the consequences of an accident." Osius quotes Tony as thinking, "He's overdosing on confidence, on power. He thinks he's immortal. He doesn't get the idea of life in a wheelchair."

At one point, Herr's father, who had always preached self-reliance and independence, reached a point when he'd had enough. "If you don't stop, you won't climb at all," he told his son. The stern warning had its desired effect on the young climber. "I did stop my really extreme soloing," he says.

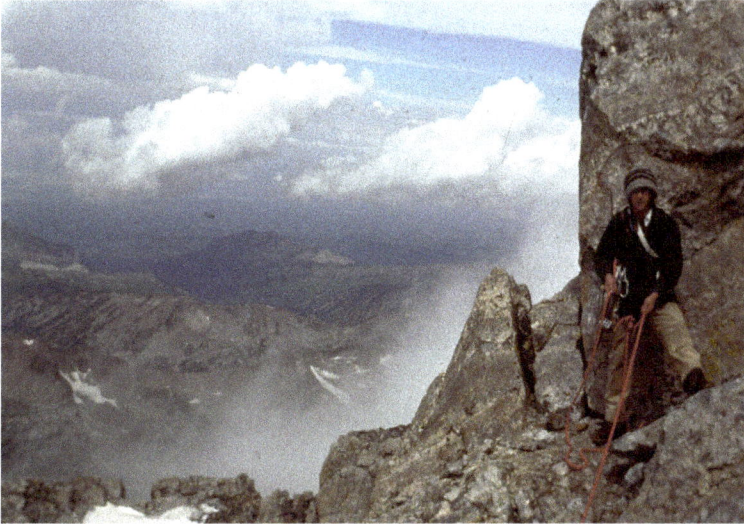

Hugh Herr, age 13, near the summit of Grand Teton on the Exum Ridge Route. The photo was taken by older brother Hans.

As Herr was responding to his family's concerns while still pushing boundaries on rock faces, Batzer was dreaming of the high peaks he encountered in the pages of *National Geographic*. "It was a bit of an awkward situation," he says, "because the world I was in was rock climbing, and I was crazy about it. I was a rock jock without any question. But I was sensing the need for a change. I was drawn to the cold weather, the higher altitude, the harder work, the endurance necessary to carry weight, and the accomplishment of getting to the top of 20,000-foot peaks. It was a natural progression in some ways. But for me as a rock climber at the time, it was seen as odd. You're not a rock jock anymore; you're more of a mountain climber. But I told myself that I was going to make that shift if I could. As it turned out, I couldn't because of what happened on Mount Washington that weekend in 1982."

As Batzer and Herr continued their long slog northward toward the Granite State, Batzer was finding it a test of his endurance. "Hugh probably slept while I was driving," he recalls. "I drove the whole

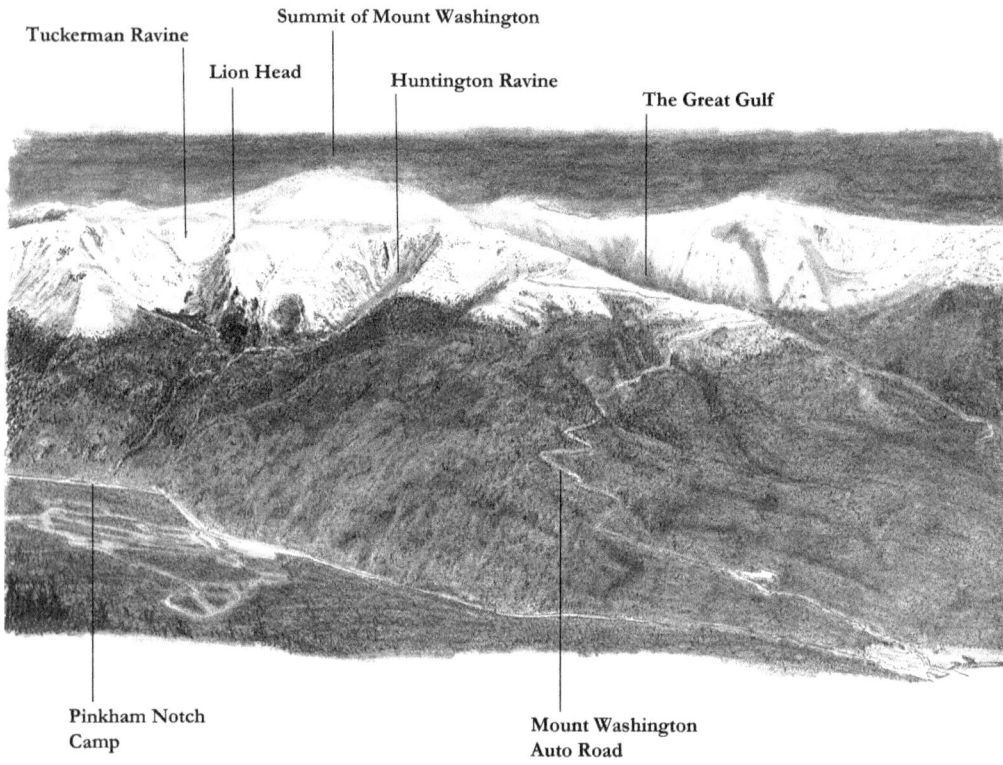

Tuckerman Ravine

Summit of Mount Washington

Lion Head

Huntington Ravine

The Great Gulf

Pinkham Notch
Camp

Mount Washington
Auto Road

time, and it was close to 30 hours without sleep."

In fact, this wasn't the first time the friends had been to Huntington Ravine and Mount Washington. One year before, on Wednesday, Dec. 31, 1980, Herr and Batzer departed Pennsylvania for their first trip to the Northeast's highest peak. They arrived at the parking lot of the Appalachian Mountain Club's Pinkham Notch Camp (today's Visitor Center) between 2:00 and 3:00 a.m. on Jan. 1 and prepared the front seats for some long-awaited sleep.

It was quiet at Pinkham at that hour. The cars and trucks of overnight guests staying at the Joe Dodge Lodge or Harvard Cabin in Huntington Ravine were parked here and there across the lot. The peaceful scene gave no hint of the urgency and sorrow that had swept through the camp some 14 hours earlier, when 19-year-old Peter Friedman became the 92nd person to be killed on Mount Washington after falling in Odell Gully on Dec. 31. Friedman's climbing partner, 18-year-old Tor Raubenheimer, was below him on the ice, belaying. He was seriously injured in the accident but was saved through the efforts of fellow climbers, who came to his aid and called for emergency medical help.

Herr and Batzer would not learn of this tragedy until their return to Pennsylvania days later. They awoke early on New Year's Day, collected their climbing gear from the back of the truck and walked directly to the Tuckerman Ravine Trail en route to Huntington Ravine, choosing not to sign in on the climbers' log located at Pinkham Camp. On arrival in the ravine, they ascended The Fan and positioned themselves at the base of Pinnacle Gully. The route they had planned up the gully is described by Laura and Guy Waterman in their book *Yankee Rock & Ice* as "the narrow, steep, dark, evil band of ice that snakes up behind the rock buttress," and is considered a full-day outing requiring winter climbing skills and involving avalanche hazard.

Herr and Batzer elected to leave behind the one backpack they had between them and climbed only with what they were wearing and the technical gear they'd brought with them. By 10:00 a.m., Herr was climbing as Batzer belayed him.

"Hugh led the whole thing," Batzer recalls. "I definitely perceived him as the leader when we climbed, and he made sure I was safe by setting an anchor and hauling me up. I remember I was moving quickly behind him, and I put so much torque on the pic of my axe that it snapped right off. He climbed down to me, held out one of his two axes, and said, 'Here, take mine.' We were 800 feet up, and Hugh finished the last two pitches with one ice axe. He was always protecting me. We worked together as a team and loved each other. Climbing was difficult on my nerves, and he helped me work through the mental side of it. He'd talk me into doing things, but it wasn't pressure; it was reassurance. That day's climb went extremely fast, a couple of hours to the top. We were done by noon."

Even though the weather was calm, and they could see the summit of Mount Washington upon topping out on Pinnacle, Batzer and Herr had no intention of continuing upward. Batzer had summited Washington in summer with his dad and older brothers when he was 12 years old. "It was beautiful weather, just a perfect day." But on this winter day, it wasn't on the itinerary. Instead, they descended to the base and retrieved the pack they had stashed behind a boulder in the snow.

Returning to the parking lot, they loaded their gear into Batzer's truck and made a beeline for Crawford Notch and the iconic—and demanding—Frankenstein Cliff, where they successfully climbed the Dracula Route. "I was so exhausted that day coming off Pinnacle Gully, but somehow I must have gotten a second wind," recalls Batzer.

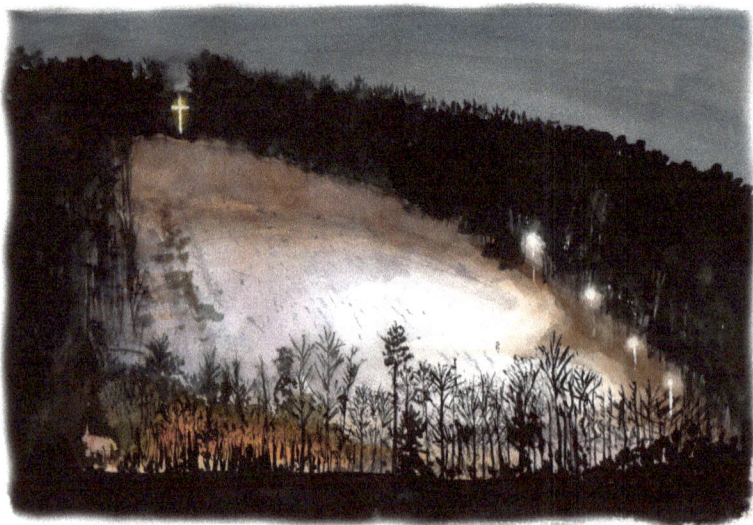

Mount Eustis Ski Area in Littleton, N.H., with its distinctive lighted cross near the summit.

After that exhausting but exhilarating New Year's Day, the pair headed home on Jan. 2. As they drove through Littleton, N.H., Batzer's eyes were drawn toward an illuminated cross that had stood atop Mount Eustis for many years. He didn't know it at the time, but it wouldn't be the last time Batzer would encounter this symbolic beacon of the North Country.

A year later, Batzer has his eyes set once again on Mount Washington and Pinnacle Gully, but this time he has other ideas on how he'd climb it, and this time he wants to summit Washington. With two seasons of ice climbing in the books, often with Herr, he feels he can now lead their climb up Pinnacle. "The sky was the limit back then," he says a little ruefully.

For the 1982 trip, though, Herr was not actually Batzer's original choice for climbing partner. Instead, he asked Eric Hurst, with whom he'd been climbing since high school and whom he describes as an excellent rock climber who'd helped him improve dramatically. But Hurst was unable to accompany him, so two weeks before he planned to head out, Batzer invited Herr, who accepted readily.

"I was kind of the older guy with a job and a truck, so I put the trip together," recalls Batzer. "Right from the beginning, I told Hugh I wanted to do an ice gully and also summit Washington, and he was right there with me. Our plan was to leave Harvard Cabin on Saturday morning, Jan. 23, and be back that same day. Then maybe we'd head over to the Frankenstein Cliff area again the next day."

Because of the pair's success the year before, Batzer is approaching the 1982 trip with confidence. But he acknowledges today that he was also recalling the experience of a friend who'd run into trouble the previous year on Washington the day after he and Herr had departed for home. "He became weak above Huntington Ravine, and they literally dragged him down the mountain because he was struggling so bad. He almost died above the ravine. The kinds of winds he talked about afterward—they were insane. I had all that in my mind as I drove toward New Hampshire, so I felt a lot of respect for the mountain. But there was also this very strong youthful sense of 'Yeah, let's keep that in mind, but let's go for it.' I didn't want to be held back by fear. I've since called it "the foolishness of youth wrapped in the beauty of youth."

During their drive to Pinkham, conversation between Batzer

and Herr has turned to their climbing plans, and Batzer speaks again of his wish to summit Washington. "It was in the back of my mind, but it wasn't a dominant passion or anything," says Herr today. "It's a walk in the park from the top of Huntington Ravine to the summit, so who cares? It's not like it's K2." They are both aware of a worrisome weather forecast but don't spend time talking about it. "I don't think we were overly concerned about that," recalls Batzer.

At 6:00 p.m., Friday, Jan. 22, after 22 hours of a drive that should have taken about nine, Batzer and Herr arrive at Pinkham Notch Camp and the eastern slopes of Mount Washington. It is now well after sunset, so they gather their gear and hike in darkness toward Tuckerman Ravine Trail to Huntington Ravine Trail and their stop for the night, Harvard Cabin.

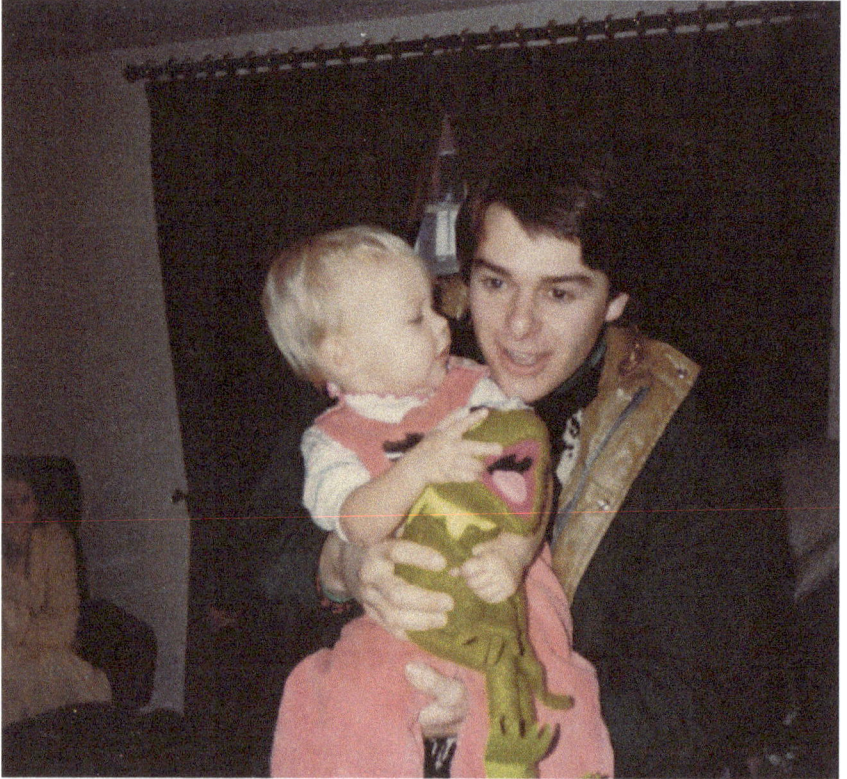

Albert Dow with his beloved niece, Amy Johnson, and her Kermit the Frog stuffed animal.

II
YOUNG RESCUER

Rescue was in my brother's blood from the time he was a little kid.
—Susan Dow-Johnson

Charles and Susan Dow-Johnson's home
Mount Lebanon, Pa.
Friday, Jan. 22, 1982
Early evening

Not long after Jeff Batzer and Hugh Herr start up the Tuckerman Ravine Trail toward Harvard Cabin, Albert Dow places a call to his older sister Susan's home in Pennsylvania. Knowing exactly who her brother really wants to speak to that evening, Susan immediately hands the phone to her daughter, Amy.

"Helllooo, Amy! This is Kermit the Frog calling to wish you a very happy fifth birthday!"

"Uncle Albuuuurrt! I know it's you!"

The only child of the Dow siblings at the time, Amy expresses regret today that her younger siblings and cousins never got to enjoy their late uncle's loving presence in their lives. "I was the only one Uncle Albert ever got to meet," she says.

Albert grew up in Tuftonboro, N.H., on the northeastern shores of Lake Winnipesaukee. In late spring, the 975 year-round residents would brace themselves for the onslaught of 10,000 or so seasonal residents flocking to their second homes and camps. In 1950, Dow's father, Albert Jr., purchased the home at "Four Corners" from his parents with money he'd earned while serving in the Merchant Marines. For 57 years, from 1948 to 2005, the family operated Dow's Corner Shop out of the barn, and over time Albert Jr. and wife Marjorie developed a national reputation for their work as purveyors of antiques.

Bea Lewis, a reporter for the *New Hampshire Union Leader* from 1979 to 1983, remembers the home and family fondly. "From their house you looked right onto Mount Shaw (2,990 ft.) and Black Snout (2,803 ft.), the whole ring dike that is the Ossipee Mountains," she recalls. "It's kind of the cradle of the White Mountains. It was a big yellow center-chimney colonial with an arc of an attached barn and a big green sliding door. I can remember as a young kid going into the barn with my mother when Marjorie—they used to call her 'Midge'— ran the antique shop. She specialized in glass. The electrified kerosene lamps were always illuminated in the barn and made you crane your head to look as you walked by. The Dows were very highly thought of, very generous, and all the local kids adored them."

Susan, 14 months older than Albert, and Caryl, five years younger than he, retain strong memories of a happy, wholesome childhood at that house. Some of their most vivid reflections reveal moving evidence of the presence of a rescuer ethos and compassion for others that animated their late brother from an early age.

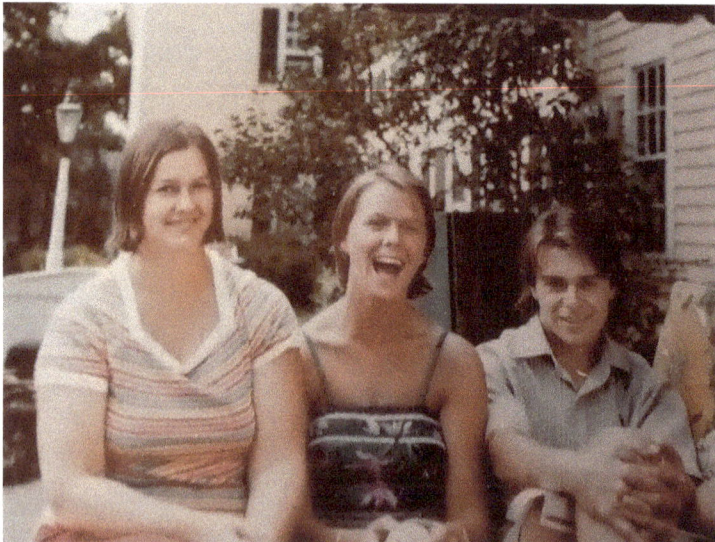

Siblings (left to right) Susan, Caryl, and Albert Dow share a light moment.

Susan remembers one afternoon when 7-year-old Albert approached her with a sense of urgency. "Can you help me get the big ladder out of the garage?" he asked. "Why?" Susan responded with suspicion, wondering what her brother was up to. Albert hastily led her across the front lawn to a spot below one of the large trees that adorned the front yard. "He had found this baby bird on the ground," she explains. "He'd gotten a shoebox and put the bird into the box. It was a little fledgling without many feathers."

Her brother was determined to return the bird back to the nest resting in a branch high above them. Susan and Albert went to the barn to retrieve the large wooden ladder, and the ensuing commotion summoned their father. Recognizing the risk to his children, Albert Jr. gingerly ascended the ladder with one hand on the rungs and the other holding the small box housing the tiny bird. Upon reaching the nest, he climbed out onto the limb and pushed the box close to the nest before descending. In the following days, they would find the box back on the ground with no bird in sight. They optimistically assumed the fledging had made his way back to the nest.

At 9, Albert used to ask his mother to make a large pail of lemonade for the public works employees who were clearing brush and long grass from the sides of the road in the stifling summer heat. Susan remembers her brother carrying the full pail and cups up the street to where the work was underway. She also recalls the son of a local pastor who had polio, which required the use of braces and crutches. "Nobody ever chose him for teams, but Albert always did."

This instinct to protect the needy followed Albert to high school as well. When Caryl suffered bullying on the school bus, which required intervention from her father, her brother arranged with his high school coaches to arrive to practices late so he could ride the bus home with his sister. "He always stood up for the person who needed standing up for," says Caryl. "Yes, I was his sister, but he would also do that for a friend."

What impresses his sisters most about the quality of Albert's altruism is not just that he displayed it at a very young age but that he didn't stop with just one offer of help—he stayed with it as long as he felt he was needed. His childhood friend and neighbor Orrin Welch recalls being a grateful beneficiary of that sustained kindness. About a year older than Albert, Welch remembers how difficult his own childhood was. "I was a little boy up the street that needed a lot of help. My dad came back from the Korean War, and he was really sick. We didn't have very much, and Albert was constantly giving me clothes and food and spending time with me. I don't think I could get any closer to having a brother than him. He was an incredible person, and I think that was because his mother and father spent so much time with him." After a full day at school or at play in the neighborhood, Welch would join the Dow family for dinner almost every night, and Albert Jr. and Marjorie later helped him get into technical school. "They were very generous people."

For Welch, his friend Albert's impact on his life remains as vivid today as it was decades ago. "In my eyes Albert was an angel flying too close to the ground," he says. "If somebody needed something, if somebody was hurting, he was the first one there. When he was just five or six years old, he'd be concerned about me getting something to eat or a warm jacket or a pair of gloves. Kids that young don't act that way, and that's why I think he was a really special person. It never surprised me that he'd later go out and try to rescue people who were in trouble in the mountains."

The young Albert was also known for being a talented athlete who relished challenging himself. At 11, he skied for the Mount Whittier Race Team along with teammate Alec Behr. Albert and Alec competed together for three years in U.S. Ski Association-sanctioned races, traveling together on weekends. Though they attended different high schools, the two met again when Albert moved to North Conway and went to work as an instructor/guide at the Eastern Mountain Sports Climbing School, where Behr held the same role. "We reconnected" says Behr, "and the friendship we'd had as young skiers was rekindled."

At Kingswood Regional High School in Wolfeboro, Albert was a three-sport athlete and a solid student. During his junior and senior years, he raced for the Waterville Valley Black and Blue Trail Smashers, commuting to Waterville Valley from Tuftonboro every day after school for practice. Skiing took him to places like Wyoming and Montana, where he competed in several Canadian American races. He graduated in 1971, and his yearbook epigraph reads, "His dislikes include being second best at anything."

When he enrolled at the University of New Hampshire, just as his father and mother had and Caryl would later, he expected to join the ski team but instead made the tough decision to focus on his studies. "Albert quickly figured out he was not going to be able to be a good student and be on the team," says sister Susan. He graduated from UNH in 1975 with an undergraduate degree in business and worked at various jobs in the Tuftonboro area.

Albert had climbed from time to time in his late teens but not with the same focus or intensity as he had skied. These were scrambles up rocky slopes, ascents of large trees or any object that allowed him to head upward. But after college, climbing became more of a passion. He started visiting local cliffs and other sites that provided vertical exposure. The family watched with interest as climbing established a firm grip on him. "One time, my husband and I were driving Albert back to North Conway where he lived, and Albert insisted we stop at Chocorua Lake because he absolutely had to solve this bouldering problem he'd been working on," recalls Susan.

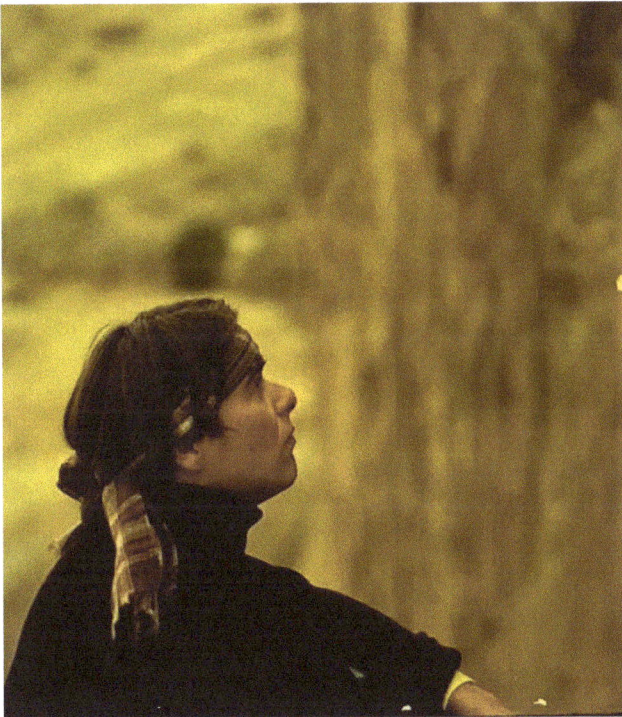

Albert Dow focused on a route during a climbing trip to Albuquerque, N.M., with Joe Lentini.

In fact, Albert had moved to North Conway to get closer to the active climbing scene in the Mount Washington Valley. He was hired as a retail clerk at Eastern Mountain Sports (EMS), which then was located inside the Eastern Slope Inn. Rick Wilcox was the store manager and the president of the all-volunteer Mountain Rescue

Service (MRS) at the time. Jimmie Dunn was director of the EMS Climbing School, and he remembers Albert fondly. "He got good enough at climbing for me to trust him guiding people," says Dunn. "He was a solid human being at all levels. He was kind. He tried hard. He was easy to get along with. We nicknamed him 'Burt.'"

Caryl says it was clear to the family that Albert was driving himself with his climbing just as he had as a skier, perhaps even more so. "He'd come home with his hands scarred, and my mother would say, 'Why do you do that?,' and he would say, 'I'm pushing myself to the limit of my ability, but I'm safe doing it.' I think he was a calculated risk-taker."

Joe Lentini began working as an instructor/guide at the climbing school in 1975 and quickly established himself as proficient climber. Wilcox asked him to join MRS, and in 1976 he took over the climbing school from Jimmie Dunn. "Albert had been working in the store doing retail, and we'd climb together some," says Lentini. "I offered him a job at the climbing school in 1978. He was really good with clients. He wanted them to get what they were looking for from the experience."

One of Lentini's fondest memories of Albert occurred while both were guiding clients. "I remember we were guiding a beginners' class together on Eagle Cliff in Bartlett. We each had separate clients. There's a slab section, and one of the clients was lying against the rock, which I could empathize with because there was no one more afraid of heights than I was when I first started. Albert said to the client—in a joking way—'Stand up! I grew up in a house in New Hampshire where the kitchen floors were steeper than this.' And it worked!"

It wasn't long before Albert proved himself to be a solid technical climber and he would soon be asked to become a volunteer with MRS. Most of the instructor/guides for EMS became volunteers. Dana Seavey, who also worked at the EMS Climbing School and volunteered for MRS, says all the volunteers felt great pride in their service. It was part of their culture. "You never looked forward to someone getting in trouble, but you welcomed the challenge to go out and help when it happened," he says.

In an off-season letter to his family in March 1979, Albert reflected on the pressure he was putting on himself as he tried to master his passion for climbing: "I am looking forward to rock-climbing and the return of warmer weather but have enjoyed the time away as I found myself quite drawn emotionally at the end of last season. At times, this crazy pursuit can be very taxing psychologically."

Albert was getting better all the time, and others were noticing. "He was poetry on the rock," Seavey says today. "He moved so gracefully, and he'd find holds that we couldn't locate. We'd go ice-climbing, and he'd always have to do mixed routes. I would go straight up Dracula in Crawford Notch or the Black Dike on Cannon Cliffs, and he would go out of his way to find sketchy one-foot-on-ice, one-foot-on-rock moves. He was so gifted, yet egoless and unassuming."

But there were quieter times in Albert's life as well. Like many in Albert's large friendship circle, Brenda Monahan, who worked at EMS with Albert and her future husband Jim, remembers the strong friendship Jim and Albert shared. "They were sympathetic souls. I'd come home from work, and they'd be sitting on the deck at our apartment amongst houseplants, listening to classical music and just talking about history, climbing, and the environment. Sometimes there wouldn't be any music at all; they'd just sit and listen to the birds singing."

A note in Albert's March 1979 letter to his family would surprise no one who knew him, including those who had witnessed his deep focus and burning intensity during rugged rock climbs: "I have put up several bird feeders at my house and am getting some great birds—even woodpeckers for the suet. The colors are splendid, and the activity in general is marvelous! I am also learning pottery on a wheel in my cellar. The wheel belongs to a friend, and several of us are learning. Much fun (have already made a bowl) and very relaxing, i.e., therapeutic."

Steve Larson, a member of MRS who met Albert in 1977, recalls the close community that characterized the North Conway scene at the time. "It was a really tight-knit group of guys who hung together," he says. Many climbers, including Albert, lived in small cottages on the property of the Eastern Slope Inn.

"The retail clerks and climbers from EMS would get together all the time for potluck supper," says Brenda Monahan. "We had good times—the kind young people have in their 20s. Life was good—we were very innocent, we didn't think anything could happen to us."

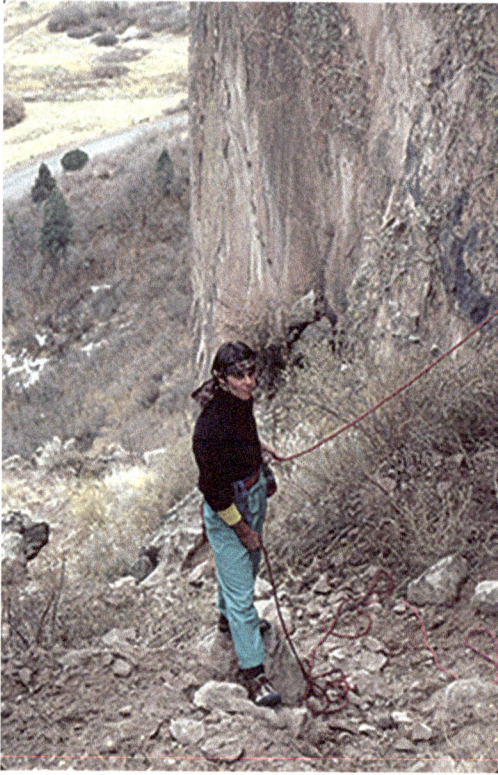

Albert Dow belaying in Albuquerque, N.M.

It was during this time that Albert and his close friends started going in search of first ascents throughout the Mount Washington Valley. Among these was Standard and Poors at the Albany Slab Rock, a challenging 5.9-rated climb that Dow, Lentini, and Michael Hartrich did together in May 1980.

It was also during this time that Albert met Joan Wrigley after being encouraged by Jim Monahan to introduce himself to her. "They became a couple almost immediately," Brenda Monahan recalls. "He was very enamored of her, and there was a time we didn't see him as much. That's what happens when you're newly in love. We were super happy for him because he was happy." Albert served as best man at the Monahans' wedding in November 1981.

A few months later, during Albert's phone conversation with niece Amy on her fifth birthday night in January 1982, his sister Susan is delighting in her daughter's smile. "You made her day Albert, thank you," she tells her brother. "Happy to do it, Sis," he replies. "Talk to you soon."

As Albert hangs up and thinks ahead to his weekend plans, he knows that weekends in the White Mountains, especially in winter, might bring an unexpected phone call from MRS and a sudden change in plans. But he is pointing toward leading a friend on an ice-climbing adventure at Cathedral Ledge in North Conway on Sunday morning, unless the forecasted extreme cold and high winds make climbing unwise. He has no idea that in about 27 hours his phone will indeed ring and he'll be called on to gather with his MRS teammates and take part in what will become one of the most memorable and tragic search and rescue operations ever conducted in the White Mountains of New Hampshire.

III
PINKHAM

A mountain region that is deemed the most dangerous
piece of real estate in the country.
—Gloria Poliquin, *New Hampshire Union Leader* correspondent,
referring to the Presidential Range of the White Mountains

Pinkham Notch Camp
Pinkham Notch, N.H.
Friday, Jan. 22, 1982
Early evening

David Moskowitz feels a bit disoriented. A seasonal crew member for the Appalachian Mountain Club (AMC), he has completely lost track of how many shifts of this 11-day stint he has worked at the Pinkham Notch Camp and how many more stand between him and a highly anticipated three-day break. Moskowitz does know for certain that it is Friday night because "it was all hands on deck" for him and for several other AMC employees who work at Pinkham. Sitting at his post at the information desk, Moskowitz enjoys the calming sounds and bursts of warmth emanating from the dry firewood as it burns in the stone fireplace nearby. He knows the solace he's basking in is ephemeral. With weekend guests expected to arrive en masse, this is the only respite he'll experience until late Sunday afternoon. Soon, the electrified buzz of the dinner bell will ricochet off the tongue-and-groove walls, and the now empty corridor will be flooded with outdoor enthusiasts seeking to carbo load at the center's dining room. Despite the sometimes overwhelming number of visitors, Pinkham Notch Camp holds a special place in his memory. "You felt like you were at the center of a beating heart," he says today. "The place really had a pulse of its own."

AMC Pinkham is what many consider to be basecamp for those intending to launch themselves upward and onto the eastern slopes of Mount Washington and points beyond. Sturdy tables crafted and shellacked in the woodworking shop are scattered throughout the main floor where hikers and climbers can peruse guidebooks and unfurl maps to plot their itinerary or fantasize about future ones. Daily newspapers hang from wooden dowels on the wall for those kept indoors by bad weather or not in a big rush to contend with it. A vending machine with first-class postage stamps and a mail drop slot help keep loved ones and envious friends apprised of epic alpine adventures in progress.

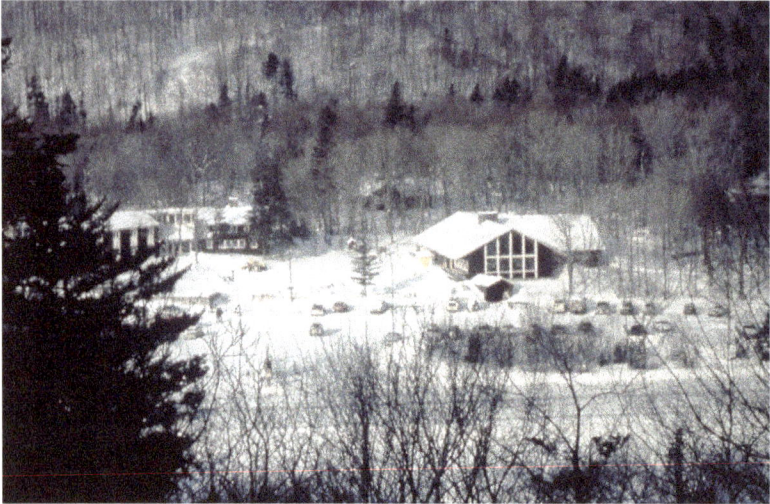

Pinkham Notch Camp in the 1980s.

With five and a half hours remaining in this shift, Moskowitz is juggling roles. He'll register guests staying in the Joe Dodge Lodge, named in honor of the legendary figure whom *New Hampshire Magazine* dubbed "the prime diplomat of the White Mountains." Dodge was instrumental in building the prolific AMC hut system. Moskowitz is also serving as backcountry concierge for anyone intending to venture uphill. "The worse the weather was, the more people would come by to talk about the forecasted reports posted at the information desk," he says.

Though clear and calm in the Notch, the weather forecast posted on the bulletin board predicts a weekend of brutally low temperatures, wind speeds that can knock you over, and copious amounts of falling and blowing snow. Moskowitz knows this forecast will keep a majority of adventurers away or, at the very least, below treeline. But he's also experienced enough to know that the ridges and ravines will still be dotted with a combination of the hardcore and the uninformed, the latter unaware of this mountain range's unpredictable and unforgiving temperament.

Outside in the waning daylight, Hugh Herr and Jeff Batzer are making a beeline for the Tuckerman Ravine Trail en route to Harvard Cabin in Huntington Ravine. Just as the pair did the previous year, they bypass the Trading Post (today known as the Visitor Center) and the Hiker Sign-In Book sitting on the front desk in front of Moskowitz. When he concludes his shift at 10:00 p.m., Moskowitz will relocate the book to the Pack Room in the basement for those arriving late.

Today, Batzer is refreshingly candid about his reasons for not stopping to register that evening. "For myself, it was cockiness," he admits. "I thought, 'Signing in isn't for us; that's for other people who aren't professional climbers.' Looking back, it was a really, really bad decision. But what I was saying was, 'I'm not concerned about that; we're here to climb.' We did sign in once we got up to Harvard Cabin, but that was probably because the caretaker, Matt Pierce, told us we had to."

Back then, as motorists on Route 16 approached Pinkham Notch from either the north or south, they were met by road signs alerting them to the risks in this area:

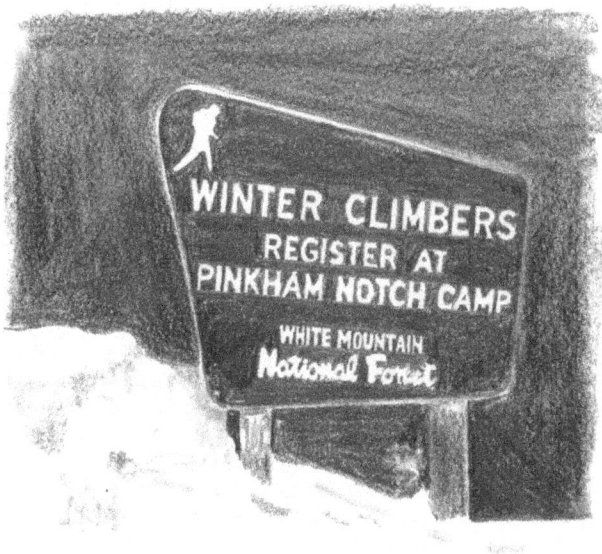

The signs, which no longer exist, were suggestions, not mandates. Today, just as it did then, the register asks for names of the hikers in a party or their leader and the size of the party. It also asks for the hike's start date and start time, the expected return date, phone number(s), vehicle information (color, make, model, state, plate number), and the planned itinerary with trails and campsites. Hikers and climbers are then asked to check out on the same sheet at the conclusion of the trip. A note on the register informs people that the record is not monitored, and that help isn't guaranteed if trouble ensues. The note reads:

> This is not a substitute for leaving an itinerary and check-in plan with a trusted friend or family member who can report you as an overdue hiker. Unless someone reports you as an overdue hiker, there will be no search.

Bill Aughton, a member of Mountain Rescue Service who worked for the AMC as the visitor services manager and search and rescue coordinator from 1990 to 1995, recalls conversations he had with hikers and climbers about the log. "I remember being asked by people who saw the road sign or sign-in sheet if anyone would come looking for them if they didn't sign out. I'd tell them that nobody here checks the book daily, but if hikers or climbers are reported missing by family or friends, then New Hampshire Fish and Game or search and rescue members check the book to see if the party did sign in, and most importantly, if a good itinerary was included."

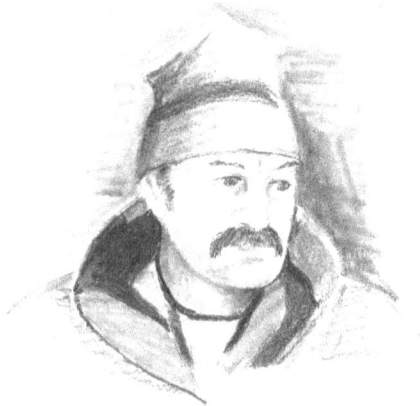

Bill Aughton

As far as Herr and Batzer are concerned on their way up to Harvard Cabin, the only people who know their whereabouts are their parents, who are several hundred miles away in Pennsylvania. Yet what they are doing is not uncommon in the White Mountains. Years later Moskowitz says, "There were many times when people just blew past the main Pinkham building and went right up the trail to either Tuckerman, Harvard Cabin, or Huntington. Hell, I did the same thing, too. You'd drive up to Pinkham from eight hours away, hit the parking lot, put on your pack and—boom!—you just went. You didn't sign in. So, I totally get that."

Tuckerman Ravine Trail
Pinkham Notch
Early evening

Herr and Batzer are roughly 30 minutes into their hike to Harvard Cabin, located about two hiking miles from Pinkham Notch Camp. Their original plan to arrive with enough daylight to do reconnaissance in Huntington Ravine has been stymied by their driving mistake and the short winter day. At the 1.7-mile mark, they reach an intersection with the Huntington Ravine Fire Road and turn right for the remaining 0.3 miles to the cabin.

The pair have been hiking through a part of the forest rich with deciduous trees: American beech, sugar maple, and yellow birch. These species' survival, especially in winter, is due to their location at the lower, more sheltered levels of the forest. Somewhere between 1,500 feet and 2,000 feet, the hardwoods slowly begin to yield to the more robust and resilient conifers: red and black spruce and balsam fir. This transition from taller trees with naked branches to smaller ones thick with needles and their calming aroma is the signal Herr and Batzer have been waiting for. They are reaching the gateway to the high terrain they've been anticipating all day.

Behind this forested landscape lies some of the most awe-inspiring and imposing terrain east of the Rocky Mountains: to the left, Tuckerman Ravine; to the right, Huntington Ravine. These two massive geological amphitheaters are among the six glacial cirques (along with Oakes Gulf, Gulf of Slides, Great Gulf, and Ammonoosuc Ravine) that encircle Mount Washington. They were plucked and

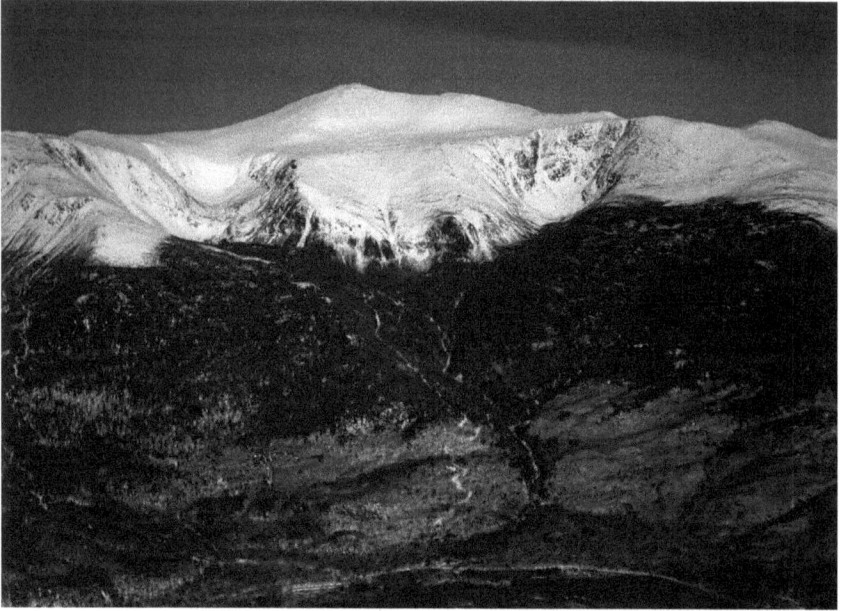

The Cutler River Drainage: Tuckerman Ravine (left), Raymond Cataract (center), and Huntington Ravine (right).

carved about 15,000 to 20,000 years ago by the formation and recession of massive ice sheets higher than Washington itself.

Tuckerman and Huntington Ravines are among the primary draws to this, the eastern side of the mountain. The towering headwalls and steep walls on each side surround their rock-strewn basins far below. For hiker, climber, skier, or snowboarder, there is much to be gained in this terrain—and much to lose. Tuckerman Ravine holds the distinction of being "the birthplace of backcountry skiing," and Huntington Ravine was considered by Dogarf and Wilcox in *New Hampshire Ice* to be "the ice climbing arena of New England" until the 1960s. But the interaction between steep terrain and extreme winter weather also creates serious avalanche hazard, described by Kai-Uwe Allen, snow ranger for the U.S. Forest Service in *Avalanche Terrain and Conditions in the Presidential Range, New Hampshire, USA*: "One of the most dramatic features of the range is the presence of large glacial cirques and U-shaped basins, which flank the range. The locally termed 'gulfs' and 'ravines' serve as the catchment basin for large quantities of windblown snow and are the location of most of the avalanche-prone terrain."

Once the forecasted maelstrom arrives in about 10 hours, this threat of avalanche in the ravines is expected to ratchet up. Herr and Batzer are unaware of this emerging problem and may need to adjust their plans. But for now, 15 minutes after sunset, the frustration of the day's long drive is fading along with the last vestiges of twilight. "The weather that night was good," Batzer recalls. "It was clear, the sun was setting, and it was beautiful."

Three thousand feet above them, on the summit of Mount Washington, things are a bit more disrupted, as is often the case in this variable landscape. The temperature stands at -4°F, with winds out of the northwest at 60 mph. Yet staff on the summit, from the Observatory, WMTW-TV, and the Mount Washington State Park, are experiencing 80 miles of visibility and no sky cover. As weather observers take their hourly measurements outside on the weather tower and observation deck, they are enjoying an evening of stargazing and the glow of North Conway and cities farther south and east—that is, after ducking through regular wind gusts above 70 mph.

Though fatigued, Batzer remembers feeling good about their planned climb in Huntington Ravine the following day. "We were just exhausted that Friday night as we were hiking up to Harvard Cabin," he says today. "But I was much more confident on that trip about my endurance ability. That year I had gotten into bike racing, and I also trained a lot, so my walking ability was 25 percent better than the year before when we were there. For once, on the approach to Harvard Cabin, I could at least stay within 100 yards of Hugh. He was crazy: talk about a set of lungs and a heart that was just natural! You could not keep up with him; he was just so fast on approaches. I was pushing hard on the hike up, but I was right there."

Stepping off the fire road and onto a short spur trail, Batzer and Herr walk below an elongated cloud of gray smoke threading its way through the forest and enjoy the welcoming scent of a wood-burning stove. Through the trees they can see the muted glow of lantern light behind the single-pane, frost-covered windows of Harvard Cabin.

IV
DYNAMICS

Something hidden. Go and find it.
Go and look behind the ranges. Lost and waiting for you. Go!
—Rudyard Kipling

Harvard Cabin (3,520 ft.)
Huntington Ravine, Mount Washington
Friday, Jan. 22, 1982
Evening

Matt Pierce steps into Harvard Cabin's entryway, stomps both feet on the frozen turf, and drives each heel of his custom-made Limmer boots into the stacked pile of dry firewood beside him to dislodge snow that has packed into their burly treads during his hike up from Pinkham. He silently praises himself for selecting the perfect kit for the conditions: a thick wool sweater, heavy over-the-knee wool socks, Woolrich knickers, and a pair of Chuck Roast canvas gaiters to keep the snow from working its way into his cherished leather boots. Pierce, the cabin's winter season caretaker, is carrying a backpack filled with provisions he's brought from Pinkham in anticipation of the predicted bad weather that will likely keep him close to the cabin all weekend.

From behind the cabin door, Pierce hears the voices of guests and the familiar sounds of a winter climbing weekend in the Whites: the clang of multiple camp pots as guests position themselves for a turn at the propane cookstove, the "kalunk, kalunk, kalunk" of mountaineering boots on the cabin's hardwood floor, the snap of carabiners, and the jingling of technical gear being racked on nylon slings. Recognizing the importance of respecting the housekeeping standards he always establishes with his guests, Pierce ensures that his boots are free of snow and opens the squeaky wooden door to step inside.

Then in his early 20s, Pierce grew up in Exeter, New Hampshire when it was still considered farm country. He's spending what will be his only season at the cabin after answering a Harvard Mountaineering Club (HMC) advertisement for the caretaker job. "Even for someone who grew up mountain climbing and camping in the White Mountains in winter, it was kind of a grim existence up there," Pierce recalls today. "It was a very small, one-star upgrade from Jack London."

On Mount Washington, if Pinkham is considered basecamp, Harvard Cabin might be considered advanced basecamp. Located about a mile below Huntington Ravine's glorious amphitheater, this rustic dwelling positions climbers high on Washington's flank so they can get an early morning start and outrun the winter sun's low and rapid arc to the west. The cabin's origins date back to 1932, when the HMC built Spur Cabin, known familiarly as Harvard Hut, along the John Sherburne Ski Trail just below the base of Tuckerman Ravine and Boott Spur. Bradford Washburn, Harvard alumnus, world-renowned mountaineer, and former director of the Boston Museum of Science, was instrumental in hauling materials to the site and helping construct the dwelling. An accomplished photographer and cartographer, Washburn captured images of the White Mountains from the air and created some of the most striking maps of the region.

After the HMC constructed a new Harvard Cabin in 1962, the original was torn down. The site of this new cabin was chosen for its proximity to ice-climbing routes in Huntington Ravine. Today, the Forest Service owns the property the structure sits on and provides a special use permit to the HMC. The cabin is accessible to winter climbers each year from early December to the end of March. At 70 feet by 20 feet, it has two levels that can accommodate approximately 16 guests. Outside, a limited number of tent sites serve those who wish to rough it even more or are training for winter expeditions in other parts of the world. The logs used to construct the cabin are chinked with oakum, or what Pierce describes as a mix of, "mud, moss, rags, etcetera."

Inside are two propane lights that offer minimal illumination, requiring guests to use a headlamp for reading, finding gear, or getting to the nearby outhouse. There's no lighting in the second-floor loft, where guests roll out their sleeping pads and bags on the floor. The walls of the cabin are riddled with nails used to hang drying gear for the following day's climb. Mountaineering boots of all styles and sizes encircle the woodstove to dry out. Benches are fixed to the walls, and a dining table, cookstove, and countertops round out the cabin's sparse amenities.

Pierce arrived at the cabin in late fall to prepare it for the winter season. With the help of snow rangers in a Thiokol vehicle, he had propane tanks brought up from Pinkham and installed them for use with the two-burner stove. He also split and stacked firewood from trees cut down by the previous winter's caretaker. Before deep snow could take hold of the surrounding terrain, he felled dying trees near the cabin to dry out wood for use the following winter. As the temperature dropped, he would retrieve an axe and chip away ice that had frozen over the hole he'd cut to fetch fresh water from the brook behind the cabin.

As weeks passed, Pierce says he gradually adjusted to the cabin's "aromas of wood smoke, bachelor cooking, gym locker ripeness— and mice." Prior to his arrival, three dozen or so mice established residence inside the cabin. "The mice ruled that winter," he recalls. "That is, until 'Pop' the weasel moved into the cabin and provided nightly entertainment for me and my guests." Pop's stealth and cunning would methodically reduce the rodent population to zero by the end of the 1981–82 winter season.

For the most part, Pierce embraced the isolation of his early days at the cabin. "There was nobody telling me what to do," he says. "If no reservations had been made or no one had shown up at Pinkham and asked how to get to Harvard Cabin, I might have a night in Pinkham to do laundry or go catch a movie or go out to dinner. If I needed food, I'd go down to Pinkham and catch a ride or take my not-so-trusty Volvo station wagon into Gorham or North Conway." He'd get an occasional visit from the snow rangers, who were also gearing up for the arrival of climbers and skiers.

Once the season opened on Dec. 1, technical climbers arrived with their gear and nighttime tales of their conquests of high places. "We got daily weather reports every morning at 8:00 a.m. from the Mount Washington Observatory, and I'd post the forecast in the cabin along with the avalanche conditions when they were provided," Pierce recalls. "Guests made reservations through the desk at Pinkham back then, so the AMC would let me know in the morning and again at 4:00 p.m. how many to expect, but drop-ins were more the norm. I'd check people in before dark and give them the lowdown on the area and the rules of the cabin."

While guests were off on the mountain during the day, Pierce would tend to caretaker tasks and sometimes roam the trails on his own. "I'd shovel off the piece of plywood that covered the hole in the snow where the ladder went down to the spring and fill the bucket with water for cooking and drinking. I'd check to make sure the outhouse was OK, and then I'd head up onto The Fan to see what people were doing and hike and climb around a bit myself." The Fan is a large scree field consisting of loose rocks and debris at the base of the ravine's headwall.

As he steps into the cabin on this Friday night, Pierce greets the guests preparing their evening's stay. Sitting at the kitchen table are Layne Terrell, his then-wife Kacy (Terrell) St. Clair, and his brother-in-law, Paul Geissler. They had arrived in Pinkham late Wednesday and slept in the back of Layne's truck. "It was too late to hike up to the cabin," says Geissler. "Kacy's feet froze that night in the truck. I'd had a horrible experience with frostbite in the Adirondacks, so I knew what to do. I had her put her feet on her husband's belly to warm them up." The following morning the trio grabbed breakfast, signed in at Pinkham, and cross-country skied up to the cabin. There they

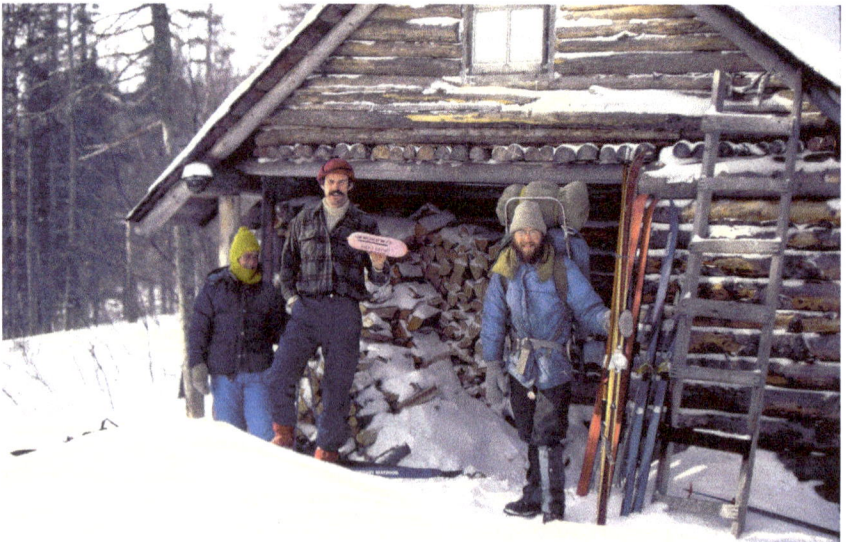

Kacy (Terrell) St. Clair, caretaker Matt Pierce (center), and Paul Geissler in front of Harvard Cabin. The sign Pierce is holding reads, "It's OK to ask for help. Harvad [sic] Cabin.

found a note written by Pierce with a warm welcome and an encouragement to "make yourselves at home."

Kacy Terrell recalls Pierce as "extremely kind and very knowledgeable." New to the sport of ice climbing and despite her bout with frozen feet, she remembers that weekend trip fondly. "I was a novice climber, so I had two days of putzing around and one climb up Yale Gully. All my previous experience was in Virginia, and it doesn't get quite as cold there."

Paul Geissler, an avid ice climber who'd climbed in New Zealand and Alaska, had traveled from Tasmania to visit his sister and brother-in-law. Layne Terrell had been climbing rock since 1975 and ice since 1980 and had been making regular trips to the Whites from their home in Virginia. "There weren't a lot of people ice climbing where I lived at the time," he says. "I'd heard Mount Washington was a good place to visit, and I got addicted to it. I love it up there." Terrell was also well aware of the risks associated with climbing on the Northeast's highest peak: "A couple of years before that trip, I assisted with a carryout to Pinkham for a climber who'd fallen out of a gully and suffered a spinal and head injury," he recalls.

The trio spent most of Thursday climbing Yale Gully. According to *An Ice Climber's Guide to Northern New England* (Lewis & Wilcox), Yale is "a slightly right leaning shallow gully to the lip. A long, varied, and enjoyable route." Prior to leaving the cabin, one of them followed the protocol outlined by Pierce and entered their planned itinerary into the log:

What was intended to be an exciting progression for Kacy proved to be a physical and interpersonal challenge. "The gully was so hard," she recalls. "There wasn't any blue ice in the gully like I was used to; it was solid and scary." Geissler led the climb and rather than using ice screws, placed rock protection (pitons and nuts) on the rocky side of the gully. As they reached the end of the climb and unroped, they headed up into Alpine Garden, where they were more exposed to the weather. "Topping out on Yale, I remember strong wind gusts and a lot of spindrift," says Layne Terrell. "Paul had a touch of frostbite on the tip of his nose, and I remember falling over when the wind gusts would subside."

Kacy's recollection of the climb is indicative of the differences in risk tolerance that existed within the group. "Our original plan was to go to the summit of Mount Washington. Once we got to the top of the gully, we decided to rope up again. I accidently stepped on the rope, and the damaged portion had to be tied off. We were up there a pretty long time. It was gloriously beautiful—and tedious—-and the wind was fierce. I remember looking down and being able to see, but when I looked up, the wind was kicking the snow up terribly. It was a whiteout. I don't think we totally gave up on the summit until I saw Paul's nose, and I freaked out a bit. His nose had gone white, and I was frightened of frostbite. The winds were picking up more, and I was the one who absolutely refused to go farther because I couldn't see, and I was scared."

On the summit of Washington that afternoon, winds were out of the northwest ranging from 30 to 50 mph. Temperatures were in the negative single digits, and visibility at the summit was surprisingly excellent at 90 miles. For experienced climbers, the weather conditions were considered manageable, but for Kacy, who was new to powerful winds and blowing snow, they were overwhelming and intimidating. Fortunately, Terrell and Geissler were sensitive to Kacy's alarm, and the group made a turbulent 7/10ths-of-a-mile traverse over to Escape Hatch, where they descended.

On Friday, the group headed into Huntington Ravine again. Kacy chose not to climb but rather to practice her axe and crampon skills on The Fan, while her husband and brother climbed Odell Gully. At the end of the day, they descended Escape Hatch as they had the day before.

Another party of three are also in Harvard Cabin that Friday evening, preparing for an early start the following day. Henry "Hank" Butler, Jim Frati, and Bob MacEntee had arrived at Pinkham from the Boston area and gone directly to the Pack Room in the basement of the Trading Post, where they packed up their climbing gear, food, and bivy gear before hiking up to the cabin. Once there, they heated up a "climbers special" for dinner, Butler recalls: "A huge pot of macaroni with one can of tuna and one of cream of mushroom soup thrown in and stirred well."

Frati and MacEntee, who'd climbed together a couple of times before this trip, had picked up Butler at his home. Upon approaching Frati's car, Butler was surprised to see that his friend wasn't alone, especially when he learned that MacEntee wasn't a very experienced ice climber. "I was not happy about it," recalls Butler. "This was not part of the plan. I knew a storm was expected sometime during the weekend, and I had absolutely no idea how bad it would be. We were always training for the Alps—every climber's dream. To complete a difficult route in full conditions was the mark of a competent alpinist. We actually welcomed bad storms. But I did not want this new kid coming along. Jim assured me that the kid was good, and that they had climbed together previously, so I decided to trust Jim's judgment."

Both Frati and MacEntee acknowledge today that they were pretty new to ice climbing back then. "We weren't highly experienced," says MacEntee. "I had done some winter camping. and climbed some 4,000-footers in the winter. I got into technical climbing with Jim. I tried to make good decisions, but I was also capable of making mistakes."

Two additional guests were sitting on one of the benches, talking quietly and preparing their gear. Hugh Herr and Jeff Batzer had arrived after the Terrell/Geissler party and before Frati and his companions. "I was a little perturbed because they had gotten into some of my food," recalls Pierce, though Herr and Batzer have no recollection of this. "They were 17 or 18 and probably somewhat entitled at that age."

Pierce asked the pair if they had registered in the cabin's log, and they hadn't. He then asked each to pay the $2.50 per head required for the night's stay, but they had left their wallets in the truck, not realizing they were required to pay. After dealing with previous climbers who didn't feel the need to pay the lodging fee, Pierce was keen on collecting it. "A number of climbers would try to squirrel out of paying. There were times I could barely get $2.50 out of a group of two or three. More than a few climbers argued with me over the fee. There are always some who feel their pursuit of fun should be free." Batzer and Herr assured Pierce they would pay before heading back to Pennsylvania, and after several more proddings, they finally signed in to the log.

Layne Terrell recalls that the tension level in the cabin rose as the evening progressed. "When the boys came in—they were younger than us, and we were young at the time—it was like a comedy of errors. Matt was a little put off because they couldn't pay. Everybody assumed that these two guys were pretty novice. It was an odd night."

Batzer says today that he regrets their youthful behavior that night. "It got more awkward as the evening went on. But everyone was very patient with us, and Matt had to do his job."

Herr, too, remembers their exchanges with Pierce. "I'd describe him as a prickly guy. We were young, rough around the edges, and he was the caretaker. He felt we didn't follow protocol as he wanted us to."

Taking the hint that their presence is causing some tension in the small cabin, Batzer and Herr turn in early and retreat to the second-floor loft, where they stay to themselves and listen to the lively conversation below until Pierce signals that it's time to call it a night. "We had a 10:00 p.m. lights-out policy, kind of a courtesy rule: quit yapping, quit drinking, and get in your sleeping bags," says Pierce.

The following day's weather forecast has everyone taking a wait-and-see approach. They know an update will arrive by radio call from the Mount Washington Observatory at 8:00 a.m.

Before turning in himself, Pierce prepares a thermos of hot tea and ensures the gas burners on the cookstove are off. He douses the two propane lanterns, rendering the cabin pitch black, and uses his headlamp to ascend the ladder to the landing, where he crawls through a window frame and into the "rabbit hutch" above the porch, a 10-by-4-foot space that serves as the caretaker's quarters. "There wasn't enough room to stand up straight," says Pierce. "It was just a place to sleep." He makes sure his headlamp is close by in case he's rousted during the night by trouble inside or out. Given the cabin's close proximity to the ravine, Pierce can be called upon for search and rescue-related matters. Occasionally, he is asked to select guests who appear trustworthy and competent to form a so-called "hasty team" to respond to an incident in the ravine or beyond. He's hoping that won't be necessary this weekend, but with an ominous weather forecast and the many human factors at play in the cabin already, he's not optimistic.

V
MARGIN CALL

The dangers of life are infinite, and among them is safety.
—Goethe

Mount Washington Observatory Surface Weather Observations (7:00 to 8:00 a.m.): Temperature -7°F; winds out of the south averaging 50 mph; visibility 2 miles, snow; windchill -21.2°F; peak wind gust: 68 mph.

Harvard Cabin
Saturday, Jan. 23, 1982
7:00 a.m.

Matt Pierce is waking up slowly within the confines of the "rabbit hutch" and the two sleeping bags he's encased in. "It was a cold winter that year," he recalls. "If it was a particularly nice day. I'd turn the sleeping bags inside out, take them outside, and beat the frost out of them." He feels around inside the sleeping bags for the thermos of hot tea he made before going to bed. It's part of his nightly ritual to store the thermos inside the bags because it adds some additional warmth and ensures the beverage isn't cold when he takes his first sips in the morning.

It's rare that anyone sleeping in the second-floor loft adjacent to the caretaker's hutch rises before Pierce has had the chance to descend the ladder to the main floor and reignite the woodstove. "Unless it was a balmy 25 degrees, I'd have a fire going in the morning," he says. He lights the burner of the cookstove, heats a kettle of water, and recharges his tea. He knows that the aroma of woodsmoke will rouse guests seeking a rapid infusion of hot caffeine.

The 7:12 a.m. sunrise is still a few minutes away, but guests begin to rise and stand at the cookstove heating oatmeal and coffee or warm themselves up by doing jumping jacks. Each checks out the view from a window to gauge the weather. The Terrells and Geissler look at the muted gray skies and light snowfall swirling across the terrain and immediately decide, "Nope, not today." They know the mountain is in the early throes of forecasted bad weather, and with two days of climbing already behind them, including Thursday's epic in the Alpine Garden, they have no interest in braving another tough one today.

Hank Butler, Jim Frati, and Bob MacEntee are hesitating. Before making a final decision, they elect to wait for the 8:00 a.m. weather forecast from the Observatory. "We had all day," says MacEntee. "We were in no rush to get out."

While Jeff Batzer is still lying in his sleeping bag, gearing himself up to face the cold loft, he listens with trepidation as the winds buffet the cabin. He isn't reassured when he glances out a window after rising. "I could tell before we went out the door that conditions were bad," he says. "I thought, 'Oh, man, we're not going to get to the top of Mount Washington.' I was kind of dejected, but I hoped there'd be some way to work it out so we could make it to the top of the mountain."

Batzer joins Hugh Herr, and the two prepare to go out and up. Sitting on a bench, they align their gear with their chosen route. Their plan is to climb Pinnacle Gully, the same route they climbed the year before. "Pinnacle was called Pinnacle because for a lot of people that was the feather to collect—bragging rights or whatever you want to call it," says Pierce. When they have readied the single backpack they'll take with them, the two friends make breakfast with their freeze-dried food. The other guests quietly go about their business and wonder if these two young guys truly understand what they might be getting themselves into. No one is ready to vocalize their concern, however, as they await the weather report.

In fact, the weather had deteriorated while the would-be climbers still slept during the hour before dawn. Visibility on the summit of Washington had taken a nosedive from 90 miles down to 2 miles, the average wind speed had increased by 12 mph, the windchill factor had dropped 6 degrees, and it had started snowing.

At that time, there wasn't a Higher Summits Forecast as exists today. Until the mid-1990s when a more simplistic version of the current forecast was first posted on the Mount Washington

Observatory website, those engaging in mountain pursuits consulted local forecasts and considered their own experience above treeline to determine how arriving weather systems might affect Washington's mood and whether it made sense to test the mountain's tolerance for visitors. In 2014, a comprehensive 48-hour Higher Summits Forecast, accompanied by a Forecast Discussion, was introduced and is still in place, updated twice daily.

Dr. Peter Crane, curator at the Mount Washington Observatory and a Harvard Cabin caretaker from 1977 to 1978, worked for the AMC for 10 years before joining the Observatory. "In 1982, the weather forecast was broadcast to all AMC facilities and Harvard Cabin on a shared radio frequency via an 8:00 a.m. broadcast," he says. "The forecast came from the National Weather Service and included the valley forecast for that day, that night, and the next day."

As the guests at Harvard Cabin gather around, the radio crackles to life, and everyone leans in. As they expect, current conditions on the summit of Mount Washington are not great, and the day's forecast calls for a rapid deterioration of weather involving snowfall, shifting high winds, and cold temperatures that will continue throughout the weekend.

Given the snow and the speed and direction of the winds, Pierce knows the risk of avalanche in Huntington Ravine will build over time. "All in all, with the winds that high, it didn't matter where you went, wind slab was going to form somewhere that weekend. I was of the mindset that we were getting snow, and it was going to blow hard and be nasty out. If you're in a gully you have to assume the possibility of wind slab. Sometimes it's fun, fluffy stuff, and sometimes it isn't."

Rene LaRoche, a snow ranger from 1966 to 1994, recalls today that the avalanche forecast for the start of that weekend was not alarming. "I don't remember observing any avalanche hazard on Thursday, Friday, or Saturday before the storm arrived," he says. "The hazard began to develop later on Saturday and over the following days."

After hearing the forecast, Pierce takes a few moments to process the information and then offers his assessment to the group. "I told everyone it was a good day to stay down low and warm," recalls Pierce. "Not weather to climb in unless you had a good reason to."

He knows there's only so much he can do to influence anyone's decision to go out, especially given the varying appetites for risk among climbers. Still, when he sees Herr and Batzer moving ahead, he feels the need to step in. "They were talking about going up Pinnacle, and I said, 'You know, it's going to be bad today, really windy, maybe blowing 75 and gusting higher. Whatever you go up, it's not going to be good once you top out.' My impression was they weren't totally green, but it just didn't seem like it was in their best interest to do what they talked about doing."

Herr and Batzer definitely sense the worry they are causing among the other guests and are open to discussing the advisability of their plans. "I was aware of the concern for us from the older people in the cabin," recalls Batzer. "There wasn't a lot of talk, but I could sense definite concern for us because we were so young. I don't think anyone would have known it was Hugh Herr with me. They had no idea how experienced and gifted he was."

MacEntee says he recalls Batzer and Herr asking the others what they thought. "There was talk about it not being a great day to climb, and maybe that's why they tried to go early," he says. "My impression of Hugh was that he had a lot of good high-level rock-climbing experience, but it seemed to me that neither of them had a lot of alpine experience in winter, maybe some but not a lot. But Hugh had so much confidence."

Herr says today that he and Batzer made their decision to go out with full knowledge of the conditions they were facing. "I was aware of what the weather was going to be, and the weather conditions were listed at the cabin," he says.

In fact, at this early hour, with the storm still in its infancy, the weather is not so serious as to unduly alarm Herr and Batzer, especially given their experience in high places. Accepting the fact that they are still resolved to climb, Pierce tries another tactic aimed at reducing some of the risk he anticipates the pair will face. "I was trying to steer them away from Pinnacle because people had been blown off pitches there. First and foremost, it was wind concerns. If you're going to go fast and light, which they were talking about doing, Odell Gully presented a lower risk for that day's conditions and forecast. You could tell by how much stuff was in their pack that they weren't planning on an evening out."

Pierce's good counsel ends up persuading Herr and Batzer to

change their plans, and they decide to climb Odell Gully rather than attempt Pinnacle. Eager to get started, they take up their pack and their rope and head out for Odell. "We left one pack at the cabin and carried one between us to stay light," says Batzer. "Our pack held a camera, a canteen of water, dried food, a bivy sac, a headlamp, matches, and a compass. We decided not to take a sleeping bag to

Odell Gully

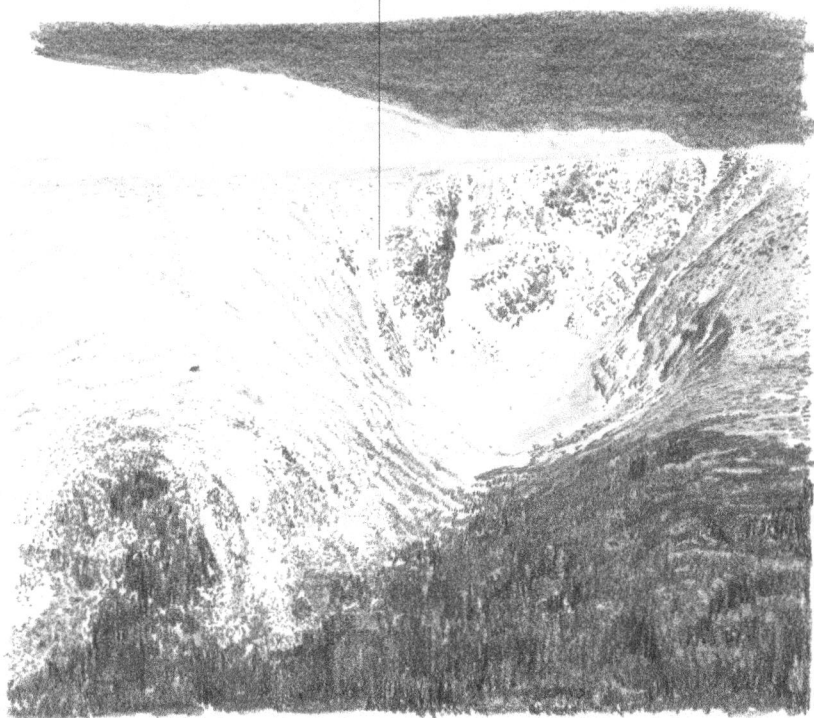

Huntington Ravine

keep things light."

Pierce says today that Herr and Batzer's decision to go fast and light was not uncommon back then. "Few people brought bivy gear with them, and only some of those who did would bring it with them climbing. Others would leave some or all of it at the cabin. It was the rage to go light and fast, especially for the young climbers. It was just a hill in New England, after all. Very cavalier. Older climbers tended to be better prepared."

Given their technical climbing skill, Herr and Batzer's decision to go up early and descend before the weather turns is a reasonable undertaking. They're familiar with the ravine and the Escape Hatch from the previous year's visit. Odell Gully lies just to the left of Pinnacle. In addition, by packing a compass that each knows how to use, they've included an important tool in the event that high winds and blowing snow compromise visibility. Yet despite their skill and knowledge of the area, Batzer acknowledges today that he and Herr underestimated what they were heading into. "It was a lack of understanding about Mount Washington," he says. "We knew the conditions, but we didn't realize we were dealing with an absolute giant when it comes to weather."

Before they leave the cabin, Pierce reminds the young duo to clean up the remains of their breakfast and write their itinerary in the log. One of them jots down:

1-23/82

Hugh Herr, Jeff Batzer: up odells down escape hatch.

No one remaining in the cabin is aware of Batzer's hope to summit Washington, which remains in play. The pair step onto the short, well-packed spur trail and begin their one-mile trek into Huntington Ravine.

Shortly after their departure, three more guests exit the cabin and head for the ravine. The ominous forecast and concern for Herr and Batzer are not enough to deter this trio from getting after it. The ravine in all its alpine grandeur and the likelihood of "full conditions" are just too enticing. Below Herr and Batzer's log entry, they write:

1-23

Henry Butler, Jim Frati + friend up to Hunts, whatever's feasible.

VI
DARK RAVINE

When you invent the ship, you also invent
the shipwreck.
—Paul Virilio, philosopher

Mount Washington Observatory Surface Weather Observations (8:00 to 9:00 a.m.): Temperature 7°F; winds out of the south averaging 54 mph; visibility 0 miles, snow/blowing snow/fog; windchill -21.9°; peak wind gust: 66 mph.

Huntington Ravine Trail
Saturday, Jan. 23, 1982
8:30 a.m.

Hugh Herr moves over the hiker's trough, a narrow channel in the snow created by foot traffic, and Jeff Batzer is right there with him. Batzer smiles as his legs and lungs reap the reward of the hundreds of miles he's logged on his road bike back home. Small clouds from their rapid exhalations appear and disappear as they work to steal time from this short winter's day. When the tops of the trees reach shoulder level and the terrain before them widens, they're eager to see what the conditions look like high on the mountain. Will the door to the summit of Mount Washington be open wide enough for them to squeeze through it later this morning?

Batzer's goal of reaching the summit after the technical climb of Odell, which Herr doesn't fully aspire to, remains unspoken. For Batzer the desire is more pressing because the top of the mountain represents the start of his progression onto much higher peaks. For Herr, it would be merely a long walk for a trusted and loyal friend.

Thus far, all indications point toward an expanded itinerary. "I was very excited," Batzer says today. "We were trying to get going early because we needed all the time we could get for whatever was ahead of us. The sun was coming up and it was gray out, but I don't remember any wind or snow up above us. It actually seemed like conditions were somewhat calm compared to what they were at the cabin." Batzer is so enthusiastic about how the morning is rolling out that he likely doesn't realize that his favorable perception of the conditions is strengthening the confirmation he seeks for what he wants to achieve.

Huntington Ravine is named in honor of geologist Joshua Henry Huntington. With New Hampshire State Geologist Charles Hitchcock, Huntington co-led the 1870–71 winter occupation of the summit of Washington. This high-mountain weather station was the precursor of the Mount Washington Observatory, founded in 1932. The ravine is, in the words of Guy and Laura Waterman's *Forest and Crag*, "stark and menacing, but also beautiful beyond compare on the right day and in the right frame of mind." The first winter ascent here occurred on Feb. 23, 1927, when John Golden and Nathaniel Goodrich successfully climbed what is known today as Central Gully. The flagship route, Pinnacle Gully, which Herr and Batzer climbed successfully the year before, was first ascended on Feb. 8, 1930, by Samuel Scoville and Julian Whittlesey. In the years that followed, other well-known routes were established, and new variations in the ravine are still being climbed today.

Herr and Batzer's new objective this morning, Odell Gully, was first climbed on March 16, 1929, when Noel Odell led four members of the Harvard Mountaineering Club and three from the AMC on a successful winter ascent of the gully that would ultimately bear his name. Odell chopped every step in the ice and snow for himself and his companions from the bottom all the way to the top. In March 1982, Phil Kukielski, a reporter for the *Providence Journal*, aptly described Odell Gully as "a scar in the south side of the ravine's headwall. In summer, it's a natural storm drain. In winter, it's an ice sculpture. Groundwater from the plateau above forms long ribbons of blue-green ice that stretch 800 feet to the base of the ravine."

When Odell arrived in Huntington Ravine he was already known in the annals of mountaineering as a member of the 1924 British Mount Everest Expedition and was the last person to see George Mallory and Sandy Irvine high on the ridge of Everest before they disappeared in the high cloud cover. Mallory and Irvine's position on the mountain and subsequent disappearance sparked an international debate that remains today as to whether Mallory and Irvine were the first to reach the summit of the world's highest peak. Odell comments on that fateful day in "Mallory and Irvine—1924":

> At 12:50, just after I had emerged from a state of jubilation at finding the first definite fossils on Everest, there was a sudden clearing of the atmosphere, and the entire summit ridge and final peak of Everest were unveiled. My eyes became fixed on one tiny black spot silhouetted on a small snow-crest beneath a rock-step in the ridge; the black spot moved. Another black spot became apparent and moved up the snow to join the other on the crest. The first then approached the great rock-step and shortly emerged at the top; the second did likewise. Then the whole fascinating vision vanished, enveloped in cloud once more.

In keeping with their established routine, Batzer carries the single pack they have with them while Herr totes the technical gear. Herr has a new climbing rope slung over his head and sitting on his shoulder "like a Swiss alpinist," recalls Batzer. With the assistance of nylon slings, he carries a rack of assorted protection: carabiners, ice screws, cams, and chocks. Although they've packed for a rapid ascent of Odell, the two are well equipped for the day's plan. Both have rigid crampons, glacier glasses, a climbing harness, and two ice axes each. "We had the best technical equipment there was," recalls Batzer. "At least I did because I had money. Hugh was in high school but still had good stuff. But we didn't have Everest-caliber gear, the kind you take when you expect to be out for days."

The pair arrive at the point of the trail where the terrain expands before them in a manner that's difficult to comprehend. Freezing fog spanning the entire color palate of gray hangs just below the ravine's rim like a giant cornice. When combined with the steep walls of the ravine and their elongated striations of dark ice runnels and gullies choked with snow, it's as if Herr and Batzer are drifting in a small boat at the base of a gigantic rogue wave in the Antarctic Ocean. They're in the alpine zone now.

As they reach the end of the tree-lined trail and it breaks out into open ground, they take in the conditions at the top of the portion of the ravine they're able to see. The decision about the summit quest is immediate and shared: they will not go for it. "It was a brief interaction," recalls Batzer, "and it was the way Hugh and I operated with each other. We would talk deeply and at length about life and everything else when we weren't climbing. But when we were climbing, we'd make a fairly quick decision."

With a summit bid now off the table, Herr and Batzer decide there's no need to bring the backpack with their bivy gear. They have reduced their risk by not choosing to advance to the summit and believe it will be safer to climb Odell without the weight of their pack, as light as it is. "It was an important piece in our psyche," Batzer recalls. "This was the mindset of two young climbers. Fast and light could be dangerous, but we felt it was safer from a technical standpoint because you're not carrying much weight. We put a lot of emphasis on safety with the technical side of climbing, and we thought by going light we'd decrease our chances of falling off our routes. That was the thing back then: you'd leave your pack behind, attack, and come down."

Their decision to leave their pack behind is identical to the one they made a year earlier when they stashed the pack before climbing Pinnacle and retrieved it after descending Escape Hatch. Everything worked out then, so why should this year be any different? They're confident in this minimalist approach, and it aligns with their intent to climb and descend fast. Jeff Fongemie, director and avalanche forecaster for the Mount Washington Avalanche Center and a member of Mountain Rescue Service, understands the logic Herr and Batzer used in 1982. "I'm not big on stashing packs, but it makes sense in the situation they were in. It's kind of protected there, and you can look up and see your climb."

But by stashing the pack are Herr and Batzer narrowing their safety margin rather than widening it? Do they realize there are differences in the weather system this year, that there are new variables in play? The weather the previous year was clear and calm; today it will worsen. On that previous visit, they did not consider advancing to the summit of Washington. As of now, they've canceled their planned summit attempt, but will they be able to resist that temptation at the top of the gully?

After caching the pack behind a large boulder, Herr and Batzer focus their attention on Odell Gully. They don their crampons, unholster their ice axes, and start up The Fan, a steep slope riddled with rocks that, when covered by snow, makes the going a bit easier, but no less dangerous. Herr says today that his concern about avalanche hazard was growing at that point. "I knew avalanche dangers would increase as the day went on, so I was in avalanche-avoidance mode: go early, go really fast." Batzer doesn't possess the same level of experience as Herr and will rely on him for guidance through the terrain.

Today, they are pleased to find ankle-to-shin-deep snow covering a still discernable trail. Bill Aughton, a former member of the British Special Air Service and a member of Mountain Rescue Service, says that although The Fan is not a technical gully, it is to be respected. "With The Fan, the steep snow comes down from the gullies, and people think they can just walk up those things. I've seen people on The Fan without crampons and just a long ice axe. It's an inherent danger before you get on to the climbing, and to me it's actually safer in the gullies."

Having reached the top of The Fan without difficulty or incident, Herr and Batzer arrive at the base of Odell Gully just before 9:00 a.m. It's finally time to climb.

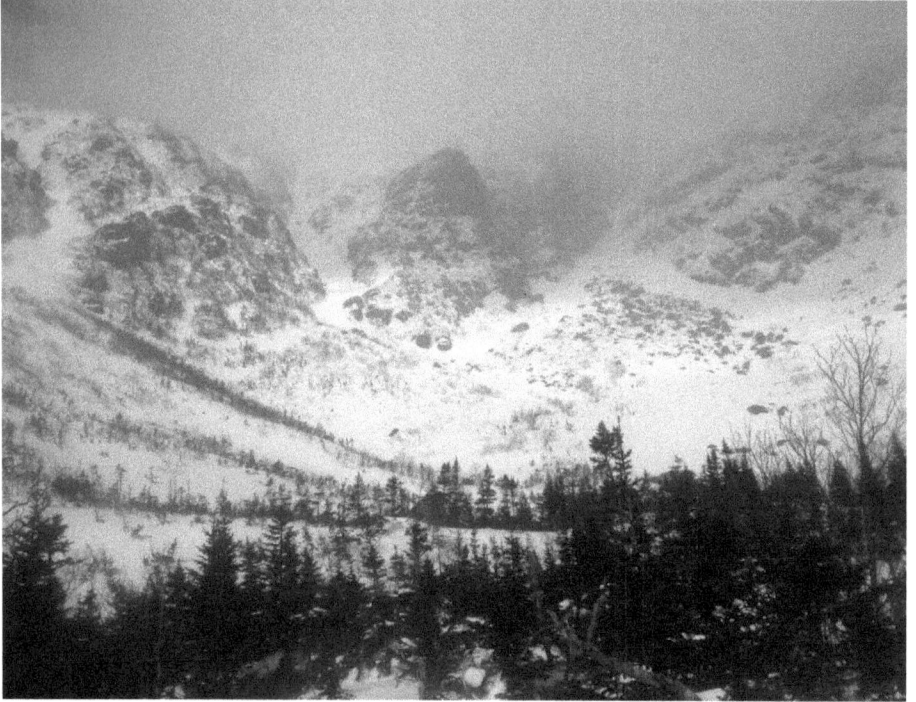

Huntington Ravine in low cloud cover and frozen fog.

VII
PUSH

If you're not young and brash between 17 and about 24
you might as well shoot yourself because that's when people
are young and brash.
—Alan "Hevy Duty" Stevenson, noted climber

Mount Washington Observatory Surface Weather Observations (9:00 to 10:00 a.m.): Temperature 1°F; winds out of the south averaging 59 mph; visibility 0 miles, snow/blowing snow/fog; windchill -31.5°F; peak wind gust: 69 mph.

Huntington Ravine
Saturday, Jan. 23, 1982
9:00 a.m.

Matt Pierce stops at a point on the Huntington Ravine Trail where he can take in as much of the towering amphitheater as possible. He has been drawn here by a combination of concern and curiosity. "I remember it was low visibility," Pierce says today. "I could see somewhere between a half to a third of the way up the wall of the ravine, and then things disappeared into the blowing snow. I went up there because I wanted to see what conditions were developing and how cold it was."

Pierce sees Hugh Herr and Jeff Batzer at the base of Odell Gully readying themselves to climb. As he looks on, his worry eases somewhat because they've remained committed to their altered plan of bypassing the more technical Pinnacle Gully. Pleased that his warning earlier that morning seems to have influenced the pair, he crosses his arms, jams a Dachstein mitten-covered hand into each armpit, and stiffens his upper torso. "It was really cold," he recalls. "The wind was blowing, but not super hard, and then all of a sudden you'd get hit with a pretty good gust. When you're at the bottom of the ravine, you get the rollover effect of really strong downdrafts or the williwaw winds that come pouring down a gully and hit you. In those conditions, the higher up the gullies you go, the more you get exposed to the wind. Then at the top, you stick your head up above the edge of the ravine and you're completely in it."

Pierce is fixated on watching Herr and Batzer and doesn't see Hank Butler, Jim Frati, or Bob MacEntee, who are heading up The Fan. At the time, Frati was a teacher for an outdoor program in Brockton, Mass., and in his second year of climbing. "We left the cabin shortly after Jeff and Hugh, and they were just ahead of us," he recalls. "It was so windy, and the snow was blowing so much while we were hiking up the trail that I really couldn't make them out very well, and then I just couldn't see them at all. We separated from them in The Fan and went to do our own climb."

The three are also mindful of Pierce's concern about the escalating avalanche hazard, so they choose their route once they see where Herr and Batzer are headed. "We were going to do the gully that Hugh and Jeff weren't doing," Frati recalls. "We knew they were in Odell's, and the conditions were so bad when we got into the ravine

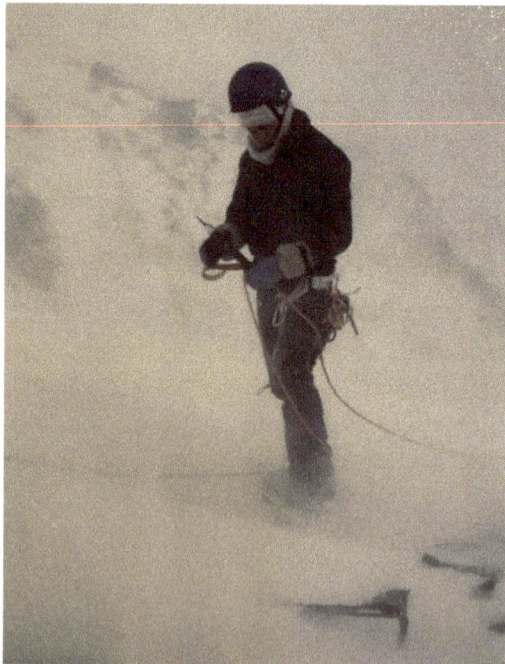

Bob MacEntee stands on The Fan amid blowing snow and low visibility as he prepares to climb Central Gully with Jim Frati and Hank Butler on Jan. 23.

that we decided to climb Central [Gully] instead. The winds were just howling, and if you put your ice axe out in front of you it was hard to even see it."

Pierce watches intently as Herr is the first to start climbing. In keeping with his and Batzer's commitment to speed for safety's sake, Herr intermittently drives the sharp pic of each of his two ice axes into the ice above him and kicks the front points of his crampons into the frozen flow below him. With four points of contact to the ice, he moves gracefully up the first pitch, repeating the axe swings and crampon kicks as he goes. Pierce sees their 160-foot rope go taut as Herr, who's now out of view, establishes his first belay and pulls up the slack. Without delay, Batzer starts upward toward his friend.

The pair's high degree of hard-earned technical proficiency is on full display this morning. That is, until it's not. Using both hands, Pierce shields his watering eyes from the blowing snow and the bite of the windchill and tries to locate Batzer. He's gone, too. Absorbed by the elements, Herr and Batzer have penetrated the wafting veil of freezing fog and blowing snow.

Pebble-like snowflakes pelt Pierce's already frigid cheeks as he stares at the point where he last saw Herr and Batzer. How eerily apropos to think that Noel Odell, the first to climb this gully that bears his name, watched as George Mallory and Sandy Irvine disappeared into the clouds high up on Mount Everest 58 years earlier. It's futile for Pierce to linger any longer because, given what he knows of the seemingly boundless ambition that Herr and Batzer share, he's confident they won't call it a morning and rappel back to the base. He drops his stinging chin behind the high collar of his thick wool jacket, turns his back to the emerging onslaught, and makes his way back to the warmth and security of the woodstove at Harvard Cabin.

Central Gully
9:30 a.m.

With two figure-eight knots, Hank Butler secures to his climbing harness the two ropes that he and his companions will use to ascend Central Gully. One connects him to Jim Frati and the other to Bob MacEntee. Butler will climb up to a point where he can establish a sound anchor in the ice or snow, and then belay Frati and MacEntee as they climb side by side up to him. This is known as parallel technique. Once Frati and MacEntee are secure at the belay station, Butler will head up. This pattern will continue all the way to the rim of the ravine and allow them to move quickly.

"Back then my favorite gully was Odell's," Butler says. "Its couloirs were choked with deep-blue water ice. But because of the new guy [MacEntee], I made the call to climb Central Gully instead. Less ice in Central, less time to get up and out. Looking back now, I think that decision was crucial. With three of us climbing on one rope in Odell's, as opposed to two separate ropes in Central, we would have been topping out in the dark and directly into a raging blizzard."

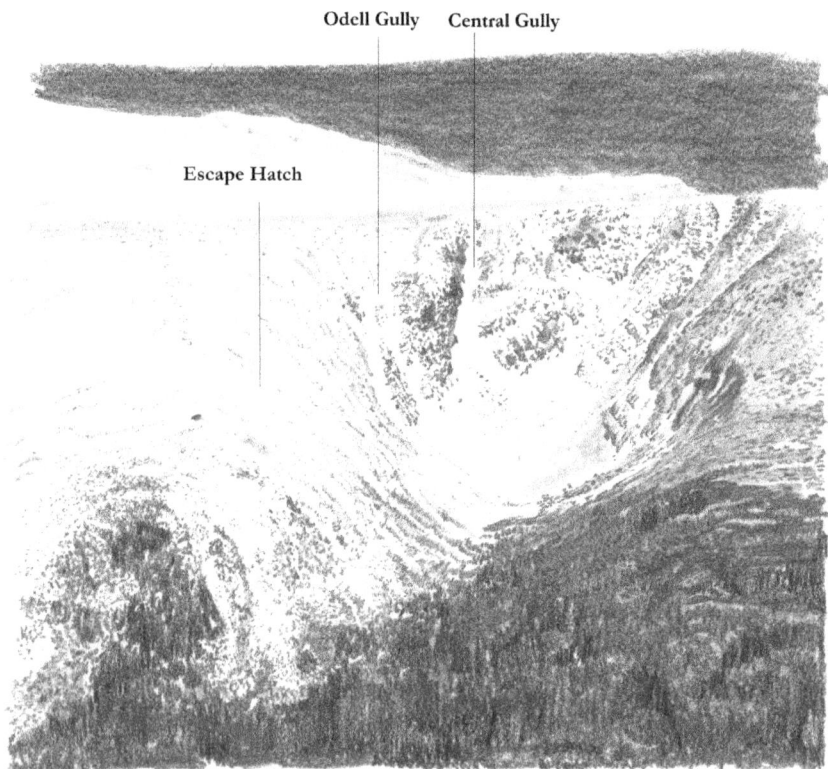

Huntington Ravine

One of the longest climbs there at 1,000 feet, Central Gully starts out as a moderately steep snow climb before arriving at a more technical ice bulge. From there, it transitions into a steeper snow climb up to Alpine Garden.

At this stage, the five climbers from Harvard Cabin are primarily concerned with completing their respective climbs before the worst of the oncoming weather system. Like Herr and Batzer, the party of three is choosing to move light and fast. "We didn't have bivy gear because we were staying at the cabin," says Frati. "We were running pretty light, but in reality, nothing was really light back then. I had lobster claw mittens with sheepskin lining. It's only after shit happens that someone says, 'You should have brought a sleeping bag with you.' You do what you go there to do and then you run away. If you don't make it, you put your tail between your legs and come back for it another day. You don't bivy in the gullies; you don't bivy on Alpine Garden. It's just too extreme."

Odell Gully
10:15 a.m.

Mount Washington Observatory Surface Weather Observations (10:00 to 11:00 a.m.): Temperature 2°F; winds out of the south averaging 63 mph; visibility 0 miles; snow/blowing snow/fog; windchill -30.7°F; peak wind gust: 95 mph.

Herr and Batzer continue to move quickly over the 800-foot route of ice and snow. Decades later, Batzer is still struck by the favorable conditions they encountered. "Odell's was almost completely ice, a beautiful, massive amount of ice, with maybe a small stretch of snow at the top," he recalls. "I was very excited, and we were trying to really get going because we knew that time was of the essence. We were lightning fast because we'd worked a lot together, and we knew in that situation we had to watch our backs and make the most of the time we had. Our adrenaline was definitely pumping, but we always took great care."

Herr surpasses the last vertical ice bulge in the gully and moves past the point where Dartmouth College student Peter Friedman fell to his death the year before when Herr and Batzer were last in Huntington. He is running out the pitch, which means he's trailing a rope without the added safety margin of placing ice screws and clipping into the rope so Batzer can belay him if needed. If Herr falls, he'll plummet unimpeded down to Batzer and then past him until the rope becomes taut. They're hoping the two threaded Chouinard screws anchoring Batzer to the ice can withstand the force of a potential fall by Herr.

"I wasn't going to spend time placing screws," Herr says today. "I didn't need the security. I was really experienced technically, and just to entertain myself, I rope-soloed Odell that day. I would climb 160 feet and trail the rope and belay Jeff up. And because of that, we moved so fast. I knew that with potential avalanche risk you want to get through the danger zone really fast. The gully was actually fine on the way up. There wasn't a lot of conversation at belay points."

Batzer also recalls the discipline with which he and Herr executed their craft. "It was businesslike on the way up." he recalls. "I wasn't as fearful on that climb as I had been on the other ones. Hugh was calm; I felt calm. Technically, the climb went smoothly. We weren't struggling with it. We were just trying to keep things as quick as possible for whatever might come up."

As uneventful as the climb up is at this point, a simple mishap on Batzer's part will complicate their day later on. "Halfway up the climb, we were rushing," Batzer recalls. "I had these straps around my wrists that went through a Velcro strap on the Thinsulate insulated Gore-Tex mittens. I was relying on the Velcro to hold the straps so I could take my mittens off and let them hang as I was working with ice screws at the belays. As I was doing that, one Velcro strap let go, and that mitten came off and was gone. I was like, 'Oh brother, that's not good.' Underneath the mittens, I was wearing silk liner gloves and over those Millar Mitt angora wool gloves that came only halfway up my fingers so I could have more dexterity. The liner and wool glove were the only things I had on my one hand, and I knew that wasn't great. But my hand was staying fairly warm because I was switching my remaining mitten between my two hands. I still thought, 'We'll get up, we'll get down.' The weather wasn't too bad from our perspective. We weren't going to the summit, so I wasn't overly concerned. But later on, I would certainly regret dropping that mitten."

The two reach a point where the ice flow breaks left and right. They elect to do "Odell Right," the hardest of the two options and the one that will provide more ice to climb.

Central Gully
11:30 a.m.

Mount Washington Observatory Surface Weather Observations (11:00 a.m. to 12:00 p.m.): Temperature 1°F; winds out of the south averaging 64 mph; visibility 0 miles, snow/blowing snow/fog; windchill -32.4°F; peak wind gust: 80 mph.

Hank Butler, Jim Frati, and Bob MacEntee are two hours into their climb in Central Gully. Butler is using a combination of Lowe Snargs, which he pounds into the softer ice as anchors, and Chouinard ice screws, which he screws into the harder ice. Where there's only snow at belay stations, Butler digs a deep seat into the slope, sits in it, and belays Frati and MacEntee as they climb to him. When they reach the gully's ice bulge. Frati and MacEntee climb it one at a time for increased safety. Years later, Butler recalls how pleased he was with the performance of the team that morning. "All of the ice climbs in Huntington Ravine face east, and most of the bad weather arrives from the west. While climbing in the gully, you're actually ensconced in the somewhat protective steep wall of the ravine. The conditions were excellent, and everyone climbed well, and quickly."

MacEntee, who readily acknowledges his novice status on ice and in gullies back then, enthusiastically leaned into his companions' experience during this phase of his progression. Yet his memories of the climb are less rapturous, and he acknowledges the sketchy weather that others seem to have taken in stride. "We were on the climb and the snow was shooting down on top of the ice as we were going up, and we probably shouldn't have been there," he says. "The weather was deteriorating during the climb, and it was really the beginning of the rapid deterioration that happens up there. But we were like, 'Oh yeah, it's not too bad,' so off we went."

Odell Gully
11:45 a.m.

Herr and Batzer simul-climb the final snow pitch in Odell as they approach the three-hour mark of a climb that has included four pitches of ice and two of snow. They move past the apex of Pinnacle Buttress, where they had originally planned to emerge from that day.

Batzer shakes off the mild disappointment he feels as he leaves the buttress behind him. He drives the toes of his cramponed boots deep into the Styrofoam-like snow, pauses as he grips the head of each ice axe, leans into the steep slope, and looks between his legs at the void below him. Thin runnels of loose snow funnel down the gully and disappear into the low cloud cover that has seemingly embedded itself to the terrain. He looks up toward the rim of the gully where it meets the plateau of Alpine Garden.

"As we approached the top of Odell's, the skies were gray, and I could see it was snowing harder up above us," he recalls. "You could also tell the wind was blowing more up there. It was snowing a little down below us, too. It was really cold, and we could tell it was getting wild. It wasn't yet, but it was definitely getting there. As we reached the top of the gully, it was becoming more obvious that the conditions were changing for the worse the higher we went."

VIII
IMPULSE

A lot of people don't believe it can be that bad,
and when it is that bad, they say this is what we came for—full conditions.
But then some people overextend themselves, and it happens pretty quickly.
—Steve Larson, Mountain Rescue Service

Mount Washington Observatory Surface Weather Observations (12:00 to 1:00 p.m.): Temperature 1°F; winds out of the south averaging 62 mph; visibility 0 miles; snow/blowing snow/fog; windchill -32°F; peak wind gust: 79 mph.

Rim of Huntington Ravine (approximately 5,300 ft.)
Saturday, Jan. 23, 1982
Early afternoon

Hugh Herr and Jeff Batzer untie the knots in the rope that connects them to each other and to their climbing harnesses. Herr winds the rope into an alpine coil and slings it over his shoulder while Batzer continues swapping his remaining mitten between hands to keep them from freezing. Standing just below the rounded rim of the ravine, they tuck into a pocket on the leeward side of a large rock formation. The cleft in the rock is confining but comfortable and shelters them somewhat from the tenacious 60-mph winds.

Crouching next to one another, they welcome the brief respite after three hours of splendid exertion in the ice-choked gully. A small gap of about six feet in diameter forms a window between rock and terrain, allowing them to look out onto the barren plateau of Alpine Garden. Conditions a quarter of a mile across the garden are full, rendering the summit cone of Mount Washington imperceptible. A seemingly endless mass of frozen fog blocks the summit from view, for the moment acting as a trigger guard against Batzer's urge to head up there.

They have reached their goal of ascending Odell Gully with time to spare. Sunset is still more than four hours away. On any other day, Herr would be perfectly content to conquer a technical route and leave its summit to others. But today, shoulder to shoulder with his teammate, Herr feels they have unfinished business. Batzer had expressed such enthusiasm for reaching Mount Washington's summit on this trip, and his uncharacteristic silence on the matter now feels like a void Herr needs to fill. For him, continuing to the summit wouldn't be about checking another box. It would be his opportunity to honor his friend and climbing companion. Herr knows that Batzer is often engaged in a knock-down, drag-out battle with fear on their climbs and yet still follows him upward, maintaining the belays that have allowed Herr to push himself into higher technical realms. So as they huddle in that rock cleft, the idea of going for the summit is back on the table.

"It was kind of like two kids looking at a snowstorm," Batzer recalls of that moment. "We thought, 'This really doesn't look that bad.' So at that point we had the discussion."

"Why don't we go for it?" Herr asks.

As he has so many times before in moments like this, Batzer feels his stomach contract, a physical reaction he often experiences when an alarm bell in his brain signals perceived risk. "It's probably not a good idea to go to the top," he replies.

Herr recognizes this response as his friend's modus operandi. Whenever Herr suggests they do anything outside Batzer's comfort zone, Batzer is quick to stall the process. It's a familiar dynamic and doesn't cause tension between them.

"I knew Hugh was trying to honor me," Batzer says today. "We had different opinions at the top of the gully, but I wasn't thinking Hugh was crazy or anything like that. Though he didn't communicate it in words, I knew he was committed to trying to get me to the top that day. It was typical of me to hesitate. Hugh was always optimistic, and I was always fighting to stay with him. I was the brakes, and he was the gas."

"I think we can do this," Herr says encouragingly, understanding Batzer's fear and seeking to ease it.

Batzer is quick to say that Herr would never intentionally place him in danger. In fact, quite the opposite. The two young climbers may have arrived here without a backpack, but they are carrying with them the security of strong friendship and an impressive cache of shared struggle and success. "Hugh did unusual things to keep me safe on other climbs, and because of that, there were times when I had put him in jeopardy," Batzer says. "He was always protecting me, and all of it was cushioned by our work as a team—and by the fact that we loved each other."

The two have about a quarter of a mile on relatively flat ground to reach their planned descent of Escape Hatch. There's no direct trail leading from Odell to Mount Washington's summit. They could follow the Huntington Ravine Trail to the Auto Road and ascend, or take the Huntington Ravine Trail to Nelson Crag Trail and up, or go across Alpine Garden to Lion Head Trail and then on to the summit. But they're unaware of these options because the map of the mountain is inside the backpack they dumped down in the ravine. In any case, all of these routes would have taken more time than they were likely willing to spend.

"It was a mixed-bag decision," Batzer recalls. "There wasn't absolute certainty as to whether going for the summit was the right thing to do. We'd go back and forth, doing a kind of a risk assessment. You could tell it was storming some, but it wasn't as bad as we thought it was going to be, and going to the top didn't look completely out of the question. Hugh was confident, and I was pretty easily convinced to go for it. It was an intricate discussion, but it took only about a minute. Once we made the decision, it was full throttle for us."

In quick order, they move out of the cleft to take what they believe to be a straight shot to the top. The summit is about six-tenths of a mile away and includes 982 feet of elevation gain. In favorable conditions, it's not uncommon for well-oriented winter hikers and climbers to use the firm snow, scuffed down by the winds, to take a path of least resistance to the summit without following established trails. What is uncommon is topping out on a climb in Huntington Ravine and then heading to the summit from there. *An Ice Climbers Guide to Northern New England* contains this caveat: "Few parties who spend the day climbing in Huntington Ravine ever make it a point to press on to the summit of Mount Washington. ... A number of rescues have ensued as a result of "going for the summit" in bad conditions. In situations of poor visibility, it is the better part of valor to head down."

At the start of their sprint to the summit, the pair find the terrain ideal. The snowpack is solid and offers no resistance. The points of their crampons biting into the crust sound like plastic cracking beneath them. Although the high winds from the south are buffeting them from the left (at their 10 o'clock) as they walk across Alpine Garden, they are undeterred and feel confident in continuing their way upward.

There's no conversation as the winds rush through the undulating terrain, and soon the pair are having trouble keeping their bearing. "We were flying by the seat of our pants back then," says Batzer. "As far as navigation goes, we would have gotten an F. We knew the technical routes, but we thought we'd figure out everything else as we went. It was a disaster in the making."

At 12:20 p.m., the Mount Washington Observatory—less than 850 feet above them—notes that the light snowfall that began at 8:00 a.m. is now falling at a moderate-to-heavy rate. Because the consistency of the snowfall is light and fluffy, the high winds are making the already poor visibility above treeline even worse.

Meanwhile, Herr and Batzer continue to feel their way up the mountain, and the weather conditions begin their freefall. "As we ascended, it got worse and worse and worse," Herr recalls.

Ryan Knapp, a senior staff meteorologist and weather observer at the Mount Washington Observatory since 2005, recognizes the deteriorating situation Herr and Batzer are experiencing. "Given similar scenarios I've seen in my time here, when you have moderate-to-heavy snowfall and tropical storm-type winds, the visibility will be significantly poor, less than one-sixteenth of a mile. As they ascended the mountain in those kinds of conditions, it was only going to get worse. In the case of Mount Washington, you get more exposed the higher up you go because there are fewer and fewer trees and rocks to block the wind."

Herr and Batzer approach Ball Crag, a section of jagged rock named in honor of Benjamin Ball who, in October 1855, survived three days and two nights on the mountain in full conditions using only scrub growth, his overcoat, and an umbrella for his bivouacs. Ball's ordeal is well documented in his book *Three Days on the White Mountains: The Perilous Adventure of Dr. B.L. Ball on Mount Washington*.

For their part, the two young climbers are barely coping with the conditions they're encountering. "After about 25 to 30 minutes, Hugh and I were screaming at each other, 'This is ridiculous!'" Batzer, recalls. "The wind was blowing harder than anything I had experienced in my life. You couldn't see more than 10 or 15 feet in any direction. As we walked up, the conditions kept intensifying. They were tolerable and then, all of a sudden, they were intolerable. We didn't know where we were going. The gusts were so strong that had I jumped up in the air I would have flown about 10 feet and then kept flying. I remember screaming at the top of my lungs. I have a really loud voice, and I'm sure Hugh could barely hear me."

Once they top out on Ball Crag they're at Homestretch, the final section of the Auto Road and the last half-mile before the summit. But they have no idea they're on the road or where the summit is. "My experience was technical and mountain ascents across North America," Herr says today. "Navigation in a whiteout and moving across relatively flat terrain were not in my tool set. I'd been in a whiteout before, but when you're in a whiteout in Huntington Ravine, who cares? You know exactly where you are—you're in a gully. You know what up is, you know what down is, and you're funneled to exactly where you want to go. The problem is when the gully becomes a flat region, and every direction is identical, and wind is changing direction. That's just impossible. It's a white maze. I hadn't experienced that particular phenomenon in all the climbing I'd done out West. That risk is dominant in the Whites; it's not as dominant in other ranges, and that was not in my calculation."

Herr acknowledges today that the key mistake he and Batzer made that day was to go above Huntington once they had climbed Odell Gully. "Tragedies happen in a sequence of errors," he says. "We're going light and fast to beat the weather and get out of the avalanche zone, so we stash the pack and plan to grab it on our way down. We get to the top of the ravine knowing Jeff wants to go to the summit, and we mistakenly think, 'Oh well, we'll just walk five minutes longer to the summit.' Had we stuck with our plan and just descended, it would have been completely fine. But even though we only walked a short distance toward the summit, it was game over."

After walking about four-tenths of a mile to an elevation of 6,150 feet, the friends reach a point where they realize they're in way over their heads. "We checked in once with each other, and we were like, 'Let's get out of here!' says Batzer. "So we turned around and started heading down."

Herr targets Central Gully in the middle of the ravine, where Hank Butler, Jim Frati, and Bob MacEntee are nearing the top. With the raging winds now mostly at their back, they use the gusts they've been fighting as an escort back to the gully and what they hope will be safety.

IX
PERIL

Visibility was often marginal at best, the snow cover obscured the usual landmarks, and there were no cairns on the homestretch of Carriage Road; and the wind—the always present, all-pervading wind—would press the traveler into submission.

—William Lowell Putnam, *The Worst Weather on Earth: A History of Mount Washington Observatory*

Mount Washington Observatory Surface Weather Observations (1:00 to 2:00 p.m.): Temperature 1°F; winds out of the south averaging 63 mph; visibility 0 miles; snow/ blowing snow/ fog; windchill -32.2F; peak wind gust: 86 mph.

Rim of Huntington Ravine
Saturday, Jan. 23, 1982
1:00 p.m.

Hank Butler, Jim Frati, and Bob MacEntee are on their knees as an agitated Mother Nature greets them. Once they cleared Central Gully's ice bulge lower down, the trio simul-climbed the last steep pitches of snow before breaching the rim and colliding head-on with Mount Washington's fury. They share absolute clarity about their next move. They will quickly abandon this small parcel of real estate which, ironically, is where Hugh Herr and Jeff Batzer are now working so hard to reach.

The ropes connecting them flail through the air as the strong, tropical-storm winds do their best to send the ropes tumbling down to the floor of the ravine. Knots frozen by continuous spindrift and subzero temperatures require ungloved hands to thaw and untie them, a painful and tedious exercise. "A brutal blizzard was raging," Butler recalls, "and we still had to hike across the fully exposed Alpine Garden to get to our descent route, appropriately called the Escape Hatch. I knew this was the only safe way down, and that we had to get down right away!"

A traverse of just under half a mile separates them from their planned descent route and the reassurance it offers. *An Ice Climbers*

Guide to Northern New England describes the kind of situation they have found themselves in: "If the weather is bad or rapidly deteriorating, you'll be looking for a quick way to drop down into the woods. This shallow snow gully allows a hasty descent back to the bottom of Huntington Ravine during inclement weather. Use good judgment here, since this gully has at times avalanched, and at times has been hard ice."

Butler reels in the rope connecting him to MacEntee, and Frati does the same with the rope connecting him to Butler. Frati traps the tangled mess of his rope between his thighs, gingerly removes his daypack, and stuffs the rigid rope inside it. Butler does the same with the other rope. Once back in the calm confines of Harvard Cabin, where they can thaw out the ropes, there'll be plenty of time to wind proper coils. The windchill feels like hundreds of pin pricks on their faces. Having perspired from their exertion in the gully for over three hours, they are at risk for hypothermia and frostbite. "You couldn't see anything at all," Frati remembers. "When I held my backpack at arm's length, I couldn't even see that. At the time I was wearing all my army surplus gear. The climbing industry wasn't as it is now with the lightweight equipment and clothing that's available today."

With the frozen ropes now secure in their packs, the three lean into the southerly onslaught.

As if the headwind isn't bad enough, the air is also choked with falling and blowing snow being lifted out of the eastern snowfields and off the ramp of Ball Crag. Driving each leg forward, they're forced to multitask in an environment where even one task takes supreme effort. Each of them must be mindful of foot placement, drop down to avoid the relentless haymaker gusts of over 80 mph, and keep his teammates in sight while ensuring they can see him.

"We had to walk into this; there was no other choice," Butler says. "The going got really tough. We were pretty well protected, except for our faces. Our hats were wool balaclavas, which cover everything except eyes, nose, and mouth. McEntee and I had ski goggles to protect our eyes, but our faces started to freeze. The whipping snow would hit your face, melt, and then freeze. My balaclava was quickly encased in ice and my left cheek was frozen."

Their occasional screaming to communicate is muted by the roar of what sounds like a succession of locomotives barreling north across

Alpine Garden before launching off Chandler's Ridge and into oblivion. They've only been walking a few minutes, and Frati is already in trouble. "I didn't have goggles. I rarely wore them because they freeze up. But that day, when I would blink, my eyelashes would freeze together."

During brief stops between the higher gusts, Butler can see that the conditions are putting Frati in a precarious situation. "Jim was hurting. His eyelashes had frozen and fused together. It took all our strength to keep heading directly into the blizzard. You had to ignore your natural survival instinct, the one that told you to turn the other way, out of the wind. Every five meters, I would spin around and drop to my knees to remove my hands from the double mitts and over-gloves. I would briefly warm my face with the palms of my hands and pull the accumulating ice off my cheek. That didn't work for very long, and I knew my cheek was gone."

This appears to be the point where the three friends' recollections diverge, an understandable occurrence 40 years after the event. At the conclusion of one attempt to defrost, Frati and MacEntee recall losing visual and verbal contact with Butler. "Hank took a couple of steps, and we couldn't see him," MacEntee says. "And we just couldn't regroup. I remember trying to bring him back in, but we also couldn't go on a search for him. We gave it some time but quickly realized he'd taken a few steps away, out of sight. We assumed he was heading down. We knew he had more experience than we did and would know the way down."

Frati also remembers the immediate concern he felt after Butler is enveloped by the storm. "We'd gone less than 50 yards when we got separated. Hank just went faster, and the storm swallowed us. Hank was about four or five years older than me, and he'd been climbing for years, so he kind of took me under his wing and was teaching me. So when we got separated, I thought, 'Holy shit, now what?' But I'd been up there in winter before and knew about the Escape Hatch. To this day I don't know how we got separated because he was a half-step from me. That's how bad it was."

But Butler himself does not recall becoming separated. In his memory, the three continued together.

Frati and MacEntee remember passing by Odell Gully and crossing over the route Hugh Herr and Jeff Batzer took to the summit less than half an hour before, their boot tracks long since erased by the prevailing winds. "I can't imagine anyone making the decision to press on to the summit that day," MacEntee says. "There's no way. You couldn't even stand. Hugh and Jeff may have hit the top of Odell a little sooner than we did because they were the first ones out of the cabin. Maybe when they got to the top, the wind wasn't quite as strong. When we got up there, we knew the area well enough to be able to get down, but it was still challenging."

Lion Head (4,900 ft.)
Mount Washington
1:30 p.m.

Joe Lentini is in his element. The director of the Eastern Mountain Sports Climbing School and a team leader for the all-volunteer Mountain Rescue Service grins as he stares into the face of the building storm during a guided climb. Lentini and his clients left Pinkham that morning and hiked up Lion Head via the Winter Route. Because of landslides that significantly increase the avalanche hazard, the U.S. Forest Service relocated this route in 1995 to its present location. Members of Lentini's group are packed for almost any contingency. In addition to wearing base and mid-layers made of wicking materials from head to toe, they're wearing winter mountaineering boots, crampons, and ample protection for their hands, head, and face. Each carries an ice axe, a headlamp, chemical heat packs, and extra food and fluids.

Lentini packs his food next to a water bottle filled with hot water to keep the food from freezing. When guiding, he also brings a first-aid kit, a bivouac sack, an expedition-weight down parka or sleeping bag, a map, a compass, and a shovel. "I always carry a shovel," he says. "I demonstrate to people how easy it is to quickly dig a snow hole that you can get into if needed."

The approach Lentini is using with his clients is slow and heavy in contrast to the fast and light approach that was growing in popularity at the time and is still prominent today. "I would be lying if I said I never went fast and light," Lentini says. "But I tell my clients and any of my climbing friends that a bivy sack and an extra insulated jacket weigh a little more than a pound or two, and that any climber must always be prepared to spend the night out or for someone with them to spend the night out."

As Lentini's gaze shifts between the tempest before him and his exhilarated clients, he is not surprised at the conditions. But his experience is in sharp contrast to that of Hank Butler, Jim Frati, and Bob MacEntee roughly eight-tenths of a mile northwest. "We were right at Lion Head, and a little above treeline," Lentini says today. "I knew we were going to feel the strong winds there. For my entire career, I've gone to that point in bad weather just so clients can step over and feel the wind's power. I'd explain to them that it was going to get much stronger if we kept on going. Unless you've felt that, you can't imagine it. I knew a storm was coming that day. I followed the weather and said to my clients, 'Look, if we keep going, we might be able to get to the summit, but it's not worth it because who knows what could happen. The mountain is always going to be here, and we can come back.' So down we went."

Lentini recalls that conditions were worsening as the group descended, with a lot of blowing snow and snow and ice on the trail below Lion Head. "But as far as avalanche hazard is concerned," he says, "there wasn't a wind slab—yet."

Alpine Garden (5,300 ft.)
1:45 p.m.

Gusts of wind force Frati and MacEntee down on all fours. They drive the pic of their axes into the ice and pull themselves forward. "We couldn't even talk to each other," says MacEntee. "I had to put my mouth to Jim's ear. It was that wild. I'd seen a few wild days up there on Presidential Traverses, but this was one where I said to myself, 'We can't stay in this very long.' We were almost breaking our ice axes as we crawled across Alpine Garden. We crawled almost all the way to Escape Hatch. Jim and I were both really strong. He was a bodybuilder, and I was a cyclist. We had the ability to drive forward. When we climbed together, we could really push. We just had to keep our wits about us and move slowly to find the route down. We knew which way to go, but the most unnerving part was getting separated from Hank. I kept wondering if he was OK."

Following the rim of the ravine, they drop down to investigate each gully in hopes of finding Escape Hatch. It is a smart strategy. "I shouted to Jim, 'Stay left and keep the cliff to your left,' MacEntee recalls. "We kept dropping down because you couldn't see anything, so our plan was to just go left and every so often drop down. If it wasn't the right spot, we'd climb back up and follow the line of gullies. I can remember going down gullies and stopping because it was straight down—it just dropped right off. We were huddled down and tried to keep the high terrain to our right."

Finally, they spot the sign they've been looking for. "There was a handle of a shovel sticking out of a cairn marking the Escape Hatch," Frati recalls. "When I saw it, I knew we were headed in the right direction. I hadn't been down Escape Hatch many times. It was really by luck that I found the shovel handle and entrance."

They sit in the snow and begin to glissade down the 600-foot chute, which is already clogged with fluffy snow. Escape Hatch faces northeast and loads and cross-loads snow when winds are transporting it from the south. "It was so bad at one point that I was sitting in the snow, and the only way I knew I was making any downward progress was because the snow was building up in front of me," says Frati.

At this point, the snowfall is moderate to heavy. But strong southerly winds are extracting snow from Raymond Cataract, a shallow gully between Huntington and Tuckman Ravines, and loading Escape Hatch and the adjacent South Gully, which is contributing to the rising avalanche hazard on Mount Washington.

On reaching the base of Escape Hatch, Frati and MacEntee return to Harvard Cabin. "We probably made a not-so-good decision to climb that day, just as Hugh and Jeff did," MacEntee acknowledges today. "For whatever reason, we felt we could climb, top out, hit Escape Hatch, and avoid the severe weather of the summit. I will admit that had I known what I know now or had a better picture of how rapidly the weather was going to deteriorate, I would not have climbed."

Frati and MacEntee believe Butler crossed the Alpine Garden and descended the Winter Route on Lion Head. Although he remembers his descent route differently, Butler aptly summarizes the seriousness of the situation they were all in as they headed down: "We were very lucky to escape with our lives. I doubt we would have lasted another 10 minutes on the Alpine Garden in those conditions."

Northeast Ridge (5,300 ft.)
Mount Washington
2:00 p.m.

Mount Washington Observatory Surface Weather Observations (2:00 to 3:00 p.m.): Temperature 3°F; winds out of the south averaging 65 mph; visibility 0 miles, snow/blowing snow/fog; windchill -29.6°F; peak wind gust: 88 mph.

Hugh Herr and Jeff Batzer are wasting no time as they bail out. Heinous wind gusts provide a stern escort down the mountain. "We were keeping close enough so we didn't lose each other," Herr recalls today. "We had to scream because the noise of the wind was so remarkable and crouch because of its speed at our backs."

They are attempting to use wind direction to return them to Huntington Ravine. It is the same technique Phil Labbe employed six weeks earlier when he got separated from his WMTW-TV Thiokol, which sparked an immediate response by Mountain Rescue Service volunteers, including Albert Dow. The stark difference here is that Labbe had experienced 32 winters on Mount Washington, compared to the two winter days over two seasons that Herr and Batzer have spent here. Labbe understood the winds, the nuances of the mountain, its unpredictable moods, and the twists and turns of the Auto Road. Herr and Batzer have never been on this side of the mountain and don't even know they are there.

The additional vulnerability in Herr and Batzer's plan lies in their assumption that wind direction remains static. Huntington Ravine lies to their east, but they don't realize the wind is running south to north. They contended with winds from their left on the way to the summit and therefore believe that by keeping the wind directly at their backs on the descent, it will bring them back toward the middle of Huntington Ravine. But in fact, the southerly winds will move them northward, and the wind direction will shift as it interacts with the terrain. In addition, the strong gusts of wind will shove them off their direct line. With near-zero visibility and no physical reference points, map, or compass, it is quite easy to see how they deviated significantly off their intended course.

Today, Batzer recalls the moment he noticed indications of what he later realized was the Auto Road, but the signals did not register with him at the time. "We hit the road after 20 minutes of descending, and I remember seeing tracks and thinking, 'That's interesting.' We knew they were tracks from a machine but didn't equate it to the Auto Road." For his part, Herr doesn't recall seeing any signs of the Auto Road. "Everything was covered," he says.

The 22nd edition of the *AMC White Mountain Guide* indicates how easily one can miss what is an unmistakable road in good weather: "During whiteout conditions terrain features vanish, including such a seemingly obvious landmark as the Auto Road."

As they move farther into the lee of the summit, winds are beginning to decrease in strength.

Herr is out front and moving with urgency. He has a singular focus on getting himself and Batzer to safety. "I was getting concerned that we were getting too far apart," Batzer says. "A couple of times I was screaming, 'Hey, slow down, let's stay close!' I was really afraid we'd get separated. Hugh had his back to me, so he didn't have a sense of how far away from each other we were getting."

The two are a half-mile from their turnaround at Homestretch when they reach what Herr believes to be the rim of Huntington Ravine. "We were frightened," he admits today. "But we hit what appeared to me to be Central Gully. I was like, 'OK, great, we're fine.' And then it became very clear we were somewhere else."

X
LAND OF SHADOW

There are no safe paths in this part of the world.
Remember you are all over the Edge of the Wild now.
—Gandalf, *The Lord of the Rings*

Mount Washington Observatory Surface Weather Observations (3:00 to 4:00 p.m.): Temperature 6°F; winds out of the south averaging 66 mph; visibility 0 miles, snow/blowing snow/fog; windchill -25.4°F; peak wind gust: 89 mph.

Great Gulf Wilderness (5,200 ft.)
Thompson & Meserve's Purchase
White Mountain State Park
Saturday, Jan. 23, 1982
Midafternoon

Hugh Herr and Jeff Batzer pause briefly at the crest of what they believe to be the gateway back to the floor of Huntington Ravine. Having extricated themselves from the chaos on the windward side of the mountain, they feel a wave of relief as they take stock of their favorable position. What they don't know is that Huntington Ravine, and more specifically their intended target of Central Gully, is almost four-tenths of a mile to the southeast. "Had we not abandoned the rucksack, which held our compass, we could have found our way back to Huntington Ravine and to our descent path," Herr says today.

Batzer says his anxiety level at that point was still low. "I thought we were getting out of there," he recalls. "I was thinking this would be over soon. We thought we were on the right side of the mountain and that it wasn't going to be hard to find our way back to the trail in Huntington. We'd retrieve the pack we stashed and head back to Harvard Cabin."

The low visibility reveals only a slice of the terrain downslope from them. On a clear day, they'd take in almost all 5,500 acres of the remote wilderness, and the high peaks of the Northern Presidentials that flank this massive glacial cirque. Today, however, these helpful indicators of their actual location have disappeared inside dense, frozen fog, and the frenetic movement of snow. Still, they agree they've hit their mark, so Herr starts down the slope and Batzer follows.

The pair trudge down the center of the snow-filled drainage, and Batzer is relieved to find that Herr is setting a much slower pace than he did near the summit. The drainage lies to the southwest of the Wamsutta Trail. This trail, named for the first of the six husbands of Weetamoo, Queen of Pocasset, starts just above the six-mile mark on

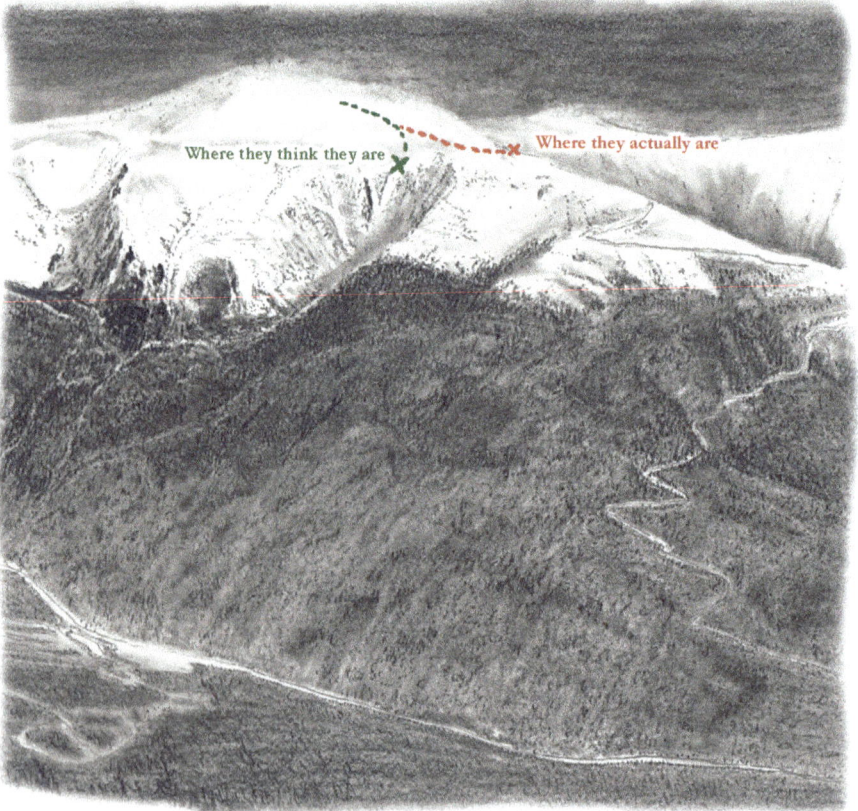

Where they think they are

Where they actually are

When Hugh Herr and Jeff Batzer arrive at the rim of Great Gulf, they are approximately a half-mile from their intended target of Central Gully in Huntington Ravine. The natural drainage they choose to descend is similar to that of Central.

the Auto Road and follows a spur down Chandler Ridge, where it intersects with the Great Gulf Trail and the Six Husbands Trail on the floor of the gulf itself.

Although winds are more tempered here in the lee, Herr and Batzer are still stalked by copious amounts of wind-transported snow coming in from as far away as Lakes of the Clouds on the south side, Boott Spur to the east, the summit cone, and Ball and Nelson Crags. Snow began falling between 8:00 and 9:00 a.m. amid southerly winds strong enough to haul it to Great Gulf, which is acting as a gigantic collection bowl. As snow continues to accumulate, gravity and calmer downslope winds allow the snow to settle on the slopes and floor of the Gulf. Herr and Batzer are also using gravity to speed their way down. When they arrive on the floor, they will have left almost 2,000 feet of elevation in their wake.

The average slope angle of their escape route is a gradual 21 degrees and, at its steepest, 35 degrees. It is on these steeper sections where avalanche hazard can materialize. A majority of avalanches occur on slopes of 30 to 45 degrees, the steepness of a black diamond ski run. But avalanches are not on either of their minds right now. "The descent was pretty cool," Batzer recalls. "We thought we'd hit Huntington and were in a snow chute. We knew we'd gotten to the edge of something, and we knew we had to be careful because we thought there'd be ice below us. We started moving very slowly, and it was actually really good: hop, sink down in, hop, sink down in. We were covering a lot of ground. Visibility was poor, but Hugh was always six to eight feet in front of me. It was beautiful."

Fortunately for Herr and Batzer the slope, though filled with snow, holds firm as the two bound through it. Their enthusiasm is high, but what they cannot know is that the farther away they get from the top of the drainage, the closer they will be getting to a winter hellscape. Michael Hartrich, then a member of Mountain Rescue Service, recalls the "No Man's Land" reputation this part of Mount Washington carried back then. "Great Gulf is an area that, especially at that time, was infrequently visited because there's nowhere to go. Occasionally, groups would winter camp in there and then come back down, but there's no safe access anywhere in there, so you very rarely ever saw anyone there in winter."

Mike Pelchat, the Mount Washington State Park manager for 24 years before retiring in 2018 and a longtime member of Androscoggin

Valley Search and Rescue, which he helped organize in 1988, describes the challenges concealed behind the grandiose beauty of this area. "Even though at times one may hear loud vehicles traveling the Auto Road or the Cog Railway whistle floating in the breeze, the Great Gulf feels as wild and pristine as it likely did when the first hikers tramped through in the late 1800s. I don't believe the area has ever been logged because of its remote location and less-than-desirable lumber, which mainly consists of twisted black spruce and balsam fir interspersed with birch and mountain ash clinging to old avalanche scars. To try to hike across the Gulf without a trail would be an incredibly dangerous bushwhack through krummholz so thick it would be a superhuman feat to come out the other side unscathed."

Great Gulf was added to the National Wilderness Preservation System in 1964 as part of the original Wilderness Act. Today, its reputation as a place of striking desolation still holds. Lt. Mark Ober of New Hampshire Fish and Game is the district chief for District 1, which includes the Gulf. Ober has been assigned to District 1 since 2006 and has served in a supervisory capacity for a decade. He's been a member of the Fish and Game Advanced Search and Rescue Team since 2007 and has been on 200 search and rescue calls as a responder and more than 100 as a supervisor. Twenty of these missions have involved calls to the Gulf, where he has responded to six and supervised 14.

"The biggest thing about Great Gulf is that most of the people we look for there have been up on the ridge or the range and took a wrong turn, which took them down into it. Or the weather forces them down into it. There are at least three trails that go off the Auto Road and into the Gulf. Most of these are very steep and not well traveled or well marked. They're not meant for the faint of heart. Down toward the Route 16 end it's forested with old growth, and it's not that bad. But when you get up higher you're in thick scrub, so it's hard to maneuver, especially if there's snow involved. The snow blows off the peaks and down into the Gulf, and that's where it settles. It could be chest deep, a snow trap. During the winter, it's rare for people to be that far back there voluntarily."

When you got into trouble in the White Mountains back then, there were no cell phones for you to text loved ones, call 911, or have your phone pinged in hopes of determining your location. There were no handheld Global Positioning Systems (GPS), no devices to allow others to track your route from afar, no personal emergency locator beacons (PLB). You had only your experience and your gear. Some brought with them an ample supply of both, while others brought little to none at all. Once you'd expended all of what you had with you, you relied on luck. Once your luck ran out, it was time to hunker down and wait, if hunkering down was even an option. You'd hope you had positioned yourself in a place where rescuers could find you in time to save you.

At approximately 5,000 feet, Herr and Batzer reach treeline. "The descent wasn't technically difficult," Herr recalls. "We were plunge-stepping most of the way" The plunge step is a technique that helps keep you in balance while you descend quickly. You step down and drive your heel straight down into the snow, bending your knees slightly, maintaining a wide stance, keeping your toes up and out of the snow, holding your arms in front of you, and leaning slightly forward. "When we hit treeline," Herr says, "we only had one choice and that was to continue down what we thought was Huntington Ravine. We would have certainly died if we'd retraced our tracks."

Upon reaching the start of the resilient vegetation clinging to the slope, Batzer is surprised by the ease with which they've descended. "The chute seemed stable to us and really safe. It was still storming, and the visibility was rough, but little by little it started to clear up as we got lower. We could see about 100 yards ahead of us. Looking back up the slope, the visibility was still bad, and you could tell it was really windy, but we couldn't hear the high winds deep down where we were."

The terrain is easing, and the two continue through shin-deep snow. "We got into a flat area and thought, 'Wow, close call, but we made it to Huntington Ravine,'" Batzer says. "Now we can find our pack and get out of this area. At that point, we just thought we were in a different part of Huntington. It looked the same, there were a lot of trees around, so it didn't really hit us that we were in the wrong place. But we couldn't find our pack."

At roughly 4:00 p.m., after descending approximately a mile and a quarter from the top of the slope they followed into the ravine, Herr and Batzer reach the floor of the Gulf at an elevation of approximately 3,400 feet. The official sunset is still just over 40 minutes away, but the sun has already dropped behind Mounts Jefferson and Adams directly in front of them. They follow a small creek and eventually come to a fork where it joins a larger one. They believe they've found the Cutler River, which drains Huntington Ravine and flows toward Pinkham Notch Camp. However, this is the West Branch of the Peabody River. "It was going to be dark in about an hour, so we stopped briefly," recalls Batzer. They pause at a large, downed tree to assess their situation. Herr removes the coiled rope from his shoulder, and he and Batzer create a pad to sit on that shields them from the snow beneath them. "We considered bivying there overnight, but we still had energy and thought it was more important to keep moving to stay warm, so we decided to keep following the stream in the hope that we could break through something that night and get out."

With their decision made, they decrease the weight they're carrying by jettisoning the gear they consider unnecessary. "We dumped the rope, the crampons, our screws, the carabiners, and the harness but kept a couple of slings and our ice axes," recalls Batzer. "Anything technical came off. We thought, 'This isn't going to help us, so let's just leave it here.'"

As they start moving again with nothing recognizable around them, they begin to realize they've hiked beyond Huntington and descended somewhere else. But they are still misreading their actual location. "We thought we must have just drifted over into Tuckerman Ravine, which would have meant we'd descended to the right of Huntington," says Batzer. At this point, they expect to come out through some trees, bear to their left, and get back to Huntington, where they'll find their pack and head back to Harvard Cabin.

Not long after the pair drop their technical gear, the shin-deep snow they'd moved through with relative ease rises to knee level. From their knees it begins a subtle climb up their thighs and reaches their waists, where it holds. Now on the floor of the bowl, they hope the snow will rise no further.

Beginning to lose hope for a timely self-rescue, Herr is harboring dire thoughts that he can't bring himself to share with Batzer, whose spirits have remained high. "As soon as we hit treeline," Herr says, "I said to myself, 'We're going to die.' I thought we might survive one night, but not several nights."

XI
IN DEEP

The great booby trap of the East.
—Paul Petzoldt, founder, National Outdoor
Leadership School,
speaking of Mount Washington

Great Gulf: Temperature: 18°F; winds are low; visibility low-light; light snowfall. Note: The data provided are estimates based on conversion of summit data and observations made by Hugh Herr, Jeff Batzer, and others.

West Branch of the Peabody River (3,300 ft.)
Great Gulf Wilderness
Saturday, Jan. 23, 1982
Late afternoon

In the middle of Great Gulf, where they are not meant to be, Hugh Herr and Jeff Batzer are fighting continuous waves of snow. As they skirt the mostly frozen, heavily blanketed West Branch of the Peabody River, the snow is going for their throats. Every step they take, it ricochets from waist to shoulder to chest and back again.

"We knew this wasn't working," Batzer recalls. "Little by little, we started to realize that the snow was getting much deeper. We were getting later into the day, and my anxiety level was starting to go up. I was beginning to think we'd have an uncomfortable night out on the mountain. We felt we could make it through OK, but I knew it wasn't going to be easy."

Batzer follows close behind as Herr cuts a deep, narrow trough through the wall of snow and dense scrub brush along the banks of the Peabody. "Because they were far back in the Gulf and without a trail, following the Peabody River to get out was the right move on their part," says Lt. Mark Ober of New Hampshire Fish and Game.

The wind is loading snow into the Gulf, and Herr uses his arms and mittened hands to move aside swaths of fluffy snow and both ice axes to chop at the denser snow below. Once it's broken up enough, he drives each knee and shin forward until he's halted by the snow wall, and then he begins the process all over again.

"It was getting dark, and temperatures were very, very low," says Herr. "It was the worst bushwhacking because it was nearly impossible to move. You had the river to deal with and the average depth of snow was waist deep—and that was just the average. It often came up to our chests."

At times, as they grind forward with ice axes in hand, Herr and Batzer get on all fours. "The axes were shaped like a T and acted like snowshoes on our hands," says Batzer. "We did this to stay on top of the snow and keep from punching through, and it actually worked well. But almost right away, the mitten I'd lost in Odell's was an issue. I was rotating my remaining Gore-Tex mitt back and forth on each hand trying to keep them from getting too cold. I managed to keep things tolerable."

Without a backpack, there is nowhere to store the layers of clothing Herr and Batzer should be shedding due to the extreme level of exertion required of them. Nor can they add insulating layers during brief but frequent periods of inactivity. Herr's hooded Gore-Tex jacket creates a barrier for his upper torso, but it is containing his sweat. They have no food or water to replenish the calories and fluids their bodies are scorching through to sustain their work capacity. In the shrouded riverbed below, there are dark holes where it hasn't fully frozen over, but the risk of punching through to retrieve water is too risky. "I was eating snow like crazy," Batzer says.

Wearing polypropylene long underwear, multiple layers of wool from head to toe, and a 60/40 (cotton/nylon) Sierra Design Thinsulate parka, Batzer is sweating profusely and feeling the onset of dehydration. Herr is faring better. "Jeff was eating a lot of snow; me, not as much," he says. "He would take off his glove to eat it, and I think that's what drove the frostbite in his hands. I have this weird body that doesn't need a lot of water. Climbing in Yosemite in summer, I would go long periods of time without it. In the winter, my fingers don't go white in the cold. I have incredible circulation in my hands, and that day I never took my gloves off."

Dr. Gordon Giesbrecht, retired professor of thermophysiology and member of the faculty of Kinesiology and Recreation Management at the University of Manitoba, co-wrote the book *Hypothermia, Frostbite, and other Cold Injuries* with James Wilkerson. In considering the plight of Herr and Batzer in Great Gulf, he describes the process and effects of dehydration during exercise: "Thirst is one of the responses that usually lags behind the need to keep hydrating. By the time you're thirsty, it's too late. You need to be drinking proactively. At that point, the two of them were big-time dehydrated, and the calories required to heat the snow they were ingesting would have canceled out any hydration value."

Giesbrecht also comments on the physical price they are paying for their required exertion and lack of dry clothing. "They were wearing clothes that they would have been able to climb up into the wind with, and then they were out of the wind but working very hard in deep snow. They'd be sweating like crazy, so both sets of undergarments would be wet. They were not layering down as sweating increased, so their clothing was wet clothing. They're not eating food, so they're becoming more and more exhausted. It doesn't take much, a 5 percent decrease in hydration, to have a huge effect on muscular performance, which they both needed to survive. When stopped, shivering would be beneficial to maintain warmth, but they were malnourished, dehydrated, and experiencing decreased muscular performance."

While in motion, Herr and Batzer remain silent. During breaks, their discussions are businesslike and focused only on what needs to be done to make progress and survive. There are sections of their path where trees and snow crowd the riverbank and act as a gate that can't be opened. "There were times the snow was so deep it would meet the limbs of the trees," Herr recalls.

At times, they cannot climb over or tunnel underneath the branches blocking their way, and they must cross the river. Each time they cross, using bridges of snow or tree branches, they hear water running rapidly underneath the ice and snow. "We were trying to use fallen trees whenever we crossed," says Batzer "For snow crossings, we'd separate and cross on all fours to spread the weight out."

The effort required to lie face down or straddle the snow-lined tree trunks and pull themselves across is immense, and the risk of falling is high. During one crossing, Herr is upright and traversing an ice bridge when it collapses beneath him. The frigid water permeates his gaiters and overruns the interior of his rigid, slightly-insulated, full-shank Vasque leather boots, saturating them along with the multiple layers of socks underneath and his wool long underwear bottoms up to his knees.

"With the river, you can't see, hear, or feel if you're on land or thin ice. So of course I fell in," Herr says ruefully. "That definitely drove the hypothermia and frostbite that would come later. It was just a vicious cycle. I was wearing proper, contemporary, insulated leather boots for mountaineering. Plastic boots were just coming out and, as yet, weren't generally used. But they would have been helpful to have."

Herr rockets out of the water and onto the opposite riverbank. Batzer crosses the river unscathed, and recognizing the Herculean effort his friend has put forth, offers to take the lead in breaking trail. "We started taking turns," Herr recalls, "but overall, I think I dominated the trail breaking, which is part of the reason I ended up with far worse frostbite and hypothermia than Jeff."

Ahead of them, they spot a signal that they might actually be on an established route. "We started to see these painted blazes on the trees," recalls Batzer. "They were blue, so we thought they were trails we could follow." Neither realized that these were the blazes on Great Gulf Trail, but they were encouraged by the thought that they were heading somewhere. "Even with the blazes, though, we were really struggling to follow any sort of trail. It was unbelievingly difficult trying to get through there."

Within an hour after Herr falls into the river, it happens again. The second time, he goes through well past his waist. "It was much more desperate, and he yelled for help," says Batzer. "There was a current running under the ice, and he was afraid of going under and drowning. I extended my ice axe to him and helped pull him out. He'd been in the water for about 60 seconds at that point, so he was thoroughly wet, and I knew it couldn't go on much longer without some remedy for his situation."

Though Herr emerges without going under, he is now completely soaked from his mid-torso down. "I was wearing many layers," he recalls. "In addition to wool long underwear I was wearing gym-style pants and Gore-Tex shell pants."

Dr. Giesbrecht says that the cold effect of Herr's immersion would have been minor. "You're going to feel really, really cold, but short-term immersion in freezing water does not make you hypothermic. When you fall in the water, it's at 0° Celsius, and when you get out, your clothing is at 0° Celsius. As long as Herr is moving and his clothing isn't frozen yet, he's still OK. But when he stops, his clothing will freeze. So, the significant heat loss is going to happen over time."

In order to stay warm. Herr rightfully believes they must keep moving. "For sure, moving helped to keep us warm and stopping had its challenges, especially for Hugh at that point," says Batzer.

Batzer himself is wearing Gore-Tex pants, a pair of slightly insulated Habeler Superlight rigid ice-climbing boots with wool insoles, and a pair of brand-new insulated Gore-Tex over-boots, known as "supergaiters," which cover the boots and run all the way up to his knees. So he does not get wet when he helps Herr out of the river during his second immersion.

As moisture-wicking fabrics were becoming more mainstream at the time, climbers were transitioning away from cotton and wool. Waterproof fabrics such as Gore-Tex, invented in 1969, had found their way into the climber's toolbox, and Herr and Batzer chose synthetics for some of their hiking garments. But Dr. Giesbrecht is not convinced synthetic undergarments would have helped in Herr's specific situation. "If he was immersed, the water would have soaked his lower body completely, and once he got out, his pants would have frozen whether they were made of Gore-Tex or not," he says. "The Gore-Tex pants he was wearing will keep water from passing through to an extent. However, the major issue is that water will get in around the edges of the garment at the leg cuffs and waist. They would have quickly flooded and soaked his wool pants. Wool pants will hold water and therefore freeze if the water isn't wrung out of them. As soon as you get out of the water, before your clothes freeze, you should take them off, wring the water out, and then put them back on. This investment in discomfort will pay big dividends long term."

If Herr and Batzer were carrying extra clothing, it would give both of them the chance to change into dryer garments. They are feeling the urgent need to move on, so Herr doesn't even consider stopping to wring out his clothes. Instead, he takes the next trail-breaking shift, and the two press forward.

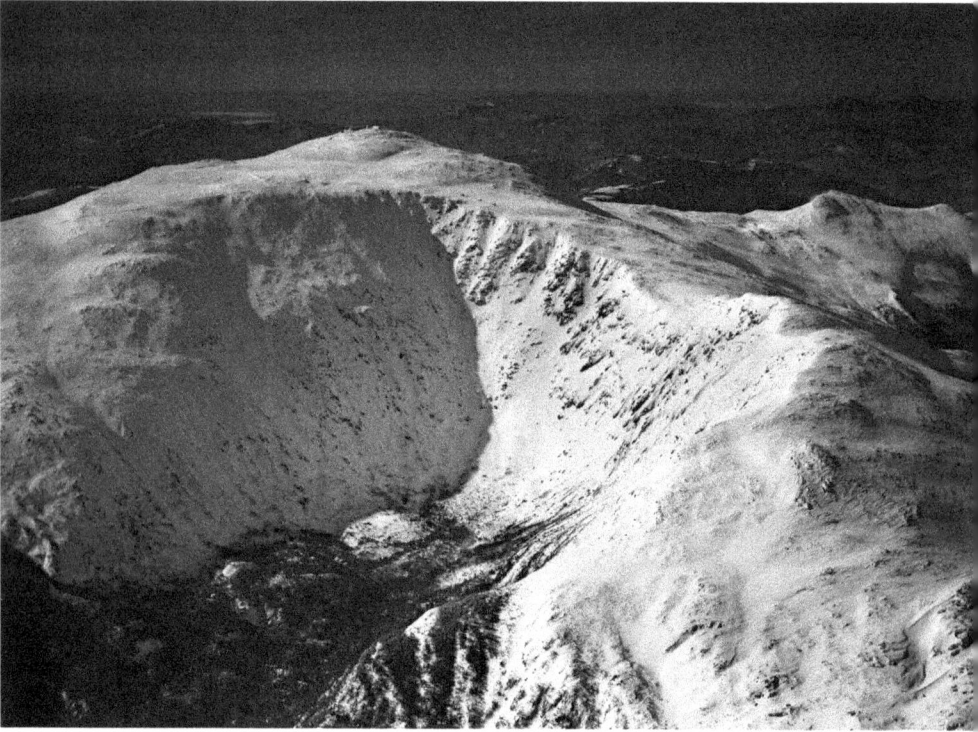

The Great Gulf

XII
CONCEALED

The cause is hidden; the effect is visible to all.
—Ovid

Mount Washington Observatory Surface Weather Observations (6:00 to 7:00 p.m.): Temperature 10°F; winds out of the southeast averaging 58 mph; visibility 0 miles; snow/blowing snow/fog; windchill -18.3°F; peak wind gust: 73 mph.

Harvard Cabin
Huntington Ravine
Saturday, Jan. 23, 1982
Early evening

Matt Pierce wants to start pacing. Nervous energy brought on by two overdue climbers is building within him. But not wanting to raise the tension level of guests from concern to alarm, he tempers the urge to move. Still, it's dark, the weather's gnarly, and it's been nine hours since he last saw Hugh Herr and Jeff Batzer on the first pitch of Odell Gully before they evaporated into the frozen fog.

The forecasted winter storm punched in some time ago and is now hard at work on the mountain. The early concerns Pierce harbored on meeting Herr and Batzer the previous evening are now fully realized. "I felt like they were in trouble," Pierce says. "If you're going to do a gully and hit the Escape Hatch and come down, you aren't going to waste any time on Alpine Garden. You're going to beat feet at that point. Once you get into Escape Hatch it's pretty straightforward, but even if you have a flashlight and some idea where you're going, it's still a lot of ground to cover. I had no idea what their climbing style was going to be that day or how experienced they were on ice, especially in extreme cold."

Pierce maintains his poker face in the dimly lit cabin, as guests take sporadic glances at the front door. Jim Frati, Bob MacEntee, and Hank Butler are already upstairs encased in their sleeping bags. Pierce had asked them if they'd seen any sign of Herr and Batzer. "No, we never saw them," MacEntee recalls telling Pierce. "We couldn't have seen them unless they were right in front of us." Pierce also asked Butler if he noticed whether Herr and Batzer had packed bivouac gear before heading out that morning, and Butler told him they had. "As I was drifting off to sleep," Frati recalls, "I heard Matt talking about the fact that Hugh and Jeff still hadn't come back."

Layne Terrell and Kacy (Terrell) St. Clair walk into the cabin after heading into town for a booze and bagel run. Both immediately sense trouble. "We picked up some peppermint brandy and were bringing it back for everybody," Terrell says. "When we hiked back up and walked in, there was a somber mood in the air. Matt said Hugh and Jeff hadn't come back, and it was dark at that point. I thought at the time that they were pretty novice, and I knew they were outside of their environment. We were very nervous about them. I didn't have a good feeling."

With the storm still raging, St. Clair recalls a harrowing trip into town and feeling a sense of relief at being back at the cabin. "The roads were scary, and I wasn't sure if we should even be driving in those conditions," she says today.

Absence of information and a feeling of powerlessness can create a vacuum for pessimism to creep in, and the guests in the cabin are likely beginning to fill that vacuum. It is a common response. From a place of relative warmth and safety, we can imagine the suffering taking place, imagine ourselves doing that suffering. We hope these morbid thoughts are curtailed by news that the lost have been found. When that doesn't happen, we try to halt our emotional downward spiral by replacing anxiety with judgment. We tell ourselves we'd never, ever do what they did, that we would make the right judgment calls to bring us back to safety.

Finally, Pierce can no longer restrain himself. He gathers his gear and announces he's heading into the ravine to look for Batzer and Herr. Hearing this, Frati and MacEntee crawl out of their sleeping bags and hear Layne Terrell volunteering to go along. The two friends offer their help as well. Pierce accepts these three offers gratefully. "In situations like that," he says today, "if there was somebody at the cabin who seemed to have their head together, I certainly would have taken them with me if they wanted to go."

The four searchers leave the cabin and take Spur Trail to Huntington Ravine Trail. "Our charge was to see if we could see any lights in the gully," says MacEntee. "We were wearing crappy D-cell headlamps."

Terrell recalls the anxiety he was feeling as they moved through the darkness. "I remember walking up into the ravine with Matt to see if we could run across them coming down or possibly see headlamps descending," he says.

Following the almost invisible trough in the snow created during earlier descents to the cabin, the four move briskly in single file. When they reach the bottom of The Fan, it is so dark and there's so much snow in the air that they can only see within the confines of the beam of their headlamps. "We were looking for lights and hoping to use our flashlights to help them get down if they were there," says Pierce. "But we didn't see or hear anything. I hollered to them but didn't get a response. I doubted my yelling would travel very far anyway, with the winds so high. We didn't know what their plans were other than that they were hoping to come down Escape Hatch."

The four men are focused on their task and likely unaware that the winds are starting a significant shift in direction that will continue well into late evening. Winds that have been blowing from the south all day are now coming from the southeast. Winds pushing 60 mph with stronger gusts have been moving copious amounts of snow throughout the entire Presidential Range. With the shift, snow is now loading from southeast to northwest. This change in direction is impacting Mount Washington's summit and Gulfside, as well as Mounts Clay, Jefferson, Adams, and Madison. It is definitely wreaking havoc in Great Gulf, where Herr and Batzer are struggling to survive.

With no sighting of two pinhole-sized lights in Escape Hatch or Odell Gully, or any sign of a catastrophic event at Odell's base, Pierce, Frati, MacEntee, and Tyrell head back to Harvard Cabin. It is about 7:00 p.m. when they return, clear the encrusted snow from their clothing and boots, and prepare to face the worried guests. Pierce can tell when they enter that the wide-eyed guests sitting at the kitchen table or on benches are eager for good news. Without a word, he looks at them wearily and shakes his head "No." Then he fires up the base radio's microphone to alert Pinkham that Herr and Batzer are missing.

XIII
RALLY

In order to get a victim off a mountain or a cliff, there have to be people who are experienced technical climbers. … It's not usually a very quick or easy process. We have to go out in all kinds of weather at all hours, and there is considerable risk on our part.

It's not uncommon for a rescue to last all night.

—Rick Wilcox, former president of Mountain Rescue Service,

in an interview with *The New Hampshire*, April 3, 1981

Mount Washington Valley
Saturday, Jan. 23, 1982
7:00 p.m.

Matt Pierce radios Pinkham and connects with Misha Kirk, who is on the overnight Notch Watch. "There is someone responsible for being in charge on any given night," Pierce says, "someone who has a good idea of what to do and who to call in an emergency."

Pierce informs Kirk that he has two climbers who departed that morning at approximately 8:00 a.m. for a climb of Odell Gully and a descent of Escape Hatch and haven't returned. He provides the point last seen, the first pitch of Odell Gully. He tells Kirk two hikers came to the cabin in the early afternoon to report hearing what they thought was yelling in Odell Gully, and also mentions that climbers who'd been in Escape Hatch that afternoon had not seen anyone. Pierce adds that he's just returned from checking Huntington Ravine as well.

Kirk asks for an approximate description of Herr and Batzer, and collects additional information on weather and avalanche conditions to provide to those within the search and rescue community he'll soon notify:

Missing Persons: Jeff Batzer, WM; 5'4"–5'6"; Weight: 130 lbs.; Dark brown hair; 18–22 years old.

Hugh Herr, WM; 5'4"–5'6"; Weight: 130 lbs; Light brown hair; 18–22 years old.

Current Weather: 20°F, windy and snowing; visibility 50–75 yards with headlamps.

Avalanche Conditions: minor sloughing all day; no major slides.

Intended Route: ascend Odell's; descend Escape Hatch.

Equipment/Experience: Matt Pierce reports they had good equipment, large rack of gear, red rope, carrying small day packs [sic] and not much extra gear; wearing tan parka.

They seemed experienced and familiar with the ravine.

It is later confirmed that Herr and Batzer had only one pack, which they had cached. The "tan parka" is the one Jeff Batzer is wearing.

Kirk contacts Peter Furtado, the assistant manager for the AMC at Pinkham, and the two work together to notify the agencies and organizations who will be involved in a search for the missing climbers. Over the next three days, four organizations will take part in this long, arduous mission: New Hampshire Fish and Game (NHFG), the U.S. Forest Service, the Appalachian Mountain Club, and Mountain Rescue Service.

Kirk initially calls Lt. Bill Hastings, the District One chief of New Hampshire Fish and Game, who is on a weekend off and refers him to Conservation Officer Sgt. Carl Carlson, also of District One. Furtado reaches Sgt. Carlson and informs him that he believes he and Kirk can recruit at least 20 searchers and will have confirmation on the total number sometime after 11:00 p.m. He adds that the plan is to gather at 7:00 a.m. the following morning at Pinkham. Carlson tells Furtado he'll contact two conservation officers from each district to respond with their snow machines. In addition to himself, Carlson will enlist six other Conservation Officers: Harold Reed, Doug Menzies, Keith Kidder, David Beyerle, Charles Kenney, and Jeff Gray.

In 1954, New Hampshire Gov. Hugh Gregg drafted an executive order, later enacted into law, giving NHFG oversight for all search and rescue operations in the woodlands and inland waterways throughout the State. On Feb. 6, 1981, the Presidential Unit Plan stated that "[b]ecause of the technical aspects involved in avalanche and avalanche forecasting, the Forest Service is the lead agency in all winter search and rescues in the Cutler River Drainage. Elsewhere, the New Hampshire Fish and Game Department is the lead agency in accord with its official state responsibility."

Because the focus of this winter search will be the Cutler River Drainage, which encompasses Tuckerman Ravine up to the summit cone of Mount Washington and over to Huntington Ravine, the Forest Service will have oversight unless the mission is expanded beyond the drainage. Until then, the NHFG will provide a supporting role to the Forest Service. With that in mind, Furtado notifies Lead Snow Ranger Brad Ray of the Forest Service, who in turn contacts Snow Ranger Rene LaRoche.

Joe Gill, AMC caretaker in Tuckerman Ravine, and AMC crew members Bill Meduski, Carol (Cullina) Cunha, Alan Kamman, and Bill Corbin are notified and asked to convene at Pinkham the next morning to assist with the search. David Warren, manager of the AMC hut system, is also notified and will assist with the multi-agency search coordination at Pinkham. The AMC was once the tip of the spear for search and rescue operations in the White Mountains. With the advent of additional volunteer organizations and the professionalism of NHFG operations, the AMC no longer plays a central role in these types of searches.

As he continues to gather rescuers, Kirk tracks down Bill Kane, a team leader for Mountain Rescue Service (MRS). Normally, Rick Wilcox, then president of MRS, would be contacted, but he is out of the country leading an expedition on Aconcagua in Argentina for the International Mountain Climbing School based out of International Mountain Equipment (IME) in North Conway, N.H., which Wilcox owns.

"I was having dinner with friends in Conway when I got a call from the guys at Pinkham explaining the situation," Kane recalls. I said, 'Why don't we give them a little more time?'" But when he hears that the missing climbers departed Harvard Cabin at around 8:00 a.m., he goes to IME and gets the call list. "Most times back then, I'd call the team leaders, and they'd go down the list. Everybody called two people, and those who could respond would call me back."

By 11:30 p.m., Kane lets Kirk and Furtado know that 14 volunteers from MRS will respond to Pinkham the next morning: Kane himself, Albert Dow, Michael Hartrich, Joe Lentini, Paul Ross, David Stone, Steve Larson, Dana Seavey, Doug Madara, Frank Hubble, Bill Aughton, Matt Peer, Todd Swain, and Tiger Burns. "I asked them all to be at Pinkham a little before 6:00 a.m.," says Kane.

Because of the extreme conditions, especially above treeline, and the complexity of the technical terrain that will encompass part of the search area, the experienced climbers from MRS will be asked to take the lead on determining the mission's parameters.

As MRS team members conclude their calls and prepare their gear, they are not only facing exposure to physical risk but to financial risk as well, and these considerations will become critical by the end of this historic mission. As the only all-volunteer search and rescue organization at the time, MRS members were not covered by workers' compensation. If a member of the team was injured or worse during a callout, they were not covered like their New Hampshire Fish and Game, AMC, and Forest Service counterparts. Some members were also without private health insurance because they were self-employed or their employers did not provide the benefit.

So, as they prepare to head into this unpredictable and unforgiving environment, these 14 volunteers are committing to a rescue mission that carries multiple levels of risk to themselves and their families.

XIV
MEASURES

A storm is threatening
My very life today.
If I don't get some shelter
I'm gonna fade away.
—The Rolling Stones, "Gimme Shelter"

Great Gulf: Temperature: 27°F, winds are low; visibility darkness; light snowfall.

West Branch of the Peabody River (3,200 ft.)
Great Gulf Wilderness
Saturday, Jan. 23, 1982
Evening

With darkness impeding their ability to navigate, Hugh Herr and Jeff Batzer are stymied. They agree to stop and attempt to establish a bivouac under a spruce tree. Quickly realizing it's not going to work, they continue plowing through the snow. Each time they stop, thinking they've found a place to bed down, the cold air stings Herr's wet clothing. He's fearful he'll freeze to death if he stops moving. "We were both terrified," he says today. "At that point, the only communication between us was what we needed to do to survive."

The two stop again at snow-covered boulders, erratics left behind by the alpine glacier that operated there thousands of years before. "We were thinking we needed to stop until morning," Batzer recalls. "We found a cleft between two rocks and slipped between this clam-like opening. We sat down and stopped briefly but decided again to keep moving. We were trying hard to hold it together and not panic, just focusing on what we had got to do next. We were being as steady as we could manage."

High above them, on the summit of Mount Washington, the fierce weather is taking a brief respite before winds shift west and ratchet the intensity level back up. Overnight, temperatures on the summit will rise to a high of 21°F before dropping sharply after 2:00 a.m. Temperatures in the Gulf will also rise, but unfortunately won't hold.

At last, Herr and Batzer locate a suitable place to set up their emergency shelter. "We found very large granite boulders and dug snow away from the edges," Herr says. "We created a cave with a granite roof and a snow shelf for a floor." Surrounding them are thick clusters of spruce and fir trees, and Batzer suggests they take advantage of the insulative properties they'll provide. "We broke off the branches and made an insulation barrier between us and the snow shelf," he says. "Years before, I had been on a backpacking trip and

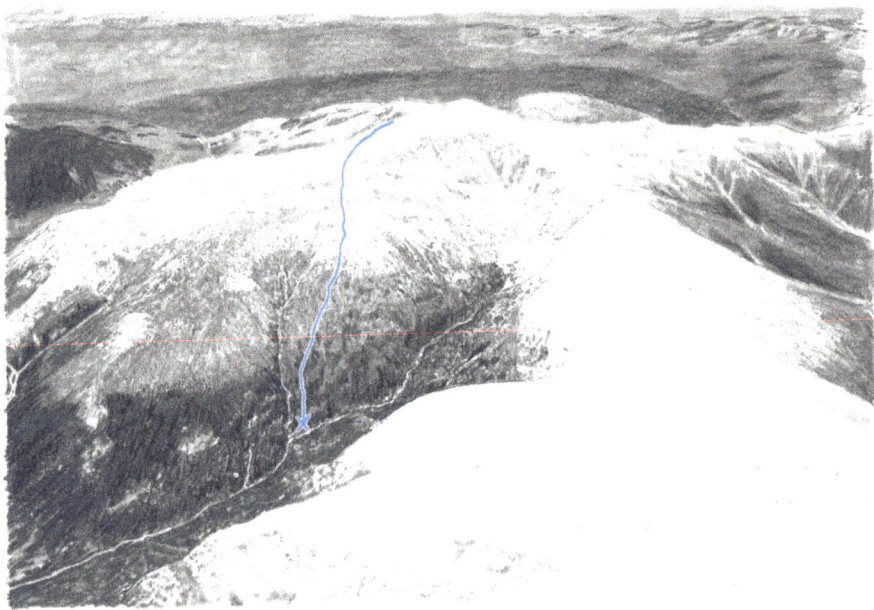

The actual descent of Herr and Batzer into the Great Gulf and where they bivouaced on the night of Jan. 23.

used leaves under and on top of my sleeping bag because I was desperately cold, and it worked."

With more than three feet of spruce branches atop the snow, they turn to Herr's situation. "The layers Hugh was wearing below the waist were soaked and frozen," says Batzer. "Before we got in the cave, Hugh stripped everything off from the waist down, except for his wet socks. He was pretty miserable and cold, but he was still holding it together. I gave him the virgin wool cycling tights I'd been wearing, and he put his wet and frozen windpants on over them. They were already pretty stiff. That left me with a thick polypropylene wicking layer, wool cycling shorts, and my Gore-Tex pants."

The pair crawl into the cave onto the spruce bed they've created and make what will be a critical decision: they remove their boots. Herr's leather boots are completely soaked, and Batzer's are damp from perspiration. "We put our boots at the back of the cave, safely away from the weather," Batzer recalls. "We thought that keeping our boots on and not wrapping our feet in something dry overnight could lead to frostbite. We wrapped our legs and feet in my parka."

Their reasoning, though understandable, will prove to have serious consequences. Dr. Gordon Giesbrecht, a cold-weather injury expert, says, "When you get hit in the foot by a puck playing hockey, you keep your skate on if you want to keep playing because once you take it off, you'll never get your foot back in. If you're in a tent with a sleeping bag, it's a good idea to take your boots off and put them inside your bag. But in a survival scenario like the one Herr and Batzer are in, without sleeping bags or a fire, you should take your boots off only to wring the water out of your socks and put them right back on because even if your feet freeze in them, they'll still allow you to walk."

After lying down on their nest of branches, Herr and Batzer cover themselves with a thick layer of spruce and fir. "The rock we were wedged in was 10 feet by 10 feet, and we were underneath in this nice little cavity," says Batzer. "It protected us. It wasn't really snowing that night. It was glowing, and you could see across the river. Up above, it was overcast. It was dead quiet, no snapping of trees or anything. I had this idea that we'd certainly get out in the morning."

They lie face to face, hug one another, and overlap their legs to try to keep warm. "I wasn't feeling the effects of cold initially," says Herr today. "But I was worried we wouldn't last the night. That might have been true if either of us had been alone. What I didn't take into account was the power of two people hugging each other. You collapse your surface area, and you increase your heat output by a factor of two. It's very powerful for keeping the major organs alive."

Giesbrecht agrees with this strategy for preserving scarce body heat. "If you've got two freezing bodies, there's no question that hugging is a good thing. You're not hugging a boulder; you're hugging a body whose surface area is cold but is providing some insulation. You'll continue to lose heat to that body, but at some point, it will equilibrate. You won't be losing as much body heat as you would if you moved away from the body."

But Giesbrecht adds that Herr and Batzer have complicating factors that are compromising their ability to stay as warm as they need to be: "With wet clothing, the insulation value of hugging is not optimum. When they lie down, their clothing will freeze, which will suck more heat out of them. They were in a very tough situation."

Batzer senses that Herr is sleeping for short intervals, but he himself does not sleep at all. "I wasn't desperately cold, but I was pretty miserable waiting for morning to come," he recalls. "We talked from time to time, but it was business talk. Nothing normal or fun. There was a lot of maneuvering to keep warm, and that was helpful. We still had a lot of strength, and we were stable, but we couldn't wait to get out in the morning and have the situation fixed. I had this idea that if we fell asleep, we'd never wake up."

Giesbrecht says that Herr and Batzer's situation serves as an important lesson for anyone who ventures into the backcountry today. "Anytime you walk away from safety and into the wilderness, you should ask yourself the question, 'Do I have the equipment and experience to survive until tomorrow morning in good health?' If you can survive one night this way, you can survive several nights. The most important survival aspect in winter is to be able to light a fire. Shelter is great, but fire is most important. If you can light a fire, you can keep warm, dry out wet clothing, melt snow for water (if you have a metal container), keep busy (a great psychological advantage), and make a signal for searchers. Had they had fire-starting capability, all they would have had to do was stop, not panic, and realize the most important thing was to dry the wet clothing and boots. But they didn't have anything to light a fire with, so they were in trouble from the start."

Since leaving Harvard Cabin more than 12 hours earlier, Herr and Batzer have traveled a total of 3.75 miles. The distance from the top of Great Gulf to where they finally lay their heads for the night is just under a mile and a half. It has been quite a struggle. Neither of them is wearing a watch, but official reports indicate that they reach the floor of the Gulf at 4:00 p.m. and arrive at their bivy sometime after 7:30 p.m., traveling only 0.37 miles and losing 200 feet in elevation during all that time through waist- and chest-deep snow.

The two have no idea that a search for them is in its infancy. If they knew, they would also realize that no one imagines they are in Great Gulf, which is nowhere near where they expected to be.

"We were not talking about rescue," says Batzer. "At that point I wasn't even thinking that Matt Pierce would be concerned about us. I thought he might think we'd just decided to stay out for a few days. There's that grace period when people tell themselves that these things happen, and it sometimes takes a while for climbers to get back. So all we were thinking at that point was that we had to get out of there on our own, and we believed we could."

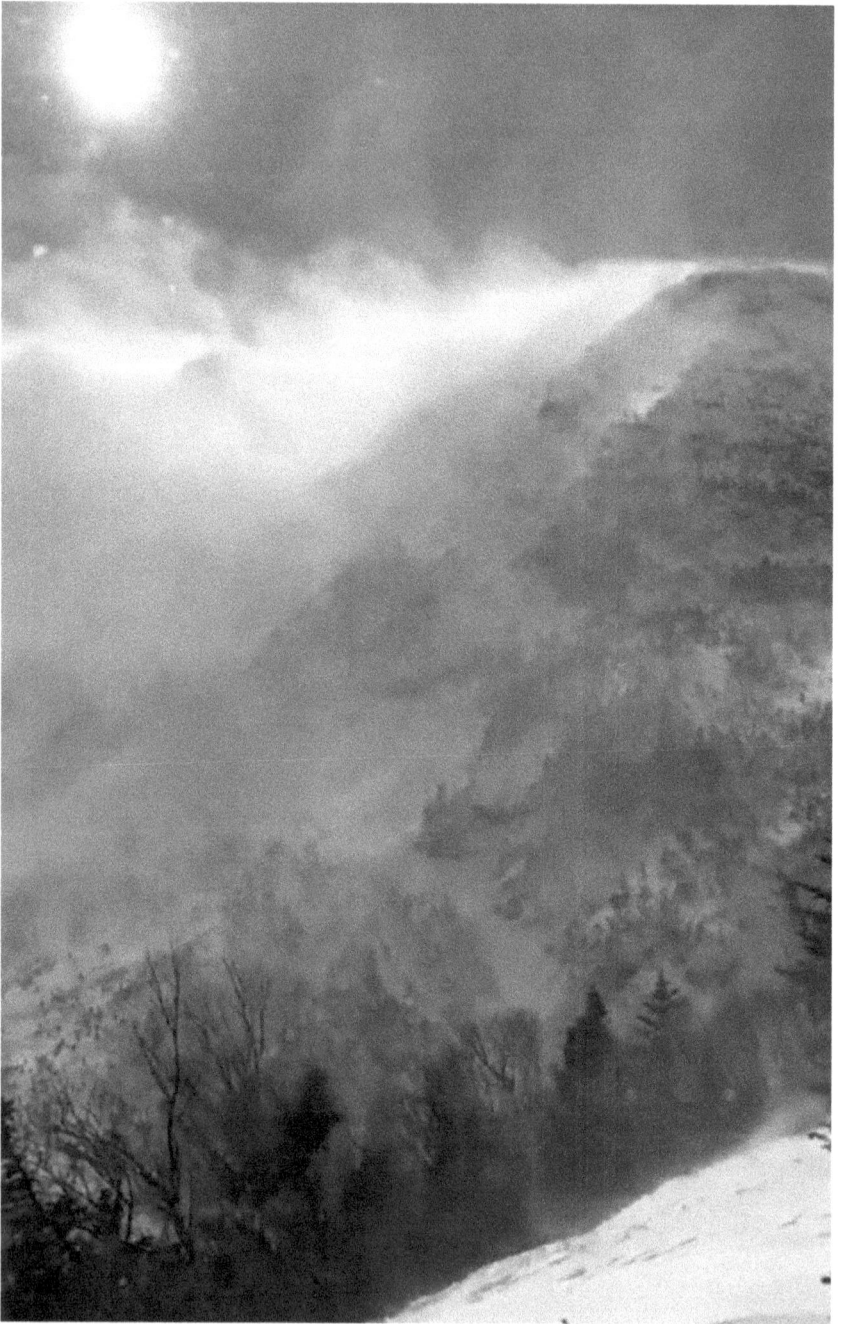

Plumes of snow being sloughed from Boott Spur in Tuckerman Ravine and deposited at lower elevations on the eastern slopes of Mount Washington.

XV
PRECURSOR

Mount Washington's legendary winter weather … is not accompanied by enormous snowfall, although the accumulations in Tuckerman Ravine are world famous. This mecca for spring skiers owes its snow to the winds, which sweep most of the precipitation from the west and northwest slopes of the Presidential Range and drop it in the calmer eddies on the eastern basins— of which Tuckerman Ravine is merely the most favored by this process.

—William Lowell Putnam, *The Worst Weather on Earth*

Mount Washington Observatory Surface Weather Observations (10:00 p.m. Saturday, Jan. 23, to 4:00 a.m. Sunday, Jan. 24): Lowest temperature 9°F; winds out of the west averaging 47mph; visibility 0 miles; snow/blowing snow/ fog; lowest windchill -17.7°F; peak wind gust: 65 mph.

Presidential Range
Saturday, Jan. 23, and Sunday Jan. 24, 1982
Late evening/Early morning

As Herr and Batzer ride out their cold and fitful bivouac and rescuers are alerted to their absence, winds that have whipped across the higher summits from the south and southeast make a rapid shift west. The three storm tracks that converge on the Presidential Range—south to north, southeast to northwest, and west to east— move snow all winter long. This ever-changing dynamic creates a snow load that is extremely hard to read because it is so variable across the terrain, ranging from a few inches of walkable snow to chest-deep dunes that are exhausting to plow through.

By midnight, Mount Washington will have logged a total accumulation of 7.1 inches of low-density snow, the type that's easily moved by the wind. In the North Country of New Hampshire, 7 inches of snow is just another weekday. But above treeline, this amount of accumulation, when pushed around by with high winds, is a disaster in the making.

"As winds shifted to the west, all the snow that had loaded during the day into or toward Great Gulf sloughed off and, like a giant comb-over, was blown back in the other direction, toward

Tuckerman Ravine," says Ryan Knapp of the Mount Washington Observatory. "You had seven inches of snow loading and then another two or three more inches that fell later added to it. All of that snow is blowing and accumulating elsewhere at higher depths because above treeline there's nothing holding it in one place. That's partly why in the wintertime the summit might be reporting only one to two inches of snow. Most of it has gotten blown off and has accumulated in other places."

The snow loading in the Presidential Range is so significant that evidence of it is often seen long after the winter months have ended. "Tuckerman Ravine will still have snow in June and sometimes into July because basically all of our snow on the summit loads the eastern faces of the mountain and the northern faces of the Great Gulf," says Knapp.

The current shift in wind direction from southeast to west is a critical factor in all that happens next, because the winds will catapult prolific amounts of snow to the east. This will set the stage for the fateful, catastrophic events that will soon befall those who are lost and those risking their lives to find them.

XVI
FIRST WAVES

The mountains are calling, and I must go.
—John Muir

Mount Washington Observatory Surface Weather Observations (4:00 to 5:00 a.m.): Temperature 7°F; winds out of the west averaging 43 mph; visibility 0 miles; snow/blowing snow/fog; windchill -19.7°F; peak wind gust: 54 mph.

Great Gulf: Temperature: 17°F; winds are low; visibility darkness; light snowfall.

Tuckerman Ravine Trail
Sunday, Jan. 24, 1982
4:30 a.m.

Note: On Oct. 2, 2001, Misha Kirk died suddenly at age 50 of a neurological seizure. Following his participation in the search and rescue mission for Hugh Herr and Jeff Batzer, he had journaled extensively about his experiences over the course of those three days. Information from his journals is being shared here with the permission of his partner, Patrice Mutchnick.

Misha Kirk moves across the frozen terrain with an efficiency forged in the U.S Army. Too amped up to sleep and unable to remain flat in his bunk for another 90 minutes, when search teams will gather, he wants to do something now. Kirk is a nationally registered emergency medical technician and a former Green Beret medic and weapons specialist assigned to the 10th Special Forces Group (Airborne) based at Fort Devens in Massachusetts. With his mountaineering background and familiarity with the unforgiving nature of this range, he knows Mount Washington is in control of whatever situation Hugh Herr and Jeff Batzer have gotten themselves into, and he'll do whatever he can to regain some of that control on their behalf.

Kirk was on Notch Watch at Pinkham the previous night when he received a call from Matt Pierce at Harvard Cabin reporting that Jeff Batzer and Hugh Herr were missing. He'd spent a good part of the night working with Peter Furtado, also of the AMC, to notify the appropriate authorities and search and rescue teams for the mission that will soon be launched. He has no idea how critical a role he will play in that mission over the next few days.

"I remember stumbling out of bed wishing that Jeff and Hugh had walked into Harvard Cabin after I had gone to sleep, so I could just stumble back into bed. But no," he wrote in his journal.

Kirk fine-tunes the gear he began preparing the night before, soon after search teams called in their final numbers at 11:30 p.m. He expects this will be a full-day outing, given the current and anticipated weather conditions on the summit. Then he leaves Joe Dodge Lodge

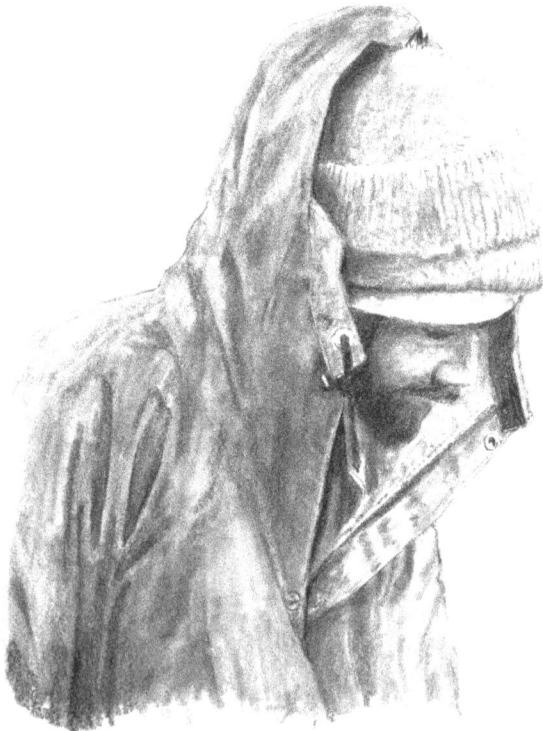

Misha Kirk

and heads over to the cafeteria at the Trading Post, where he makes himself a small breakfast and fills his thermos with hot coffee. By 4:15 a.m., he has boots on the trail.

In addition to his winter gear, Kirk is carrying a high-band radio under the call sign Unit 17. He wants to get into Huntington Ravine by dawn for a hasty search before crews start arriving at Pinkham at 6:00 a.m. Sunrise is a little after 7:00 a.m., so he's relying on his bulky, D-cell battery headlamp to guide him up the trail.

"I had always liked hiking in the dark, but after only four hours of sleep and arising at 3:30 a.m., this morning was hard to take," Kirk wrote. "I was on the start of the Tuck Trail, a one-head-lamped, half-awake zombie. ... If by chance they were sitting at the bottom of Odell's in Huntington Ravine, I wanted to be there at first light. I knew a huge search squad would assemble at [Pinkham], and I thought: no sense in having people spread all over the mountain if Jeff and Hugh were in Huntington's."

Kirk arrived at the AMC in 1978 and quickly made a name for himself for his alpine rescue acumen. "Misha had recently been discharged from the army and was working for the AMC until he could get into medical school," says friend and former Mount Washington State Park Manager Mike Pelchat. "He was an army medic and an accomplished rock and ice climber." A cancer diagnosis in the 1990s upended Kirk's goal of becoming a physician, and at the time of his death in 2001, he was a nationally registered paramedic and studying to become a registered nurse.

"The climb began to soothe me, and soon I was awake," wrote Kirk. "My load felt lighter, my pace steadier. Since I only had the visibility of my headlamp, the weather was hard to read. I couldn't see the stars, and as I climbed higher, the wind began to howl."

Before heading into Huntington Ravine, Kirk takes the Spur Trail over to Harvard Cabin to check in with Matt Pierce for any updates. "By the time I got to Harvard Cabin, I couldn't tell if it was snowing or if the wind was just blowing the snow around," he recalled. "The beam of my headlamp was completely filled in with a blizzard. I leaned against the door and walked into the dark, cold cabin. I could hear snoring as I called Matt's name out. Fifteen minutes later, I left the Harvard Cabin. As I closed the door, everyone was up and preparing for the day's search. They were to wait until they heard from me or the base."

With Kirk heading into the ravine and essentially kicking off the mission, Matt Pierce asks some of the guests who'd expressed interest in helping in the search to start preparing themselves and their gear for what he knows will be challenging conditions for even the most experienced among them.

When Kirk regains the Huntington Ravine Trail, he continues upward into the storm. "Plowing through calf-deep, unbroken snow, I was encased in a black box with my light bobbing up and down ahead of me. But day began to dawn, and soon the black box turned dark gray, then gray. I was in a thick cloud of snow swirling and roaring in a million directions. At times, it would break, and I could see 150 feet ahead of me, then suddenly, nothing again."

He enters the massive amphitheater but is unable to see the high walls before him. Fortunately, he's well versed in the terrain and some of the natural and man-made markers there. "As I approached the first-aid cache [since named the Albert Dow First-Aid Cache], at the base of The Fan, I shivered, both from the cold and from the strange eeriness I felt around me."

At the time, the first-aid cache housed a wooden toboggan, steel stoke litters, splints, wool blankets, a sleeping bag, foam pads, and other first-aid supplies. Remote caches are still used to position rescue supplies in higher terrain for rapid access in the event of an emergency.

The point last seen is a critical component in the early stages of any search, so Kirk heads directly to Odell Gully, where Matt Pierce was the last to see Herr and Batzer a little over 20 hours earlier. His journal offers a vivid description of the conditions he is experiencing:

> I could only see a few feet ahead of me when I began to climb The Fan. Whenever I lifted my head to look up above me, the wind would ram blowing snow down my clothes, nose, and mouth. I could only proceed on all fours, looking down at my feet. I reached the base of Odell's, or what I thought was the base, barely able to see anything. Feeling a little ridiculous, I climbed back down. When I reached the base of The Fan again, I stood up only to be lifted and slammed down by the wind I thought must be over 65 mph. I ducked behind a huge boulder to recover and rest. This was the first time that morning I really thought about Jeff and Hugh. I shuddered to

think they might be out there in this weather. I could barely keep warm, and I had all four layers of clothing on. It felt like it was -100F. I doubted they could have survived the night if they were stuck somewhere in Odell's. Wherever they were at this point, I wished them luck.

With no sign of Herr or Batzer at the base of Odell Gully, Kirk shifts his focus to searching the snow-covered, boulder-strewn Fan. Herr and Batzer could be bivouacked there, or they could have been swept out of the gully by an avalanche or a catastrophic fall.

"I began to search the boulders as systematically as possible in the obscurity," Kirk wrote. "Just above the Griffin-Stadtmueller Boulder, I saw the pack. A chill ran through me, and I stopped. The way it lay there with the snow piling up around it, I could've sworn a body was under it. I approached it and kicked the pack; it popped out and over. Whew…, no body."

Kirk picks up the green alpine pack and is immediately concerned by what he finds—or what he doesn't find—inside. "The pack contained bivy-gear but no ID," he told his journal. "I couldn't be sure if it was Jeff and Hugh's, but if it was, I thought these guys are in trouble." Kirk reports his findings to base, where searchers are beginning to gather for a pre-mission breakfast, and then continues his search.

Several press accounts and some official reports indicate that in addition to the contents Kirk cites in the cached pack, there was also a sleeping bag. But Batzer and Herr both confirm that this is inaccurate. "We did not bring a sleeping bag," Herr says today. "I packed a Gore-Tex bivouac sac in the event we were delayed and had to spend the night. We felt it was fine to stash the pack, but we needed to be damned sure to stick to our plan and descend quickly. Our decision to go to the summit, seemingly innocent at the time, was the mistake."

The location where Kirk finds the pack is eerily coincidental. At the time they stash it, Herr and Batzer are unaware that they're placing it near the site of a memorial. The first avalanche fatalities in Huntington Ravine took place on April 4, 1964, when John Griffin and Hugo Stadtmueller were killed by a massive slide. They were the 50th and 51st fatalities on Mount Washington and only the third and fourth avalanche fatalities. Like Herr and Batzer, their plan had been to climb Odell Gully. The mountain had received considerable snowfall over the course of two days, and the ravine experienced heavy snow loading from the high winds. The avalanche that killed Griffin and Stadtmueller was not witnessed, but at some point during their ascent of The Fan or Odell, they were caught in it and suffered traumatic injuries as they were swept down the talus-congested slope.

After the tragedy, a memorial plaque was placed by friends on a large boulder in Huntington Ravine, where it remains today. "We chose the spot because it's on the Huntington Ravine Trail," says John Porter, a renowned climber, author, and friend of Griffin and Stadtmueller, who discovered and reported the avalanche debris that killed them. "It is sheltered and not far from where the bodies were found. We felt everyone would see it, and it was less exposed there being on the overhang of the boulder."

IN MEMORY OF
JOHN GRIFFIN AND HUGO STADTMUELLER
KILLED IN AN AVALANCHE
APRIL 4, 1964

Prior to the deaths of Griffin and Stadtmueller, the Forest Service limited avalanche forecasting and ravine closure to Tuckerman, where the first Mount Washington avalanche fatality occurred in 1954. After the 1964 tragedy, they included forecasting and ravine closures in Huntington as well.

Kirk himself is focused on his search and does not yet see the uncanny coincidence of finding Herr and Batzer's pack at this very spot. He decides he'll hunker down and wait in the ravine for his fellow rescuers to arrive for the start of a comprehensive search of the eastern slopes of the mountain. "When I had picked over the entire bottom of The Fan, I went back to my original boulder," he wrote. "I huddled in the lee of the boulder and did jumping jacks to keep warm."

Soper Residence
Wolfeboro, N.H.
5:30 a.m.

Mount Washington Observatory Surface Weather Observations (5:00 to 6:00 a.m.): Temperature 7°F; winds out of the west averaging 43 mph; visibility 0 miles; snow/blowing snow/fog; windchill -19.7°F; peak wind gust: 54 mph.

Great Gulf: Temperature: 17°F; winds are low; visibility darkness; light snowfall.

Bruce Soper is suspended in a deep sleep when he's shocked awake by the phone on his nightstand. Searching in the darkness for the receiver, he answers with a hint of trepidation. Calls at this early hour are never good news. On the other end of the phone is Albert Dow, who apologizes for calling so early.

Soper and Dow have planned to meet later that morning for some ice climbing at Cathedral Ledge in North Conway. But Dow tells his friend, "Something urgent has come up, and I can't climb with you today."

Soper had recently taken a position at the superintendent's office at the Governor Wentworth School District in Wolfeboro, the same district Albert Dow had attended years ago. After he developed an avid interest in ice climbing, he asked friends whom he should contact to help him get better at it. "Albert's name came up immediately, and so I contacted him," Soper recalls. They felt an instant rapport and began ice climbing together, including a few times at Cathedral Ledge. "This was a learning experience for me," says Soper. "I purchased the necessary safety equipment on Albert's advice."

In the true spirit of Mountain Rescue Service's desire to work quietly behind the scenes, Dow offers Soper no additional details about the "something urgent" that is forcing him to postpone their planned day together, and Soper probes no further. He thanks Dow for calling, and they agree to reschedule their climb soon.

Today, those early January outings with Dow and his willingness to invest time in helping him improve still resonates deeply with Soper. "Albert was the kind of person we all should aspire to be," he says.

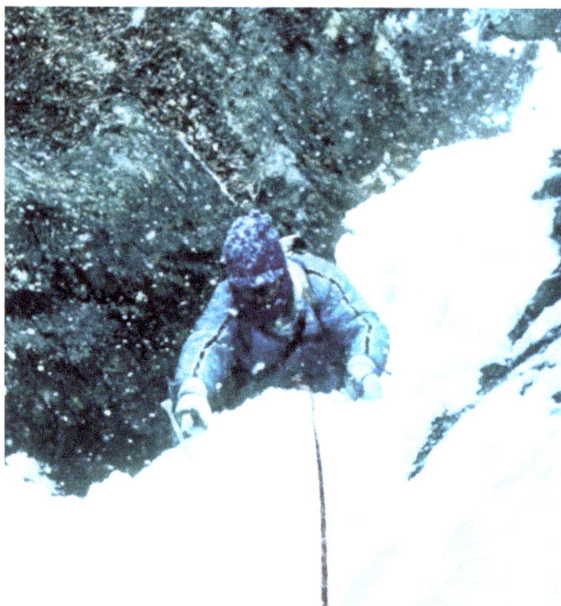

Albert Dow on a first ascent at Frankenstein Cliff in Crawford Notch, N.H.

Odell Gully
Huntington Ravine
6:00 a.m.

Mount Washington Observatory Surface Weather Observations (5:00 to 6:00 a.m.): Temperature 7°F; winds out of the west averaging 43 mph; visibility 0 miles; snow/blowing snow/fog; windchill -19.7°F; peak wind gust: 54 mph.

With the two empty sleeping bags belonging to Hugh Herr and Jeff Batzer in the loft and high winds raging all night, a restful night's sleep is out of the question for anyone at Harvard Cabin. By morning, Jim Frati and Hank Butler have flipped a switch. Here for the weekend to climb strictly for pleasure, both are now firmly entrenched in rescue mode. "We really thought we could find them up in the gully," says Frati today. "When they found the stashed pack, we thought, 'They're still in Odell's!' We felt we would be able to find and help them."

"Jim and I were hopeful we could find them bivouacked in a protected spot somewhere in the lee of the headwall," adds Butler. Because Frati and Butler anticipate extreme conditions, they agree that their less-experienced companion, Bob MacEntee, should stay behind.

As Frati and Butler enter Huntington Ravine, the narrow beams of their bobbing headlamps reveal a wall of wind and blowing snow. "It was so cold!" recalls Frati. "The cabin is pretty well sheltered, but when we rounded the turn, the wind was really blowing down into the ravine." Visibility is so appalling that Frati and Butler never see Misha Kirk hunkered behind a nearby boulder awaiting the search team, nor does Kirk see them.

The pair ascend The Fan and set up at the base of Odell Gully. Frati looks up into the gully and even with limited visibility, he is alarmed by what he sees. "You could see that the snow was piling up quick," he says. "I wasn't that experienced, but it looked to me like avalanche conditions were pretty high."

Butler takes the lead as Frati belays him. Spindrift pouring down the gully assails them as they get higher. "We searched every possible nook and cranny along the way," says Butler. "The whole time we were screaming 'JEFF! HUGH!' We found no sign of life. No sign of anything."

The windchill and untethered snow are wreaking havoc on Butler's face and Frati's ability to see. "I didn't have goggles," says Frati. "I would blink, and my eyes would freeze together."

They are one pitch up, having climbed approximately 160 feet. With no sign of Herr and Batzer, their level of concern reaches its peak. "Back then, we climbed on 50-meter ropes," says Frati today. The high winds and freezing temperatures are stacking layers of unstable snow into the narrow gully. The two are perilously positioned in the alpine version of a minefield. An axe placement or boot kick from either of them could trigger the release of a slab of snow capable of sending them tumbling out of the gully and onto the scree-filled Fan below.

"Hank said the avalanche conditions were high, and that we should descend, and I trusted his judgment," says Frati. Ever so carefully, they down-climb out of Odell leaving over 600 feet of the 800-foot gully unsearched.

Frati and Butler hike out of the ravine and onto the Huntington Ravine Trail. As they near the Spur Trail, they find a parked Forest Service Thiokol, and inside Harvard Cabin they meet the first group of searchers preparing to head into the ravine. Butler drops onto a bench and sits next to one of them. "I was having a conversation with a member of the rescue team about the weather conditions," he says. "He told me I got burned really good, but I didn't know what he meant. I'd forgotten all about my face. He pointed at my cheek and told me I had a bad case of frostbite and to seek medical attention as soon as I got down."

XVII
GLOOM

When you are going through hell, keep going.
—Sir Winston Churchill

Great Gulf: Temperature: 12°F; winds are low; visibility twilight; light snowfall.

Emergency Bivouac Site (3,200 ft.)
Great Gulf Wilderness
Sunday, Jan. 24, 1982
6:00 a.m.

Jeff Batzer is feeling buoyant and blissful. Although he's dehydrated, hungry, cold, and tired, his semi-conscious state has temporarily disconnected him from his physiological plight. Swaddled in a thick bed of vegetation that feels to him like he's cradled in his mother's arms, and soothed by the aroma of balsam fir, Batzer floats in a sea of illusion. Am I home? Is it Christmas morning? I wonder what we're having for breakfast.

His body recoils when Hugh Herr initiates one of the countless readjustments he and Batzer have made throughout the night as they huddle together in their tiny, cave-like shelter. This latest disruption feels to Batzer as though he's been grabbed by the shirt collar and yanked into the present. Now mostly alert and oriented, Batzer's body aches … everywhere. Blood circulates through his poorly insulated outer extremities, where it cools and makes an unwelcome return to his heart. His brain, sensing a problem, takes the role of traffic cop and directs the veins and arteries in his hands and feet to constrict. That's good for his core but not for vulnerable hands and feet. For Herr, who never dried out after his partial submersions in the Peabody River, the regression toward life-altering cold injuries is already well underway.

Batzer feels the warmth of Herr's exhalations across his chilled face. Their arms and legs intertwine like the needled boughs they're encased in. They are engaged in a primal and essential intimacy, as each understands his only hope for survival is to keep the other alive.

We're used to assuming that a thermometer's mercury will rise as daylight approaches. But that's not the case today, nor will it be anytime soon. An area of low pressure to the north is traversing Quebec and pushing a cold front into New England. The ambient temperature in Great Gulf and on the summit of Mount Washington has dropped 6°F over the last two hours and continues to backslide. Windchill values on the higher summits will reach life-threatening levels as westerly winds increase steadily in speed and strength.

Searchers responding to the callout will have to deal with the more than seven inches of blowing snow that's fallen above treeline over the past 24 hours and continues to fall. High-speed winds are scuffing the light, easily transportable snow from acres and acres of exposed terrain and moving it east, reducing visibility to arm's length. The eastern aspects of Mount Washington, where the search for Herr and Batzer will focus, continue to load with snow. The higher the wind speed, the farther down the slopes it will reach. The dynamics of this storm system and the terrain it's interacting with will create significant instability in the snowpack.

While extreme conditions above treeline tend to garner more attention, Ryan Knapp of the Mount Washington Observatory says that even beneath the canopy of trees, weather conditions for Herr and Batzer are unforgiving. "It's even really cold at the bottom of Great Gulf," Knapp says. "At the base of the headwall it's still the equivalent of a 4,000-foot mountain. There's very limited daylight, because the ravine is so deep, and at that time of year, you have a low sun angle. They may not have seen any daylight at all that day."

Herr is now fully awake. Without a word spoken, he and Batzer untangle and roll onto their backs. Like sea turtle hatchlings emerging from the sand, they dig themselves out from under their heavily-weighted blanket of tree boughs. Their shoulders and triceps, sore from hours of swimming through chest-deep snow, are protesting this violation of a normal range of motion. Before exiting the cavity of the boulder, each feels for his boots buried within the snarl of branches.

Sitting motionless on a small pile of spruce and fir, they are smacked by a wall of below-freezing air. If they remain static, they're certain they'll freeze to death where they sit, so they immediately get to work donning their boots. Batzer finds his cold and somewhat stiff, but still malleable. He removes his one remaining mitten and quickly loosens the boot laces to create a wide opening to jam his feet into. "I remember thinking, 'These boots are hard to get back on,' he says. "But they still weren't terribly frozen on the inside at that point."

Herr's boots are still soaked. "Getting my boots on was nearly impossible that morning," he says today. "They were leather, and they were wet. So they were like ice blocks. I had to pry them open." As he tries to make the stiff leather pliable, he is further diminishing his already waning energy stores.

Once inside their boots, the two gather their ice axes and prepare to move. In a brief, unemotional conversation, they speculate that a search for them might be underway. Neither feels a surge of optimism at the thought, however, and they still don't know where they are. But they sense that if they keep descending by following the river, they might be traveling in some type of drainage that will lead them to safety.

At this point, they are still at least 4.5 miles from Route 16 and plowing through deep snow and gnarly scrub brush. Batzer recalls limited dialogue as they make their slow, grueling way forward: "Let's go this way. Let's go that way. It's my turn to break trail. I'll pull to the front."

Feeling parched, they risk a steep downhill drop to drink from the river. "We stopped once at the creek to take in as much water as we could," Batzer recalls, "It was an awkward process, because it was so hard to get down to the water to drink without falling in."

With each punishing step, Batzer grows more concerned with the toll this ordeal is taking on Herr, who seems detached. "What a tough time for Hugh," Batzer says. "He was not talkative at that point. He would only talk because he had to do business in order to survive, but there wasn't a whole lot of it. Frankly, I wasn't talkative, either, because there just wasn't a whole lot to talk about." So each is in his own head as they contend with a seemingly infinite wall of snow and the fear of falling through the ice during river crossings.

Herr says his silence was driven by a combination of painful exertion and the stark reality of his deterioration. "I wasn't panicking," he says. "I understood that our survival was dependent on a very efficient use of our energies, and panicking is not efficient. The only way I could help Jeff was to do a lot of the post-holing and leading and not share with him my prediction of what could happen to us."

XVIII
EN MASSE

You start thinking about it when you're still in bed and your eyes are closed.
You can hear the wind, and you can hear the pelting of the snow or rime crystals
that rap upon the window. ...You're accumulating information all the time.
—Lead Snow Ranger Brad Ray, quoted in *Mountain Voices:*
Stories of Life and Adventure in the White Mountains and Beyond

Mount Washington Observatory Surface Weather Observations (6:00 to 7:00
a.m.): Temperature 1°F; winds out of the west averaging 58 mph; visibility 0
miles; snow/blowing snow/fog; windchill -31.3°F; peak wind gust: 68 mph.

Appalachian Mountain Club administrative offices
Pinkham Notch Camp
Sunday, Jan. 24, 1982
6:30 a.m.

On this early Sunday morning, David Warren, manager of the hut system for the AMC, is in crisis management mode. Today he's donned a different hat, that of search and rescue coordinator.

"I had a black and white framed photo of the whole search area taken from Wildcat Mountain hanging in my office," he says today. "It had all of Tuckerman and Huntington Ravines and the ridge. I took that off the wall and propped it on one of the sofas in the main office area. We had a black grease pencil and used it as our 'whiteboard' to identify and mark areas we had searched."

Warren, who grew up in Exeter, N.H., spent much of his childhood hiking in the White Mountains with his father. At 6 years old, he summited Mount Washington for the first time, and 10 years later, he began working part time for the AMC. After graduating from Wesleyan University in 1978, he returned in a full-time capacity in various roles. "It remains one of the best jobs I ever had," Warren says.

The administrative office area will serve as ground zero for the coordination efforts. Located in a building that sits between the Joe

Dodge Lodge and the Trading Post, at the time it was often transformed into what Warren refers to as the "center for operations" for alpine accidents and searches in Cutler River Drainage and beyond. As he awaits the arrival of other planners who will assist in search-related tasks, Warren prepares the cubicles and side offices for their work, powers on the Xerox machine, and stokes the woodstove. But the most important accoutrement in the room is the base radio, which will become the communications hub for the duration of the mission. "The AMC would coordinate rescues at that time because we had the radio at the base," Warren explains.

Searchers arriving in the freshly-plowed parking lot walk directly to the basement of the Trading Post and dump their gear in the pack room. From there, they head to the cafeteria on the main floor where they'll await their assignments as they load up with caffeine and foods rich in fat and carbohydrates. It promises to be a long, cold day, and searchers are loading calories to fend off hypothermia. Meanwhile, the "kalunk, kalunk, kalunk" of mountaineering boots on stairs and wooden floors gives early-rising AMC guests the impression that something much bigger than a group hike is in play.

Over at the administrative building, Warren is soon joined by Lead Snow Rangers Brad Ray and Rene LaRoche from the U.S. Forest Service (USFS); Sgt. Carl Carlson, a conservation officer for New Hampshire Fish and Game (NHFG); and Bill Kane and Joe Lentini, both of whom are team leaders of Mountain Rescue Service (MRS). Because the search area encompasses the Cutler River Drainage, the Forest Service has jurisdiction, but this will be a cooperative effort for all involved.

Brad Ray was known at the time as the Dean of the Ravine. He started working as a snow ranger in Tuckerman Ravine in 1960 and was named lead ranger in 1966. Ray worked for the Forest Service for over 50 years before his death in 2021 at age 82 and had extensive training and expertise in avalanche forecasting. "He was conscientious and really devoted to his job," says longtime friend and coworker Rene LaRoche, himself a snow ranger from 1965 to 1994.

Rebecca Oreskes, who married Ray in 1995 and who also worked for the Forest Service for many years, says her husband viewed his role as a steward, not as an enforcer. "Brad really believed very deeply that people made their own choices," she says. "He also had tremendous respect for all the people who were volunteers in search and rescue missions. He saw Mountain Rescue Service team members as absolute professionals and fully trusted their judgment. His job with the public and with volunteer searchers was to make sure everyone knew the dangers they were facing."

Joe Lentini, a member of MRS since 1975, and Bill Kane, an EMT and MRS member since 1976, are serving as co-team leaders for this mission. They'll assist with determining search areas, select team members for each assignment, and brief everyone on the plan.

Sgt. Carl Carlson, a former U.S. Marine who served in the Korean Conflict and then attended the University of New Hampshire, started his career with New Hampshire Fish and Game in 1958. Known affectionately as "Sarge" and "the Jolly Green Giant," Carlson spent 31 years on the job.

Though Misha Kirk radioed Pinkham when he located a cached pack in Huntington Ravine, there is still little information that

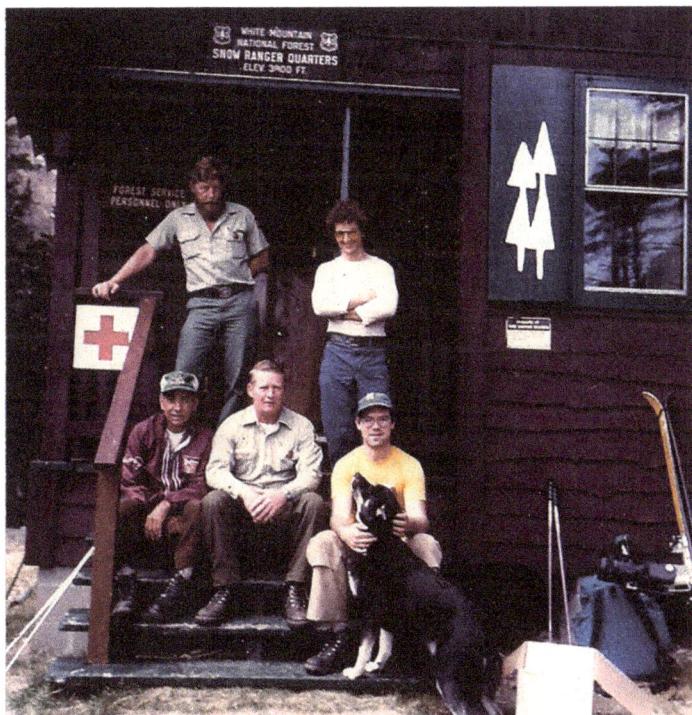

Rene LaRoche (top left), Brad Ray (seated center), Joe Gill (seated right), and Ray's dog Tuckerman, along with two visitors to the Snow Rangers' quarters in Tuckerman Ravine.

morning about Herr and Batzer's intentions, climbing habits, and experience level. So the planning team plots the day's movements based in part on what's been learned from past search and rescue missions on the eastern slopes of Mount Washington.

"We asked ourselves, 'What would you do if you topped out on Odell's and were trying to get down quickly?'," says Dave Warren today. "Most people said that if you knew the area and had any wits about you, and you knew where you were, you'd try to get over to the Alpine Garden and then come down over Lion Head. That would be the safest way. So we decided that if Hugh and Jeff were going to go anywhere, they were going to go that way."

No one has any idea that Herr and Batzer tried for the summit after topping out at Odell Gully. "Most people don't go to the summit from Huntington, because that's just a different trip," says Rick Wilcox, who was president of MRS from 1976 to 2017. Though Wilcox was guiding on Aconcagua at the time of the search, his decades of experience in this alpine arena as a climber and rescuer provide valuable insight into what was occurring on that January weekend in 1982. "That summit trip is a hike that you do some other day," he says. "In the winter months, your daylight ends at about 4:00 p.m. The only people who should be wandering higher than the ravine any time after about noon should be very familiar with the descent routes."

Mission planners also have no idea that the two lost climbers are in Great Gulf, so searching there is not included in the plan. The Gulf was visited so infrequently in the wintertime that it was rare for rescue calls to occur there. "There were callouts in the Gulf maybe a couple of times a year, at most," says Wilcox.

He adds that until the search for Herr and Batzer, there had never been a search and rescue call involving Huntington climbers who'd gotten lost and ended up in Great Gulf—and there hasn't been one since. "Most of the trouble in Huntington stayed in Huntington in one of the gullies or on The Fan," says Wilcox. "Climbers would often go up a gully in Huntington and arrive in the Alpine Garden, then have difficulty finding a safe route for their descent, which can be challenging in the harsh winter conditions that are common there."

Using Warren's impromptu search map, the coordination team identifies a scope for the search and plans how personnel will be deployed. "We decided we had three primary areas to look at," says Kane. "We wanted to get a group of us up on the Auto Road in a Thiokol to check Alpine Garden and the rim of Huntington, send teams up Lion Head and into Raymond Cataract, and send another team into Huntington to search The Fan and look for things like avalanche debris, tracks, or anything that might offer clues to their whereabouts—or their fate."

With heavy amounts of snow loading the eastern slopes due to strong westerly winds, avalanche hazard and the risk it poses are now of significant concern, both for the lost climbers and the volunteer searchers. "People have been avalanched in Huntington Ravine at the base of the climbs right down to the scree below," says Wilcox. "Then there's always avalanche danger at the top of the climbs, where you get some of the gullies filling in with snow."

Joe Lentini recalls the crucial role the snow rangers played in the planning process. "We were deferring to Brad and Rene on avalanche conditions," he says. "They were giving us an overview of what conditions were going to be like, and we were looking at what we could possibly do based on their assessment. We said we could have a team search the bottom of the ravine to look for signs of an avalanche. We also decided that teams wouldn't go up into the gullies because it had snowed a lot all night, and the wind had been blowing hard."

During a mission, if searches don't find missing climbers injured, hypothermic, or dead at the base of a climb or in Alpine Garden, or trapped in deep snow in Raymond Cataract, it is possible they are still in the gully itself. Because of the growing avalanche hazard, the planning team determines that a search of Odell Gully will have to be done from above.

After considering all their options and the conditions searchers will be facing, the planners divide searchers into the following teams and assignments:

Mountain Rescue Service/Mount Washington Observatory:

MRS team members Paul Ross, Todd Swain, David Stone, Albert Dow, and Michael Hartrich will ride the Mount Washington Observatory Thiokol driven by Ken Rancourt up the Auto Road to Cow Pasture, follow Huntington Ravine Trail and sweep Alpine Garden, the top of Raymond Cataract, and descend the Lion Head Trail.

MRS is designated Unit 21 and will use an AMC lo-band radio.

Rancourt is designated Unit 28 and will use an AMC hi-band radio.

MRS team members Joe Lentini, Bill Kane, Steve Larson, Dana Seavey, and Doug Madara will also ride the Observatory Thiokol up the Auto Road, and then split off from Unit 21 and establish a static line at the rim of Huntington Ravine and rappel into Odell Gully. This team is designated Unit 22 and will use an AMC lo-band radio.

Mountain Rescue Service/Appalachian Mountain Club/US Forest Service:

MRS team members (Unit 23): Frank Hubbell, Bill Aughton, Matt Peer, and Tiger Burns will join Bob Jaffe, David Moskowitz, and Gary Newfield of the AMC and will be transported by the Forest Service Thiokol driven by Lead Snow Ranger Brad Ray and accompanied by Snow Ranger Rene LaRoche (Unit 25) into Huntington Ravine to search The Fan.

The MRS/AMC team is designated Unit 23 and will use an AMC lo-band radio. Ray and LaRoche are designated Unit 25 and will also use an AMC lo-band radio.

Appalachian Mountain Club:

Joe Gill, Bill Meduski, Carol (Cullina) Cunha, Alan Kamman, and Bill Corbin will hike up the Winter Route on Lion Head and over to the rim of Huntington Ravine. They are designated Unit 24 and will use an AMC lo-band radio.

New Hampshire Fish and Game:

Five conservation officers will sweep the bottom of Raymond's Path and Raymond Cataract and over to Huntington Ravine on snow machines. Conservation officers will use their own radios to communicate with Sgt. Carl Carlson, who will stay at the base radio at Pinkham.

The intricacy of the planning process—the ability for all teams

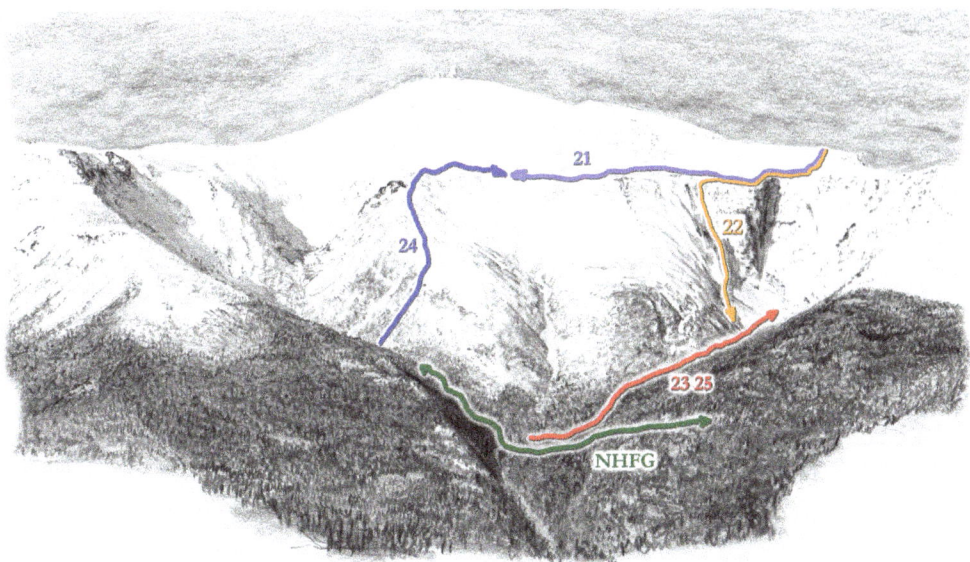

This map shows the intended search assignments by unit for Sunday, Jan. 24. Refer to page 122 for details.

and organizations to communicate with each other to maximize situational awareness—was a significant challenge back then. This is evident in the number of radio frequencies used during searches from that time period. Back then, MRS owned no radios and had to borrow them in limited quantities from NHFG, the USFS, and the AMC. "It mostly depended on who had radios to spare," says Bill Kane today. "We weren't always on compatible frequencies. When we knew the location of a rescue, one radio was enough because we stayed together going to the subject and getting them out. Searches, on the other hand, had us looking in a lot of different places. That was much tougher. We sometimes radioed a question to the AMC that they would send to Fish and Game or the Forest Service and then reverse the pathway back to us with the answer. It was not efficient, but it worked, and we did the best we could."

Dave Warren says this mission and its outcomes highlighted the difficulties that teams from different organizations encountered during such large and complex searches. "It is one of the things that changed as a result of this incident," he says.

As searchers begin to head out on their various assignments, public attention is focused elsewhere. The winter storm battering Mount Washington is also hitting the rest of the Northeast. At

Boston's Logan Airport the previous night, World Airways Flight 30, a DC-10 with 208 people on board, crashed into Boston Harbor while attempting to land on the airport's longest runway. Because of the snow and icy conditions, it skidded off the end of the 10,000-foot runway and into the harbor. No lives were reported lost, but the accident was at the top of the news throughout the weekend and beyond.

In less than 24 hours, the perilous mission being carried out in and around Huntington Ravine will also be in the public spotlight. But for now, it is still 8:15 a.m. on Sunday, the team members have been fully briefed, and all have left the warmth and safety of Pinkham on foot and in the backs of Thiokols to launch their search.

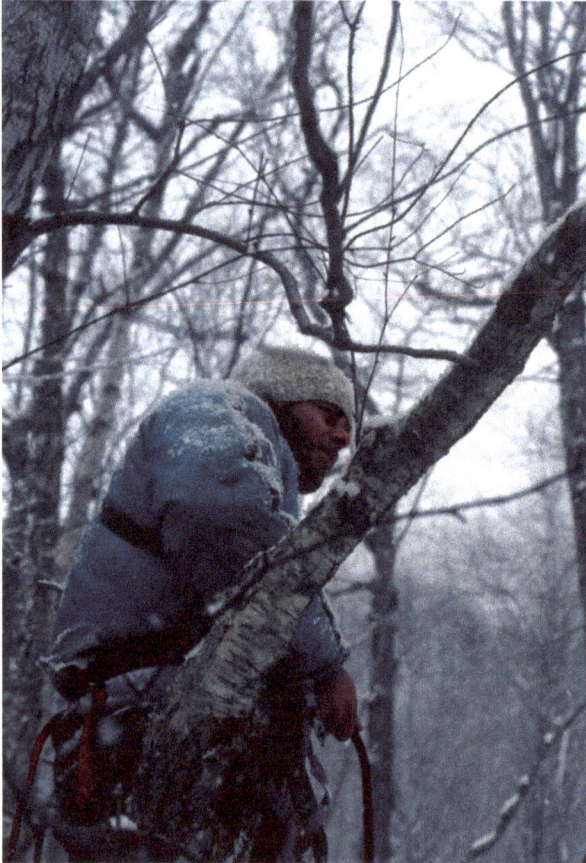

Albert Dow topping out after an ice climb on Frankenstein Cliff in Crawford Notch.

XIX
STEEPED

*The old Lion Head Route is closed for summer use due to its steepness
and severe erosion. It may be used as a direct winter route
when conditions permit.*
—AMC White Mountain Guide, 22nd Edition (1979)

*Mount Washington Observatory Surface Weather Observations (7:00 to 8:00
a.m.): Temperature -2°F; winds out of the west averaging 46 mph; visibility 0
miles; snow/blowing snow/fog; windchill -33°F; peak wind gust: 58 mph.*

Tuckerman Ravine Trail
Mount Washington
Sunday, Jan. 24, 1982
7:00 a.m.

Joe Gill, caretaker of the AMC's Hermit Lake and Tuckerman
Ravine Shelters, marches with purpose down "Tucks Trail." After
getting a radio call from Pinkham just before 8:30 p.m. the previous
night alerting him to two missing climbers, he prepared his gear and
rose early to get to his rendezvous point. He's meeting four other
AMC members of Unit 24, who are hiking up from Pinkham to link
up with him at the junction of the Summer and Winter Routes up
Lion Head.

Gill started with the AMC as a crew member in 1972 before
working his way into the hut system. In March 1977, he became a full-
time, year-round caretaker managing the shelters in Tuckerman
Ravine. That year, the AMC sent him to Jackson Hole, Wyo., to attend
the Professional Forecasting Course at the American Avalanche
Institute. His caretaker responsibilities included providing information
to those visiting this popular part of the mountain and serving as a
first responder for search and rescue missions. By 1982, he had
participated in 75 to 100 such callouts.

Gill and company are tasked with ascending Lion Head's challenging Winter Route and, if conditions permit, following the Alpine Garden Trail to the rim of Huntington Ravine. Climbers leaving the ravine frequently cross the Alpine Garden and descend by the Winter Route, so the area must be among the first searched. If everything goes as planned, Gill's team will make contact somewhere along the Garden with MRS members Paul Ross, David Stone, Albert Dow, Todd Swain, and Michael Hartrich who, along with five other team members, are piled in the back of a Mount Washington Observatory Thiokol as it crawls up the Auto Road.

The Lion Head Trail is a steep climb that is steeped in history. At one time, it was the only route up this iconic ridge. How the rugged prominence known as Lion Head acquired its name remains somewhat of a mystery. Once known as St. Anthony's Nose, it became Lion Head sometime during the mid-to-late 1800s. The 1922 edition of the *White Mountain Guide* describes the route that awaits the five searchers:

> This trail was constructed in 1920 with the approval of the U.S.F.S. in memory of Rev. William Rogers Richards, New York City, an ardent lover of these mountains. It diverges to the R. from the Tuckerman Ravine Path at the point where the Boott Spur Trail diverges to the L. Running N. a short distance to the foot of the cliffs that culminate in the Lion Head, it makes the inevitable steep climb through the scrub to tree line and thence to the lower and upper Heads. It continues with impressive views and with little grade over the open spur to the Alpine Garden Trail, which it crosses, and after passing through a belt of scrub, it ascends to the Tuckerman Ravine Path which it re-enters at Cloudwater Spring somewhat above the foot of the cone of Mount Washington. Distance, 1m Time, 1¼ hrs.

In 1966, a new Summer Route up Lion Head was established, but the original route was kept for winter use. A 1996 Mount Washington Observatory *Windswept* article explains why the 1920 route was maintained:

> That route (once the only route on Lion Head but abandoned for summer use after a 1966 relocation) had been used to avoid the most avalanche-prone sections of the standard summer route on Lion Head. The summer route crosses the

foot of the 1969 avalanche path, and also, just before it reaches treeline, traverses an area where significant amounts of unstable, wind transported snow can accumulate, sometimes needing only a trigger (such as a passing climber) to result in a significant avalanche. The winter route, while not entirely free of avalanche risk, was generally significantly less hazardous in this regard than the summer route.

(Note: In 1995, this winter route was closed and relocated following a landslide that created an increased avalanche hazard.)

"When I was caretaking, I saw some tremendous avalanches," says Gill today. "There was one morning when I went into the ravine and found a wet snow avalanche, where pretty much the whole right side of the headwall failed right down to the rock. There was a slush pile probably 18 feet deep that reached right down to the connection cache. That was the biggest avalanche I've ever seen."

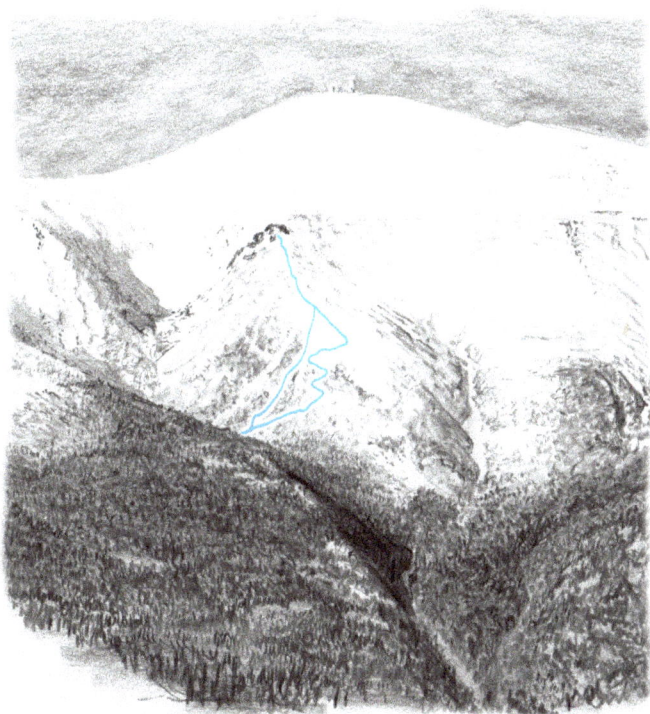

The Lion Head Winter Route (left) and Summer Route (right) as they were in 1982. The Winter Route has since been relocated to the right of the Summer Route.

Tuckerman Ravine, where Gill spent most of his working hours, was the site of the first two avalanche fatalities to occur on Mount Washington. On Jan. 27, 1954, Phillip Longnecker, 25, and Jacques Parysko, 23, both graduate students at Harvard University, hiked into the ravine and built an igloo at the base of the headwall. Before hiking in, Longnecker had been advised not to camp or climb near the headwall because of the risk of avalanche. Three feet of snow was forecast to fall that night, and an avalanche did indeed occur, killing Longnecker while he and Parysko slept in the igloo. Parysko was able to escape burial and appears to have headed out of the ravine for help. He was located the following Wednesday, approximately three-quarters of a mile away from the scene, on the Sherburne Ski Trail. Parysko was not wearing boots, socks, mittens, cap, or a parka and had died from exposure.

Two years later, the second recorded avalanche fatality on Mount Washington occurred in Tuckerman as well. On Feb. 19, 1956, Aaron Leve, 28, was killed when he and four others he was hiking with were struck by an avalanche, fully burying him.

Longnecker became the 39th fatality on Mount Washington, Parysko the 40th, and Leve the 41st.

This part of the mountain is optimal avalanche territory. Its east-facing aspect and steep terrain make it a primary catch basin for snow loaded in by strong westerly winds. Jaw-dropping snow depths linger well into late spring and summer.

Having reached the rendezvous point at the trail junction, Gill watches as his four AMC teammates—Carol (Cullina) Cunha, Alan Kamman, Bill Meduski, and Bill Corbin—approach in single file. As their warm exhalations meet the frigid air, elongated steam rises and disappears. When the five gather, there's little discussion. Each has been briefed on the situation and the assignment. Because of the cold, no one wants to stop for long for fear of cooling off after the uphill exertion.

Cunha, a member of the AMC kitchen crew at the time, remembers the "other duties as described" nature of working at Pinkham Camp. "Back then for the Pinkham crew, search and rescue was a given," says Cunha. "You were able to participate whenever it happened, and it happened fairly often. It was just a matter of who was available and who needed to stay back at Pinkham to make things work there. In the search for Herr and Batzer, it just came down to who had the equipment, and I had just bought crampons and an ice axe. I really didn't have the experience for this one, so I was just doing what I was told as we went."

Alan Kamman, who worked at the Trading Post as a front-desk attendant and did a lot of winter hiking, still recalls the atmosphere at Pinkham of Sunday morning. "I'd been working at the desk the night before," Kamman recalls. "A big storm was forecast, and that was discouraging people from going up the mountain. It was apparent there were two people missing. I was in the dining room early the next morning, and there were lots of people there getting ready to search. The mood was somber, and pretty intense."

Kamman talks of the rush he felt on learning he was given the Lion Head assignment. "At that time, I would have done anything they asked me to," he says. "I knew the route was manageable for me and that I wasn't going to be exceeding my skills, which was a good thing in a situation like that. At age 20 I was pretty darn excited about going. I thought search and rescue was super cool, and I was game for it. That winter I had dabbled in ice climbing and technical climbing, and I had a little bit of experience on Mount Rainier because my dad sent me to a five-day class there after I graduated from high school. I had been out on calls before and would be again, but this one was the pinnacle of my search and rescue involvement."

Bill Meduski, who like Cunha was a member of the kitchen crew, echoes her description of what AMC jobs included at that time. "If you were on staff, knew something about walking around the mountains in the winter, and there was a rescue to be done, they'd ask you if you wanted to go out. Being rather young and in my first full winter living in the mountains, I wasn't going to be a lead person in this mission. But those in charge knew the advantage of having a lot of eyes out there looking, and if rescue litters had to be carried, of having young, fit, and willing people available to help."

Corbin, who was not available to comment on the incident, did night watch and worked for the construction crew at Pinkham Camp. "Bill was the guy who was awake at night and kept an eye on things and would help any people who showed up in the middle of the night," Kamman recalls of his friend and coworker. "He was an avid skier, which we did a lot of together at Wildcat that winter and was also into snowshoeing and hiking. He was not an avid ice climber or mountaineer, but he would do whatever needed to be done when it came to rescues like this one."

The team members are fully aware of the terrain and conditions that await them on and above Lion Head. And the four who have just arrived know they are in good hands with Gill as their team leader. Decades later, Meduski will say, "Joe was a legend up there at the time. He could probably walk around in a whiteout and still find his way around. He'd spent so much time up there."

Ever so slowly, the various teams begin to clear terrain and close the gaps between their respective search areas in the hope that this systematic containment strategy will produce evidence of Herr and Batzer's presence on the mountain. What these five don't know as they set out together is how their experience on the Winter Route of Lion Head will become the prelude for the tragedy that will follow.

XX
SIGNS

Just when you think you've hit rock bottom,
you realize you're standing on another trapdoor.
—Marisha Pessl, *Night Film*

Great Gulf: Temperature: 8°F; winds are low; visibility daylight; light snowfall.

West Branch of the Peabody River (2,247 ft.)
Great Gulf Wilderness
Sunday, Jan. 24, 1982
8:30 a.m.

Jeff Batzer feels as though it's Groundhog Day near the Arctic Circle. "It was a cold, white hell," he says today. "It was beautiful, but I felt lost and trapped. We could barely move, and even when we could, it was atrocious. Even with the occasional trail blazes, there was still a sense of lostness."

Batzer and Hugh Herr are descending, but the reduction in grade is so subtle it's almost imperceptible. As they unknowingly reach the lower portion of Great Gulf, the nearly impenetrable vegetation slowly releases its firm hold. The pervasive 10-foot-high scrub growing in the shadow of 50-foot trees has forced them to hug and, at times, cross the river. "As we got down toward the bottom of the gulf, the density of the forest dissipated," says Herr. "Sure, snowshoes would have been helpful, but in the higher regions of the Gulf, it was just so dense."

The two are experiencing only partial relief, however, because the deep snow continues its efforts to swallow them whole. Since hitting the floor of the Gulf the previous day, the snow is holding at waist level and higher. Hidden undulations create terrain traps of armpit-high snow. When not coping with sinkholes, they find themselves walking on a layer of crust that at times collapses under their weight. The sharp edges of broken ice aggravate their already bruised and sensitive shins. Each step is a physical battle often infused with pain, and the time and energy required to move forward is exhausting beyond measure.

Meanwhile, to the southeast search teams are moving into position in the Cutler River Drainage. High above Herr and Batzer, the Mount Washington Observatory Thiokol inches its way up the Auto Road carrying Units 21 and 22 of Mountain Rescue Service. These 10 rescuers are the closest to the missing pair. But like all the others, they are relying on the scarce information available at the time, so their gaze is fixed on the eastern aspects of the mountain rather than on the area where Herr and Batzer are grinding their way toward liberation.

Herr is operating on sheer force of will. Dehydrated and exhausted, neither he nor Batzer has eaten anything since the freeze-dried meals they wolfed down at Harvard Cabin 24 hours earlier. The wool pants Batzer gave Herr the night before are now damp from perspiration, and the gym-style wind pants he pulled over them have been compromised by his two immersions in the Peabody River. The Gore-Tex outer pants he's wearing, while good for keeping the snow at bay, are suppressing the movement of moisture away from his skin. His socks and leather boots haven't been able to dry out, and his lower legs and swelling feet crave the flow of warm blood. But his lower body is not getting proper blood circulation at this point, and his legs are slowly freezing.

Though hungry and tired, Batzer remains fueled by optimism. He's miserable but convinced they'll break free from their wilderness prison. When he isn't leading their push through the snow, he switches his one remaining Gore-Tex mitten from hand to hand. Although the silk vapor liner and angora wool gloves underneath are wet, the shared Gore-Tex covering is keeping his hands warm enough to stay on the safe side of frostbite. But the line is thin.

Finally, the two get their first indication that they are in well-traveled terrain. *Is that real? Is it another downed tree? Are we hallucinating?* What they are seeing is, in fact, a long wooden footbridge spanning the West Branch of the Peabody River. The entire bridge is packed with snow from foot plank to railing, but it's *something*.

They continue forward and soon reach what appears to be a trail junction. "Seeing the bridge was encouraging," says Batzer. "But seeing the trail signs at that junction with distances to the different

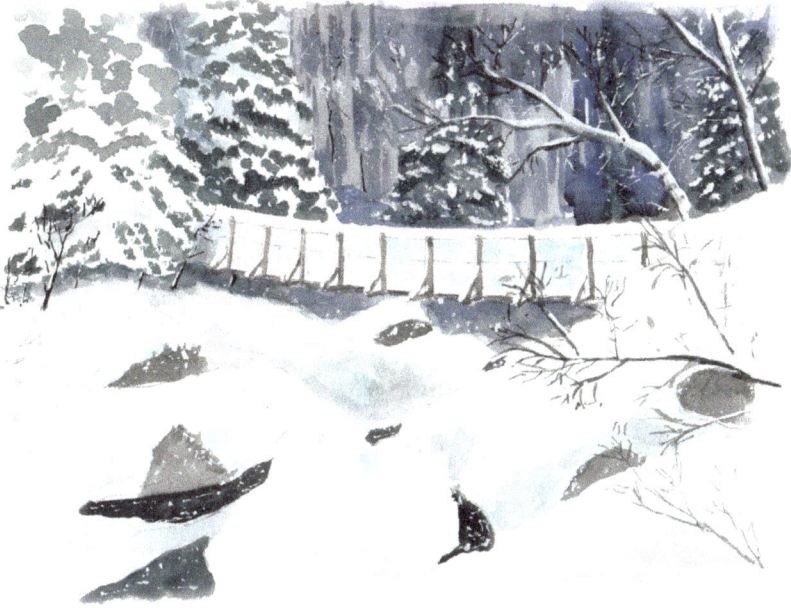

locations was where we felt tremendous relief that we could get out, that this was just going to be a close call."

Standing in waist-deep snow, the two hug one another. "I can remember us both breaking down and crying," says Batzer. "We said to each other, 'We can get out!' This would be the only time during the ordeal that we cried, because the rest of the time we were just facing the cold realities."

Their moment of tearful relief is short-lived, however, because the wooden trail signs present a series of choices, and they have to make an important decision. Which way to go? Mounted on the post are slats pointing in different directions with trail names and distances carved into each. The snow is so deep here that it reaches the signs themselves.

They have arrived at the junction of the Great Gulf and Madison Gulf Trails. Since leaving the site of their night's bivouac earlier that morning they've hiked approximately 1.54 miles and lost approximately 950 feet of elevation. The trail signs at the time indicated three possible routes: Pinkham Notch: 4.0 miles; Glen House: 2.0 miles; and Madison Hut: 2.5 miles.

The hike to Pinkham Notch Camp, where Herr and Batzer started two days before, is 4.0 miles via the Madison Gulf Trail to where it crosses the Auto Road just below the two-mile post and then continues onto Old Jackson Road to Pinkham. Had they been familiar with this side of the mountain, they would have known that, on reaching the Auto Road, a 2-mile descent of that road would bring them to Route 16.

To reach the Glen House site, Herr and Batzer would follow the Great Gulf Trail for 0.44 miles to the Osgood Trail. From there, it is a 1.56-mile hike to Route 16 and the Glen House site. That destination is approximately 2 miles away. This would have been one of the better options because the Osgood trailhead on the Auto Road is just hundreds of feet from Route 16.

Despite the sign, in 1982 there was no actual Glen House. The first Glen House was built in 1851. Between 1851 and 1967, it burned and was rebuilt four times. The structure burned again in 1967, but the site itself persisted as a destination. Today, the fifth iteration of the Glen House Hotel at Mount Washington lies on the west side of Route 16 in Green's Grant near the Auto Road. Also, in the mid-1980s the trailheads of the Osgood and Great Gulf Trails were relocated north of the Glen House site on Route 16 to the White Mountain National Forest Parking Area: Great Gulf Wilderness. So, today's hikers would find route markings that are different from those Herr and Batzer are considering.

The distance to Madison Hut, which is located in Madison Col between Mounts Madison and Adams, is one of their shorter options. But Madison Gulf Trail is unbroken, steep, and risky terrain. Herr and Batzer are at approximately 2,400 feet. To reach the hut, they would have to hike to almost 4,800 feet—and they are unaware that Madison Hut is closed in winter.

Whether via Madison Gulf Trail toward Pinkham or the Great Gulf and Osgood Trails to Glen House, getting to the Auto Road and descending to Route 16 is Herr and Batzer's best bet. Even if they continued following the West Branch of the Peabody River, it would bring them out to Route 16. But they are unfamiliar with this side of Mount Washington. Because no one has been here recently, and with

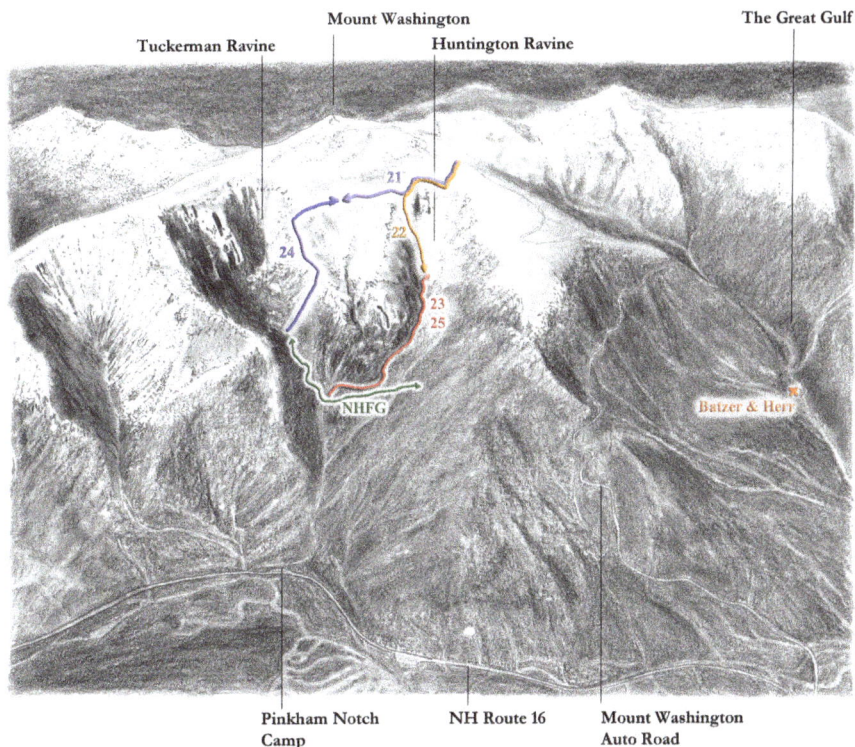

Hugh Herr and Jeff Batzer, trapped and lost in Great Gulf, are approximately 2.38 miles as the crow flies from their searchers in Huntington Ravine.

so much fallen snow, the trails are indiscernible. The landscape is pale and lacking definition. Tree blazes are hard to detect. They recognize only two destinations from the sign: Pinkham Notch and Madison Hut. Given their exhaustion, they decide that Pinkham is too far away. They believe— incorrectly—that Madison Hut will have people there who can help them.

"Madison Hut was much closer than Pinkham Notch," says Herr today. "We didn't know the hut would be locked, but it wouldn't have mattered. We would have gotten in, and it would have saved us. People have said, 'That was so stupid.' I say no; it was close, and Jeff and I were dying. So we made the attempt."

The decision Herr and Batzer make at this junction to head for Madison Hut will prove fateful. They base it on distance without any understanding of the terrain. They actually choose a wall over a floor. Had they headed toward the Glen House site or Pinkham, they might have been able to close the gap between them and those looking for them. But they don't have enough information or knowledge of the area to make the right choice.

"Even though we started out from Pinkham Notch, it seemed like it was way too far from where we were," says Batzer. "We'd never heard of Glen House before, but we did know about Madison Hut, so we thought we'd head for that. In retrospect, of the options we had, it was the worst choice. If we'd followed the trail for two miles to the Glen House site, we probably would have gotten out unharmed."

XXI
MAELSTROM

"They cared about sport deeply and had long conversations about the ethics of climbing. They had a lot of fun, but they took what they did seriously, and how that translated was they took care of each other, and they took care of anyone who went up on that mountain."
—Lin Stone, wife of late MRS team member David Stone

Mount Washington Observatory Surface Weather Observations (9:00 to 10:00 a.m.): Temperature -4°F; winds out of the west averaging 46 mph; visibility 0 miles; snow/ blowing snow/ fog; windchill -35.9°F; peak wind gust: 51 mph.

Huntington Ravine (4,200 ft.)
Sunday, Jan. 24, 1982
9:00 a.m.

Misha Kirk shudders as another wave of cold surges into his core. Time to move again. Since arriving in the ravine over three hours earlier, he has fought hard to keep warm by curling into a ball in the lee of a large boulder. At the onset of the shivering, he stands and performs calisthenics to rewarm. He's reliving his army boot camp, arctic style.

Westerly winds above him engage in a violent churn and continue showering the deep glacial cirque and the eastern slopes of Mount Washington with copious amounts of snow. Soon, the pocked scree field surrounding him will be completely covered over.

Hours earlier, in an admirable attempt to locate Hugh Herr and Jeff Batzer in Odell, climbers Hank Butler and Jim Frati bailed out of the snow-choked gully. The weather conditions are so poor that Kirk has been unaware of their proximity, and they of his. Kirk's one-man hasty search has ground to a painful halt.

"My eyelids were beginning to freeze closed, and an icicle was forming on each side of my moustache down to my beard," Kirk wrote in his journal. "I finally left the boulder to walk around and warm up. All of a sudden, I ran into a group of brightly-clothed beings, then the Thiokol. The Thiokol had been less than 100 feet from me. It had sounded its horn, but in the ferocious winds I hadn't heard it. Everybody was so bundled up that I couldn't tell who was who. But I must have looked terrible, because when they saw me, people's eyes widened, and they pushed me toward the Thiokol."

Kirk has inadvertently stumbled upon Units 23 and 25, a joint search team consisting of U.S. Forest Service snow rangers, Mountain Rescue Service (MRS) members, and Appalachian Mountain Club (AMC) staff. Lead Snow Ranger Brad Ray and Snow Ranger Rene LaRoche (Unit 25) have ferried searchers into the ravine from Pinkham. Their assignment this morning is to search the ravine's floor, and if it is stable enough, conduct a search of the steep Fan. Joining Ray and LaRoche are MRS members Frank Hubble, Bill Aughton, Matt Peer, and Tiger Burns, along with Bob Jaffee, David Moskowitz, and Gary Newfield from the AMC.

"The thought at the time was that if Herr and Batzer came down, they may not have made it back to Harvard Cabin and were bivouacked or injured somewhere in the ravine," says Dr. Frank Hubbell, co-founder of Stonehearth Open Learning Opportunities (SOLO), a wilderness medical school based in North Conway, N.H.

Bill Kane, team leader for MRS and founder of the Maine-based Kane Schools, which offer wilderness medicine and rescue training, participated in the search planning session at Pinkham. "We'd found the stashed pack, so we sent people into Huntington to see if any of the gullies had avalanched since Hugh and Jeff had climbed the day before," he says today. "We also thought they might have fallen out of a gully."

While Kirk slowly rewarms in the cab of the Thiokol, the seven searchers in the vehicle split into two groups to scour their assigned areas while Ray and LaRoche use their Forest Service-issued binoculars to scan high up in Odell and the gullies on either side of it.

Aughton, serving as team leader for the Huntington Ravine search team, brings with him a wealth of mountain knowledge. He grew up in Great Britain and began climbing at 15. A former member of the elite British Special Air Service and a local mountain guide, Aughton moved to the Mount Washington Valley and started North Conway-based International Mountain Equipment (IME) with Frank

Simon, and fellow MRS member Paul Ross, who is currently ascending the Mount Washington Auto Road with another MRS team. (In 1979 the trio sold IME to then-MRS President Rick Wilcox.)

Standing on the floor of the ravine, the seasoned mountain veteran soon realizes that he cannot ensure the safety of his teams as they search the terrain below the gullies from Pinnacle over to Escape Hatch. They definitely won't be able to move up onto The Fan. Aughton looks on with concern as low-density snow accumulates on top of the crust created by earlier snowfall and below-freezing temperatures. As this new snow layer consolidates, it will form what is referred to as "wind slab," a hazardous condition that can avalanche in this type of steep terrain. Ray and LaRoche have designated the day's avalanche hazard in Huntington Ravine as "extreme." It just needs someone or something to set it off. Aughton, who has spent much of his adult life identifying and managing threats, calls his teammates back, and the search ends soon after it began.

The Horn (3,970 ft.)
Mount Washington Auto Road
9:00 a.m.

Ken Rancourt's hope of getting searchers to the seven-mile mark on the mountain and his ability to keep the Auto Road in view are evaporating. The associate director of operations for the Mount Washington Observatory coddles the Thiokol past The Horn, a sharp left turn between miles four and five where the U.S. Army Signal Corps once operated an automatic weather station in the late 1940s and early 1950s.

Rancourt knows the relative sanctuary offered below treeline is about to end as he approaches the intersection at the winter cutoff just ahead. Once treeline is breached, the mountain's behavior will quickly transition from disorderly conduct to disobedience. As the snow-covered road's grade gets steeper, Rancourt throttles up the Thiokol, increasing the torque of its 300-cubic-inch, six-cylinder Ford engine. What this aqua colored machine lacks in comfort and aesthetics, it makes up for in raw, reliable power, especially on a long slog like this.

Unlike modern-day snowcats, which have the luxury of precision hydraulic steering and heated, enclosed passenger quarters, Thiokols back then had manual steering, and rescuers riding in the rear cargo bed were fully exposed to whatever elements the mountain chose to accost them with. "The Thiokol was filled to the brim that day, jam packed with rescuers and equipment," says Rancourt.

With the Halfway House and the Horn now concealed behind the Thiokol's two ice-encrusted rearview mirrors, Rancourt travels over a portion of the Auto Road that was first available to the public a century earlier when the road from Halfway House to Mount Washington's summit was officially opened in August 1861. Unrestrained gusts of wind pummel the machine, lifting the flailing wipers off the near-frozen and fogged windshield. As the winds send the wipers back onto the windshield, their loud slaps add another sensory stimulant that Rancourt must contend with. He is forced to stop and exit the machine with his scraper to clear the windshield of ice and snow.

As he pushes the door open wide enough to slide out of the tolerable 40°F cab temperature, he subjects himself to a windchill that drops the temperature to -40°F. But Rancourt, a seasoned winter veteran of this mountain, is wearing heavily insulated pack boots, expedition-weight long underwear, wool pants underneath Gore-Tex pants, multiple shirts, and a bulbous winter parka.

Sitting atop the fully exposed cargo bed of the Thiokol, waiting patiently, are 10 members of the all-volunteer Mountain Rescue Service. Divided into two teams at Pinkham by Team Leaders Joe Lentini and Bill Kane, each has a specific assignment. Unit 21 consists of Paul Ross, Todd Swain, David Stone, Albert Dow, and Michael Hartrich, while Lentini, Kane, Steve Larson, Dana Seavey, and Doug Madara form Unit 22.

Each team carries one lo-band radio loaned to them by the AMC. They hope they're able to stay in communication with each other and the base radio at Pinkham Camp as they separate for their respective assignments. "Because of the radio situation, we always had secondary and tertiary plans during searches," says Kane. "That's just the way it worked back then. We had one, sometimes two radios, and we were always trying to come up with ways to manage things if something changed during the mission. What would we do if somebody found them? But our radios were pretty dodgy. We could have a team on the Auto Road and also guys a half-mile away from us in Huntington, and there were times when we couldn't communicate with each other."

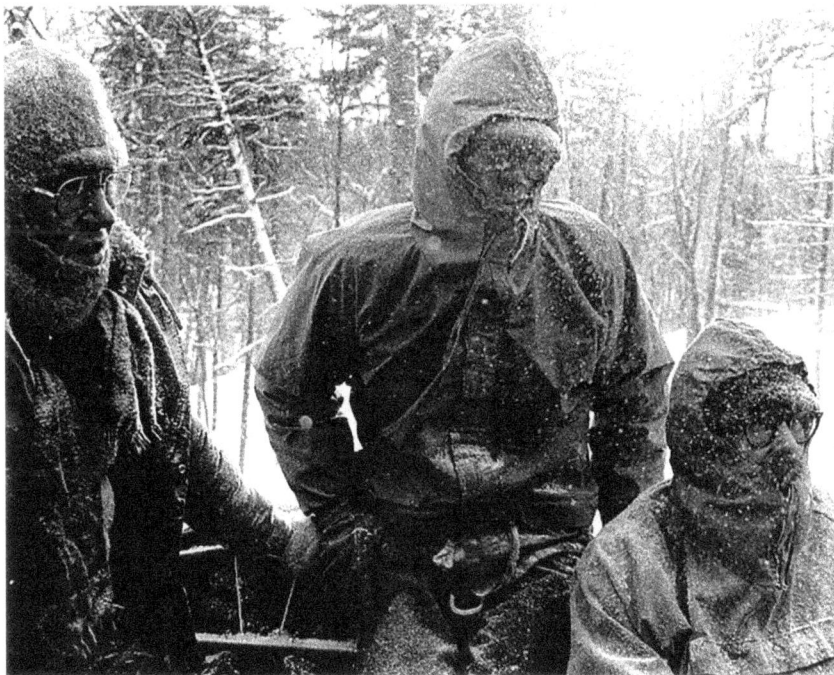

Mountain Rescue Service members Steve Larson (left), Doug Madara (center), and Michael Hartrich riding in the back of the Observatory Thiokol on the Mount Washington Auto Road on Jan. 24.

Having scraped a small hole in the windshield's ice to see through, Rancourt climbs back inside the Thiokol and resumes his forward progress, only to be stymied by the frost accumulating from his heavy exhalations. As they float onto the windshield, the spot he has just cleared refreezes from the inside. This annoying variable forces him to rub the window in a circular motion with his left, mittened hand, while he steers, throttles, and operates the plow blade with his right. Just another day of multitasking at 4,000 feet.

As the Thiokol breaks treeline and places itself and its human payload at the mercy of the wind and snow, the 10 MRS teammates shuffle themselves and their gear across the wooden bed of the tractor and toward the back wall of the crew cab. Each team member presses against the person next to him until all are seemingly conjoined. In an effort to temper the imminent onslaught of blowing snow and brutal windchill, they huddle together and use the inside wall of the vehicle—and each another—as shelter. This simple but powerful act of brotherhood provides physical and psychological safety as they prepare to move into the storm on the mountain they know cares nothing about them.

It was a month ago, on Dec. 16, 1981, that Rancourt, Lentini, Kane, Larson, Dow, and other rescuers were on this same road in similar temperatures but in much higher winds searching for lost WMTW Thiokol driver Phil Labbe. Labbe stumbled across Rancourt and the Observatory's Thiokol as he tried desperately to extract himself from the mountain's grasp. Right now, Rancourt is at almost the same location on the Auto Road where the search for Labbe reached its miraculous conclusion.

Such a rare and positive outcome won't be in the cards for Rancourt and the MRS team this morning. "The late, great Guy Gosselin, the former executive director at the Observatory, once told me, 'If you think you know where the people you're looking for are, you're wrong," says Rancourt today. "People up there are likely going to do something different from what you expect, and you're never going to be able to guess what that is."

At last, the Thiokol reaches the winter cutoff, a shortcut that charts a more direct line up the mountain near the six-mile mark. "We stopped for a couple of minutes at the winter cutoff and made the decision to bypass it, continue on the Auto Road, and try to go up to five-mile," says Rancourt. "Other than the poor visibility, the first four miles going up the road were not a big deal. But it was a heavy load, and we could hear the wind blowing and knew it was going to be bad."

It is at the five-mile mark, where the Thiokol is heading, that the full conditions will really start to show themselves. During the Observatory's weekly shift change, the go or no-go decision to continue to the summit is often made here.

"It was a good decision to try to get to five-mile that day, but it was impossible to achieve," says Rancourt. "We'd gotten to just below five-mile and proceeded up 100 to 200 yards, and it was apparent that we were not going to make it any farther in the Thiokol. If you don't know where you're going up there, you can end up in a lot of trouble really quickly."

Rancourt's experience level and wisdom fend off the potentially fatal decision his ego desperately wants to make: "Keep going," it urges. "You've got this." That subtle cognitive trap is the one Herr and Batzer fell into as they topped out on Odell 24 hours earlier. But on this morning, Rancourt's rational analysis of his situation—and his humility—win out.

"I wasn't comfortable moving forward that day," he says. "You've got a lot of people on board. You wouldn't want to go over the edge and cause more problems, so you act more cautiously. But even if I was going up alone that day, I could not have gone any farther. The MRS guys were all really well prepared, so they decided to just continue hiking up from there."

Rancourt stands at the back of the Thiokol and watches as his human cargo empties out of the truck bed. Once searchers depart, he'll need to turn the Thiokol around, point it back downhill, and inch his way back to their agreed-upon rendezvous point at Halfway House just below the four-mile mark. There he'll anxiously await the teams' return from their two search assignments.

Because of today's wind direction, Halfway House sits in the lee of the mountain. This historic but dilapidated building, razed by the Mount Washington Auto Road Company two years later in December 1984, is expected to offer Rancourt and his Thiokol some welcome respite as MRS does its hard work above treeline.

As Rancourt squints and shields his eyes from the pelting snow, the teams from MRS begin their march upward and deeper into the building maelstrom. In short order, he'll begin the process of executing a very tedious and tenuous 180-degree turn of the Thiokol. Four decades later, he vividly remembers the challenge: "As they left, I told them I'd do my best to turn the Thiokol around, which on that spot is not a fun thing to do, even today."

In dangerously low visibility, he'll attempt to turn the 16-foot-wide Thiokol around on a road that's only four feet wider. "If you do the math, there's not much room if you start doing kitty-corner turns," says Rancourt. "In the older machines you didn't have the capability to counter-rotate, so I had to make a place to turn around. It took me 25 minutes to complete."

Tuckerman Ravine Trail (2,900 ft.)
Pinkham Notch
9:45 a.m.

Conservation Officer Jeff Gray is having a "WTF" moment. Straddling his Fish and Game-issued snow machine, he feels as though he's losing the flotation battle in a raging river of snow. He glances down and briefly catches a glimpse of the handlebars his mittened hands are tightly gripping until the next wave of snow pours over the high windshield and shrouds them. The classic dark orange cowling covering the machine's Rotax engine and the steel skis protruding off the front beneath it are indiscernible.

Gray's forward progress is continuously hampered by thick pockets of snow, made obvious by his upper torso's sudden jolt forward as the machine beneath him slows almost to a stop. The raspy sound of the engine signals that it is on the verge of overheating. Acrid blue smoke sputters out of the sled, smothering Gray in a cloud of noxious fumes that later will force him to disrobe before his wife will allow him into the house.

He and four of his teammates from New Hampshire Fish and Game have been tasked with searching the lower trails of Cutler River Drainage. Looking behind him, Gray fears that one of the trailing machines enjoying the benefit of the deep trough he and his machine are cutting might barrel into him before he regains forward momentum. If only he had the time and ability to pop the cowl open and throw a handful of snow on the carburetor to cool the engine off. He presses his right thumb against the throttle lever, pins it against the handlebar, and rocks the machine side to side to free it from the snow that encases it.

"The weather conditions were horrendous," says Gray, who joined Fish and Game in 1978 and would later rise to the rank of colonel. "There was a lot of deep, heavy snow as we went up the Tuckerman Ravine Trail from Pinkham. We were on our old 'bone crushers'—Moto-Ski snowmobiles. It was a struggle just getting up there."

Their assignment is to follow the Tuckerman Ravine Trail to Raymond Path, sweep the bottom of Raymond Cataract, and move over to Huntington Ravine. Unfortunately, the depth of the snow confines them to a much smaller search area. "When we'd get off the machines to search on foot, we were just kicking and floundering with our snowshoes," he recalls. "When the snow gets really deep below treeline, you have to contend with spruce traps and you just flail around. That's what was happening to us. Because of the conditions we just couldn't do much that day."

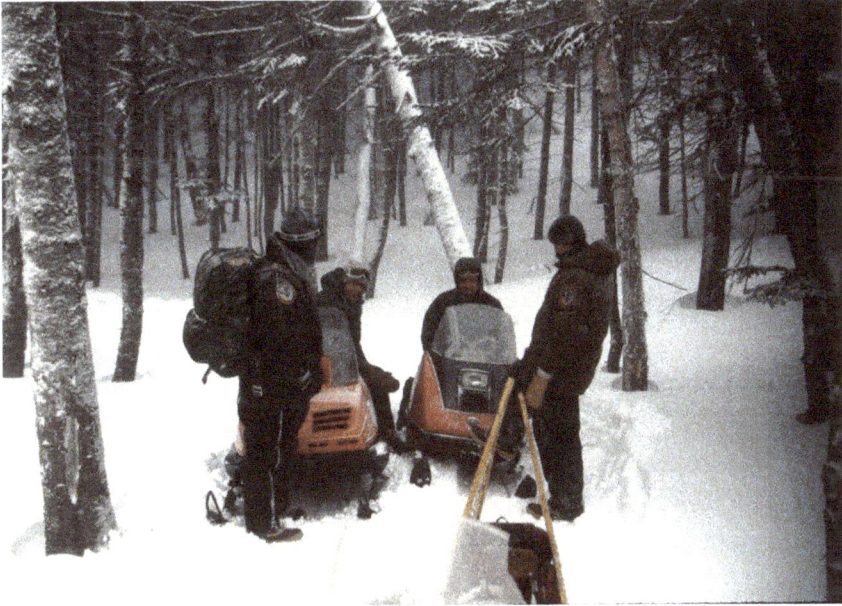

Conservation Officers from New Hampshire Fish and Game on the Tuckerman Ravine Trail during the search for Hugh Herr and Jeff Batzer on Jan. 24.

XXII
HAMMERED

There is no harm in hoping for the best as long as you're prepared for the worst.
—Author Stephen King

Mount Washington Observatory Surface Weather Observations (10:00 to 11:00 a.m.): Temperature -5°F; winds out of the west averaging 51 mph; visibility 0 miles; snow/ blowing snow/ fog; windchill -38.4°F; peak wind gust: 63 mph.

Five-Mile Grade (4,650 ft.)
Mount Washington Auto Road
Sunday, Jan. 24, 1982
10:05 a.m.

Clad in matching anoraks rendered board stiff by freezing temperatures and blowing snow, and with hoods fully compressed, the 10 members of Mountain Rescue Service (MRS) make the treacherous march toward the stretch of the Auto Road referred to as Cragway. All wear Gore-Tex pants, and mountaineering boots covered by insulated supergaiters. Some wear goggles, others wipe snow from their prescription eyeglasses, and all are fully prepared to operate here. Technical climbing gear knocks against backpacks. Beyond the standard kit, each member has gear preferences based on their own experiences in this and other inhospitable environments. They've climbed on high walls and even higher peaks far beyond the Presidential Range.

The team has decided not to bring a rescue litter along because winds are too strong to maintain control over it. What is aptly designed for patient transport over difficult terrain can transform into a mainsail or aluminum missile in winds this high. If they locate the missing climbers and they're incapacitated, each rescuer will grab on to whatever piece of Herr and Batzer's clothing they can get a firm hold of and drag the stricken pair to wherever they can get them and themselves out of the deadly windchill as quickly as possible.

As they move unimpeded in the relative calm afforded by the lee of Nelson Crag (5,635 ft.), each knows he's mere steps from the alpine version of what a firefighter faces when entering a burning structure. Just above Cragway, visibility will go from very bad to much worse, cloaking hidden hazards beneath their feet. This and other factors, such as wind speed and deafening sound that would cause an uninitiated mountain visitor to turn back, will erode the confidence of even these seasoned searchers. Unlike the firefighter who faces searing heat, these 10 searchers will experience brutal arctic cold. In an urban environment, when a firefighter is in distress he'll call "Mayday, Mayday, Mayday!," which immediately initiates a rescue attempt by a Rapid Intervention Team. Here, at several thousand feet from the nearest highway, there's no such help. They rely only on their deep breadth of experience and each other.

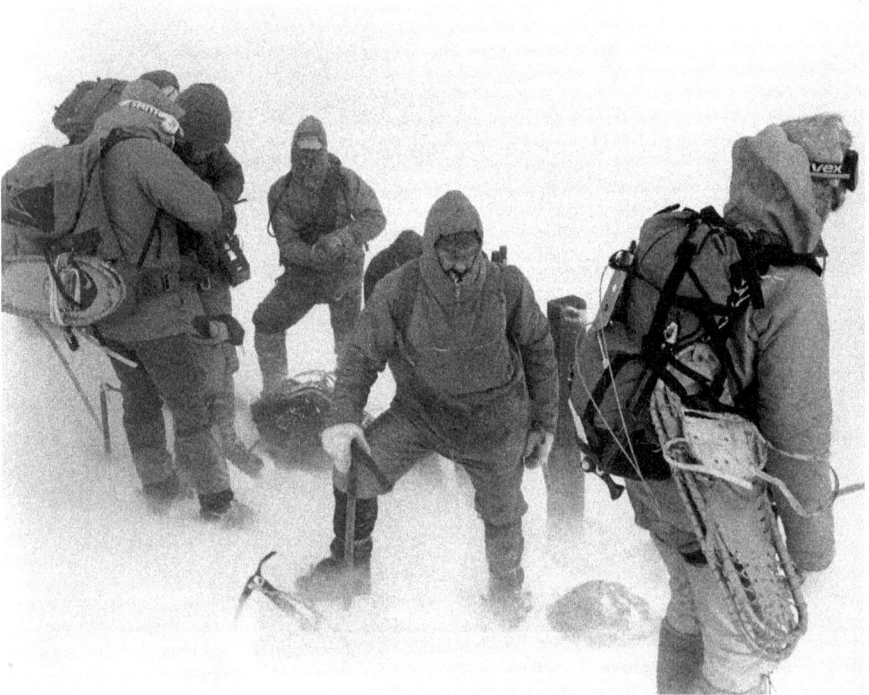

This photo of MRS at Five-Mile Post on the Auto Road was taken by David Stone on Jan. 24.

"It hadn't been planned for the Thiokol to stop where it did," says Kane. "Ken Rancourt tried to get us up and around the corner at Cragway but it was just so windy. To his credit, he did give us a four-mile head start for the search. It was on the five-mile grade just below Cragway that we really started to gear up, and at that point it can be very steep and very snow-loaded because of the high winds. It was really wild, and close enough to the edge of the road that we geared up with crampons."

As is often the case with mountain searches, MRS is adapting to the conditions and modifying their plan. Instead of taking the path of least resistance and calling it a day when the Thiokol can't get them to their intended destination, they're attempting to reach their assignments on foot. If they're able to get higher up the mountain and over to the rim of Huntington Ravine, they'll split into two groups and execute their respective assignments.

"The goal was to get up to seven-mile at the top of the Huntington Ravine Trail and then follow it over to the top of the ravine," says Lentini. "The original plan was to lower someone down Odell's partway to look for signs of Hugh and Jeff and make a decision from there. While our team (Unit 22) was doing that, the other team (Unit 21) would sweep Alpine Garden for any signs of them." Once the sweep was completed, Unit 21 would then move south toward Joe Gill's team (Unit 24), who'd be ascending the Lion Head Winter Route, and hope to meet up. The search of Alpine Garden would encompass approximately 200 of the 240 acres that comprise the Alpine Garden Research Natural Area.

Given the extreme avalanche conditions that exist in Huntington and elsewhere on the eastern slopes, the plans for Unit 22 to fix a rope at the top of Odell and rappel down into the gully was determined to present a lower risk than roped searchers ascending it from below. "That morning at Pinkham as we were putting a plan together, we asked ourselves if Herr and Batzer could still be in Odell," says Kane. "That was the point where they were last seen. The hope was that we would find them there, and everything would be good. We were feeling like these guys have got to be hurt. We had 300 feet of rope, and we thought we could get a person down there to see if they were stuck. We knew from Misha Kirk and the team that went into Huntington that they hadn't fallen down the gully. Our biggest concern was whether or not we were going to be able to get the anchors and ropes set up in those conditions."

If the Unit 22 team can reach the rim and top of Odell, they'll use shrubbery and bollards as anchor points to protect the rappel. Lentini is carrying a snow fluke on the outside of his pack to use as an anchor if conditions allow. This tool catches the eye of MRS teammate Dana Seavey, "I remember kidding with Joe before we started up that I was not going to rappel off that stupid snow fluke he had strapped to his pack."

But before any of that can happen, there's still a lot of work to do to get to Huntington Ravine. Still together, the 10 searchers round the sharp right-hand turn at Cragway Spring that leads to Cragway.

Team members Steve Larson and Michael Hartrich ratchet down their hoods even further in preparation to be punched in the mouth by the legendary westerly winds. It's the second time in 24 hours the pair has been together in the mountains. But unlike today, yesterday's outing was fun, at least at the outset. "I used to love to backcountry ski," says Hartrich. "The day before the search on Mount Washington I hauled Steve Larson out. We drove up to Crawford Notch, and there was just powder everywhere. There was a storm coming in at some point, but we weren't really thinking about it at the time. We skied from the top of Crawford Notch to Mizpah and down into Dry River. As the day wore on it started snowing, and there was quite a bit on the ground. We didn't get out of the woods until it was dark and snowing heavily. Steve had gotten his Volkswagen pickup truck stuck when we first parked, and by the time we got back we couldn't get it out and had to call somebody. We got back pretty late that night."

"Michael is quite a guy," says longtime friend and MRS teammate Steve Larson. "He was probably the first athlete climber here in the valley. His background in gymnastics brought climbing in New Hampshire to a whole new level. He is an amazing skier, naturalist, and mountain biker. I spent several years crashing on various hiking trails trying to keep up with him on skis. The day we went out before the search it was awesome snow. I'm a shitty skier, and I was a really shitty skier back then. When skiing with Michael I was just trying to get down, and on that outing I could actually ski because there was so much resistance, so much snow that day." But today is a different deal, and Hartrich and Larson are soberly focused on getting to where they need to go.

Fellow teammates Doug Madara and David Stone exchange a knowing glance as they round the turn at Cragway. Madara, who moved to the Mount Washington Valley in the mid-1970s after high school, lived what he calls the "dirtbag lifestyle" of a climber with a friend in a tent by a river until both could find jobs. "That was the dream," says Madara today. "Living on your own, climbing every day, and washing dishes at night." In between climbing and washing dishes, Madara would often hang out at International Mountain Equipment (IME) in North Conway. They gave him a job working retail, and shortly thereafter owner Paul Ross offered him some guiding work. Because of his solid mountain acumen, he was invited to join MRS as well.

Stone, a beloved member of the team and a professional photographer who died in September 2003, joined MRS in 1980 while also working for IME managing the mail order side of the business. "Once he went rock climbing that was just it," says wife Lin Stone. "He was smitten, and he took it up as he did most things, wholeheartedly. The climbing community was really close at that time. There was an English contingent: David, Paul Ross, and Bill Aughton. Much to his London friends' shock, he became a rock jock and ice climber and eventually—once he'd earned his chops—an MRS team member. He felt it was an unquestionable obligation to serve because he loved and used the mountains. He believed it was his duty, as did they all, I suspect. I never worried when David would climb with them as young men because I knew they would all give their lives for each other, and I knew that none of them risked their lives unnecessarily."

Harvard Cabin
10:10 a.m.

Caretaker Matt Pierce, along with Harvard Cabin guests Paul Geissler, Layne Terrell, Bob MacEntee, and three unidentified climbers, have just returned from an attempt to search Escape Hatch and what they could see of Alpine Garden. Before leaving the cabin, Pierce left instructions with guest Kacy (Terrell) St. Clair in the event Herr and/or Batzer came stumbling into the cabin while he and the others were away.

"Layne and Paul went out on the first day of the search, but I was too inexperienced and would have been a liability," St. Clair says. "I remember feeling frustrated and useless to the effort, but I now realize they were very smart to make sure I stayed in the cabin. Matt explained to me how to use sleeping bags and body heat to treat hypothermia in case Hugh and Jeff returned while others were out searching. I went on to become a nationally registered paramedic a couple of years after the incident, and I credit the feeling of helplessness I had while waiting during the search as one of the reasons I became one."

Bob MacEntee, who'd stayed behind earlier that morning when companions Jim Frati and Hank Butler attempted to climb Odell Gully, joined Pierce and the others for what he later recalls as a futile attempt to search anywhere. "There was a lot of blowing snow, and it was really cold," he says. "We went to Escape Hatch, and I remember we were slogging through heavy deep snow."

When they arrived at the base of Escape Hatch, Pierce quickly determined there was too much snow and avalanche hazard for them to ascend it up to Alpine Garden. "It was nasty, really cold, and really windy," Pierce recalls. "I was thinking, wherever they are, I hope they have shelter. Anywhere you went you were going to be in the wind, and the farther up you went, the worse it got. I decided it was safest to check Escape Hatch and Alpine Garden from below using my binoculars."

Huntington Ravine (4,000 ft.)
10:25 a.m.

Misha Kirk's core temperature is back in the safe zone. The search of the ravine is concluding, and the Thiokol (Unit 25) that has been helping him warm up will soon head down to Pinkham Camp with Unit 23. "I listened to the many radios we had out on the mountain and began to sort out what was happening," wrote Kirk in his journal.

Once the Thiokol has departed, Kirk will hike the Fire Road over to Tuckerman Ravine where he plans to stay at the caretaker's cabin to rest and cover for Joe Gill as he leads Unit 24 up Lion Head and onto the Alpine Garden.

Unbeknownst to Kirk or anyone else at the time, this simple divergence on his part will be the first in a series of events that will lead to the rescue of Herr and Batzer.

Cragway (5,000 ft.)
Mount Washington Auto Road
10:40 a.m.

MRS is entering the belly of the beast. The more than 60-mph wind gusts combined with falling and blowing snow have created a full-on ground blizzard. At this point, conducting a search is so dangerous that one errant step to the left or right by any one of the team members could result in a third missing soul on the mountain. The windchill, nearing -50°F, significantly limits the mobility of each searcher.

"We made it up past Cragway, but then the road turns to the northwest, and we started to get the wind straight in our faces," says Joe Lentini. "It just became a total whiteout. I can remember I'd hold my hand out and I couldn't see my fist. And then at one point I remember we were moving forward a little bit and we heard a noise and Steve Larson wasn't there. He had stepped off the edge of the Auto Road and gone off. It wasn't a big deal; he'd gone down 10 to 15 feet. But we all realized at that moment, 'This isn't going to happen. We're not going to get to Huntington Ravine.'"

Kane also recalls this as a defining moment in the search. "We stopped and Paul Ross yelled out, 'The only people we're going to save today is us. There's no fucking way we can get over to Huntington, and I'm really worried about our anchoring even if we did. This is not going to work today.'"

Ross, who like David Stone and Bill Aughton arrived in the U.S. from the United Kingdom, was working for Outward Bound in Maine and driving around New Hampshire when he says he arrived "by accident" in North Conway. He drove over to the cliffs of Cathedral Ledge and Whitehorse and moved to the valley to work for Eastern Mountain Sports (EMS) shortly thereafter. He would go on to be one of three founders of IME and the International Mountain Climbing School. "Those two lads went missing, and at first we thought they must be somewhere round about Huntington Ravine," says Ross today. "And of course the search started and there was no sign of them, and we realized they'd vanished someplace. It was atrocious conditions, and I said, "This is pointless,' because if there was anybody there, we wouldn't have seen them anyway."

Ryan Knapp, a meteorologist for the Mount Washington Observatory, describes how the wind direction and terrain was a major factor in the MRS team's inability to continue. "They're having all that snow that's blowing off of Nelson Crag and Ball Crag above them, and also the snow that's falling at the time. So there can be some pretty significant low visibility. Because those sections are our most loaded area of the Auto Road, the blowing snow is going to affect them significantly because they are located where that snow is depositing."

"We had big plans for that day," says Dana Seavey. "But once we got out of the machine and got on toward Alpine Garden, it was pretty obvious conditions were too bad. We got out right in the lee and we were just getting hammered as we moved up. I had a small, exposed gap between my mitts and outerwear, and I got some mild frostbite on my wrist within the first five minutes. I could feel my skin freezing and part of my wrist was turning gray. We didn't even know where to start. We regrouped, looked around, yelled to one another because we couldn't hear. I do remember still being ready to go if Joe and Bill had said, 'Let's start searching.' But I think our body language signaled that we were not going to be able to do much in those conditions without enduring some pretty serious suffering."

Once this piece of the search is called by the team leaders, the 10 battered searchers head back for the lee on five-mile grade and make their way down toward Half Way House and the idling Thiokol. Once they load into the back, they have a 45-minute minute descent to the Glen House site, which lies approximately two miles from where Herr and Batzer are continuing their attempt to self-rescue.

Except for the attempt by Hank Butler and Jim Frati to check Odell Gully at dawn from Harvard Cabin, most of the gully has remained unsearched. As the point last seen for Herr and Batzer, it continues to be ground zero for the search effort, and the desire to get up in there to look for the missing climbers will carry into the following day's search.

XXIII
TREMORS

The signal is the truth. The noise is what
distracts us from the truth.

——Nate Silver, statistician and author of *The*
Signal and the Noise

Mount Washington Observatory Surface Weather Observations (11:00 to 12:00
p.m.): Temperature -6°F; winds out of the west averaging 58 mph; visibility 0
miles; snow/blowing snow/fog; windchill -41.4°F; peak wind gust: 68 mph.

Madison Gulf Trail (3,100 ft.)
Great Gulf Wilderness
Sunday, Jan. 24, 1982
11:00 a.m.

Hugh Herr is on all fours because the steep, snow-clogged slope he's fighting his way up makes it impossible for him to stand upright. Emotionally, he has detached himself from the present and is now in a place where he can just continue to endure his silent suffering. From there, he can conceal from Batzer what he believes will be their demise. He's busting trail again ... still. This fruitless effort gives him something to focus on as he waits for death to arrive.

Hours earlier, at Great Gulf Trail junction, the friends had embraced and shed tears of relief, but now the stark reality of the error they made in their choice of escape route reminds Herr that this mountain gives no gifts. They had yielded to the allure of a relatively short distance to reach a landmark they'd heard of: Madison Hut. But Herr now understands that their ignorance of the terrain caused them to overrule the better options. It has not taken him long to realize that when it comes to the White Mountains, proximity can be deceptive when combined with the variables of steep terrain, paralyzing snow depths, and freezing temperatures.

"Hugh was not talking much at that point, so I just surmised he wasn't doing well," Batzer recalls. "Falling in the river twice the night before really got the best of him, and he was struggling with the cold."

The two are now grinding their way up a nightmare slope in hopes of reaching the hut located at 4,800 feet in Madison Col. They're expecting to find people there to help them. But they have no idea that last September, the hut's caretaker padlocked its front door and drove the last nail into the plywood covering the double-paned window facing Mount Adams. It will be months before the hatches of the hut are unbattened again for the season.

As they struggle upward, Batzer is fighting his own battle with the cold. The mitten he'd lost on Odell, which felt trivial to him at the time, is now poking at his psyche. The interior of his single Gore-Tex mitten is saturated from the exertion and the continuous swimming through the snow. As it had in the deeper reaches of Great Gulf, snow depths here reach their waists. Some of the snowdrifts are taller than they are. Each time Batzer switches the mitten from one hand to the other, or drives his knees into the snowpack, the harder it is for him to retain any warmth at all. "I had to really work to keep my hands from getting cold, or freezing, or developing frostbite," he says. "Even though I was wearing supergaiters, my boots were getting even more wet from perspiration."

They take turns breaking trail, just as they did the day before after the first of Herr's two unplanned submersions in the West Branch of the Peabody River. They're forced to grab on to small trees and shrubbery to pull themselves forward. Even here on the slope, they must shuffle across logs spanning ditches over six feet deep, and gingerly move over thinly-bridged water crossings as water drains off the higher reaches of the range.

Trail blazes, which sit near eye level on the trees during the other three seasons, seem to bob on the snow. These elusive markers are the only things keeping Herr and Batzer on or near the otherwise indiscernible Madison Gulf Trail. They have no sense of how far away they are from the hut above them, or when this ruthless grade will ease its grip.

By midafternoon, at an elevation of approximately 3,600 feet, they will finally submit. Since leaving the trail junction for Madison Hut, they've traveled 0.84 miles, with an elevation gain of approximately 1,300 feet. "I would contend we expended the equivalent of a fast marathon's worth of calorie burn over maybe a mile," Herr says today. "That was the level of bushwhacking we were doing. Everyone said we were lost. But, no, we were trapped in a white hell and just not able to move. And everyone said we should have been wearing snowshoes. But they wouldn't have done a fucking thing."

Pinkham Camp
Pinkham Notch
11:20 a.m.

After Conservation Officers Jeff Gray and Charles Kenney and their four fellow COs are unable to sweep Raymond Path below Raymond Cataract because the snow is too deep for their snow machines, Gray and Kenney make their way to Harvard Cabin before heading back to Pinkham Camp where search teams are regrouping. At the cabin, they retrieve the backpack Herr and Batzer stashed in Huntington as well as the one they left behind at the cabin. Inside the pack left behind are the keys to Batzer's truck.

Upon arriving at Pinkham with the gear, Gray and Kenney give the keys to Sgt. Carl Carlson of New Hampshire Fish and Game and follow him to the parking lot. Having heard from those staying at Harvard Cabin that Herr and Batzer might be from Pennsylvania, Carlson has been able to locate a Datsun pickup truck with a Pennsylvania license plate. He tried to run the plate through police dispatch, but the Pennsylvania motor vehicle computers were down at the time.

Inside the pickup truck, Carlson finds a wallet in the glovebox belonging to Batzer, and a climbing book with "To Hugh" dated 10/81 inscribed on the bookleaf. They run the plate again, and this time the Pennsylvania computers are back online. The Datsun is registered to Richard C. and Jeffrey Batzer.

With Joe Gill's team still on Lion Head, additional search assignments will be planned for Sunday afternoon. If none are successful in finding any sign of Herr or Batzer by the end of the day, Carlson will make the phone call every conservation officer dreads. He will notify Herr and Batzer's parents that their youngest sons are missing in a bad winter storm on Mount Washington.

Winter Route (4,900 ft.)
Lion Head, Mount Washington
11:30 a.m.

Joe Gill is crushing it. Like Herr and Batzer several miles to the north on Madison Gulf Trail, he is breaking trail through deep snow on the Winter Route. He's singlehandedly creating a trough for the four teammates in his wake. But unlike Herr and Batzer, who are exhausted, cold, and depleted, Gill's conditioning for mountain travel is still at its peak. He spends so much time ascending and descending this mountain that he's got plenty of fuel in reserve for what promises to be a long day ahead. "Being that the route is on the eastern aspect of the mountain, it tended to accumulate a lot of snow everywhere, and the trees generally held it," says Gill. "It was very rarely closed back then."

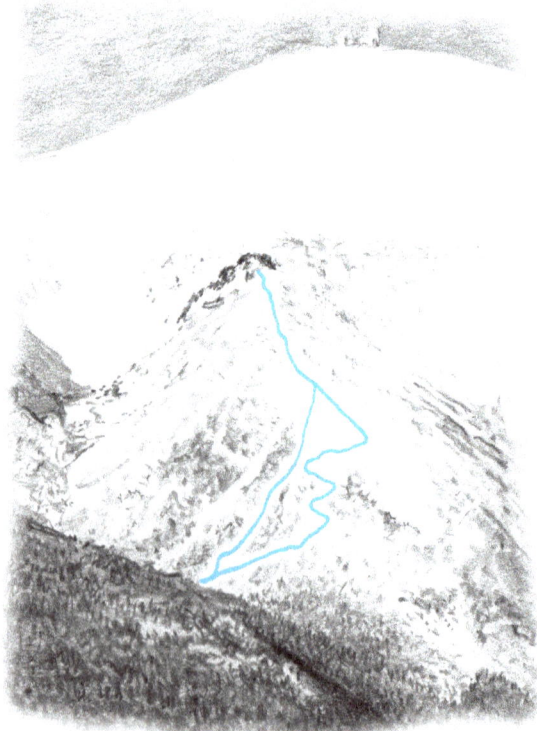

Once again, as they appear on page 127, the Lion Head Winter Route (left) and Summer Route (right) as they were in 1982.

The five members of Unit 24 (Gill, Meduski, Cunha, Kamman, and Corbin), all of whom work for the AMC, ascend this straight slope that is mostly above a 30-degree grade. In 1982, the Lion Head Winter Route was accessed from the same trailhead as the Summer Route. Located right below Shelter Four in Tuckerman Ravine, the trail led into the woods to a junction approximately 100 yards in. The Summer Route took a hard right, while the Winter Route made a very steep beeline directly up the mountain.

Although the AMC team is dealing with deep snow, the conditions here in the lee of the mountain are relatively calm. If they can reach treeline, the westerly winds will be brutal, however. Gill is intimately familiar with the route, both as a hiker and a rescuer. "People would glissade down the Winter Route without taking their crampons off first," he recalls. "We were always getting broken ankle calls."

The route is narrow, much like a single-track mountain bike trail. Balsam fir, paper birch, and mountain ash no taller than 25 feet offer a sense of security before the onslaught that awaits them higher up. "You could reach from one side to the other and touch trees most of the way up," says Gill. "The trail was often gullied out from people sliding down or walking down."

The five reach a point halfway up the Winter Route at an elevation of approximately 4,000 feet. Not far from treeline, there's still fairly significant forest cover. They are climbing in single file along the narrow swath of trail when Gill plants his Asolo leather double boot into the snowpack.

"WHUMPF!!"

He feels himself drop ever so slightly, and a release of energy travels through his ankle. The synapses in Gill's brain signal alarm and alert his body to hold in place, especially his trailing leg. He waits. Having attended a professional avalanche forecasting course in Wyoming years earlier, and frequently putting those skills to work in his role as caretaker of Tuckerman Ravine, he knows exactly what's happening.

"We'd gotten quite a bit of snow during the storm," he says. "The snowpack even in the trees was going 'whumpf' as we hiked. It was definitely doing some scary kind of settling. I was setting it off slogging up. The 'whumpf' represents a weak layer of unconsolidated loose snow with a soft slab of snow on top. That told me the snowpack was very unstable. We continued on anyway, and I made sure we stayed close to the thickest trees I could find."

Dale Atkins, an internationally recognized avalanche expert, describes the science behind the snow conditions that day on Lion Head. "Some people call that sound nature's billboard," he says. "I call it 'talking snow.' It's the sudden collapse of a weak layer buried in a snowpack. When you have a weak layer of snow, it's possible to trigger an avalanche remotely [off to the side], or from below it. All you need after a 'whumpf' is a slope steep enough for the slab to overcome friction."

At a slope angle exceeding 30 degrees, large swaths of the Winter Route on this day are at risk of cutting loose. Fortunately for Gill and the other members of Unit 24, there is enough friction present to hold the snow. "The only thing holding it in place was the density of the vegetation," says Gill. "The indicators caused me to employ all of my avalanche terrain route-finding strategies. I tried to keep us to the thickest trees just off trail because they act as an anchor to some extent. I wanted us to avoid the open slopes. I was also looking for little ridges to stay on rather than hiking in the troughs." Gill acknowledges that his appetite for risk was greater back then. "I was only what, 28 at the time? I still had a certainty regarding my personal immortality."

Although Gill has seen avalanches in Tucks during his time as caretaker, he hasn't on Lion Head. But he knows the eastern slopes are still at risk, especially during storms like this one. "One of the biggest slides in Mount Washington history was off Lion Head in the winter of 1969," he says. "It came down right across the Tuck Trail. When I first started working for the AMC in 1972, you could still see the scar. By 1982 it had grown in, but it was an interpretive sign for sure. It happened the same year that Raymond Cataract avalanched right across the Fire Road."

The biblical snow levels in the winter of 1969 remain seared in the memories of those who witnessed them firsthand, and anyone with an interest in extreme weather. Rene LaRoche, a snow ranger at the time, vividly recalls that record-setting season. "We had a hard time getting up into Tuckerman Ravine with the Thiokol," he says. "We kept making a road, but the snow kept drifting in, and finally when we did make it up and were coming back down the Sherburne

Ski Trail a few hours later, we had to stop and back up because we would bury the machine in powdery snow up to its windshield. It snowed three feet without stopping, slowed down for an hour or two, and then we got another three feet on top of that."

Even though he wasn't born yet, Ryan Knapp, a meteorologist at the Mount Washington Observatory, is well aware of the historical event. "The February 25, 1969, snowfall total of 49.3 inches is the greatest 24-hour snowfall total for the summit of Mount Washington." Knapp says. "It still stands as the highest snowfall total in 24 hours in New Hampshire history."

That winter, the city of Berlin to the north declared a state of emergency twice. According to the Mount Washington Observatory Observer's log, Pinkham Notch had 16 feet of snow on the ground on Feb. 27, Route 16 was barely two lanes wide, and no traffic was permitted in Berlin. The snow was so deep on the slopes at the Wildcat Ski Area that the gondolas had to be shut down because they kept striking the snow. Guy Gosselin, who at the time was the executive director of the Observatory, contributed to an article entitled "The Winter of '69 in the White Mountains" (*Appalachia*: Dec. 15, 1969). He wrote that the summit of Mount Washington received a total of 566.4 inches of snow (47.2 feet), and Pinkham Notch 317 inches (26.4 feet).

Because of the deluge of snow that winter, an unprecedented number of large avalanches occurred across the range. In addition to the one on Lion Head, avalanches happened in the adjacent Raymond Cataract, Ammonoosuc Ravine, Great Gulf, and Mount Madison. The avalanche on the northeast side of Madison was so big that it destroyed 38 acres of timber and left a scar on the side of the mountain that was visible from Route 16. "I saw the Madison slide as I was leaving the ranger station that morning," says LaRoche. "I was looking up at the mountain and said, 'What the hell is that?' There was a big clearing, so I stopped my car to look and saw there had been a huge avalanche. It was unbelievable."

Gill is able to lead his team safely up the challenging slope to a small 30-by-50-foot snowfield that formed each year on the upper reaches of the route. Now more exposed on the ridge, the five searchers are clenched in the teeth of sustained winds in the mid-60s, and gusts pushing 80. They huddle together at the crest of this giant rock formation. Mother Nature's assault on Unit 24 will continue if they're able to move in the direction of the summit cone of Washington, but if they can get beyond Lion Head Rock, the westerly winds will be lower in the summit's shadow.

"It was nasty and windy," recalls Carol Cunha. "I had wool pants, a windbreaker, and most of us had ski goggles because of the winds. Joe Gill was very well respected, and still is. On the Pinkham Crew you're dealing with a good number of rescues in the summer and winter, so I had been on a fair number before."

Normally steady and low-key, Gill elevates his voice to a yell so the team can hear exactly what he's saying. He checks in with each member to ascertain who is willing to continue and who, without judgment or criticism, wants to turn around. "There was a discussion about comfort level," Alan Kamman recalls. "Who's going forward and who isn't. It was snowing and snowing, and the higher we got, the windier it got. I remember summiting Lion Head, and we could barely communicate. I can remember Joe and Bill [Corbin] being right up in each other's grill just trying to hear each other."

It is decided that Corbin and Cunha will descend. Kamman and Meduski will continue with Gill across Alpine Garden. Corbin, who was not available for an interview, shared with his partner Melissa "Cam" Bradshaw that he "remembers turning back before topping out on Lion Head because conditions were grim." Bradshaw, who also worked for AMC with Gill, added, "I'm not surprised that Joe felt comfortable continuing on."

Cunha says she was not aware of the avalanche risk during the climb and was "reasonably comfortable" with what the team was doing. "But Joe was concerned about avalanche danger, and he didn't want to risk the entire team. He was the only one who knew what he was doing, as the rest of us were reasonably inexperienced, so we were following his lead. When we got up on Lion Head, he basically made us stop and very slowly turn around and head back down because he was afraid of avalanches."

Gill's concern is well placed. The seven-plus inches of low-density snow that has fallen on the mountain since the previous day remains unsettled and thus unconsolidated. Relentless westerly winds, strong enough to transport the snow to the lee of the eastern slopes, is blanketing the weak layer that's already fallen here. As the transported snow settles, the winds and cold temperatures will form soft wind slab, further concealing the weak layer below it.

This steadily increasing instability of the snowpack on Lion Head and other eastern aspects of Mount Washington has many involved in the search on edge. But for now, Gill leads the remaining two members of Unit 24 toward Alpine Garden in hopes of searching the rims of Raymond Cataract and Huntington Ravine. The MRS team on the Auto Road, some of whom Gill and his team were supposed to meet up with, has been forced to turn back by unsearchable conditions high on the mountain.

There will be other signs of avalanche risk before this day's search concludes. But amid all the noise, no one is able to see the truth in the signs: the avalanche bullet that Unit 24 dodged because of Joe Gill's caution is accompanied by other rounds waiting to fire off.

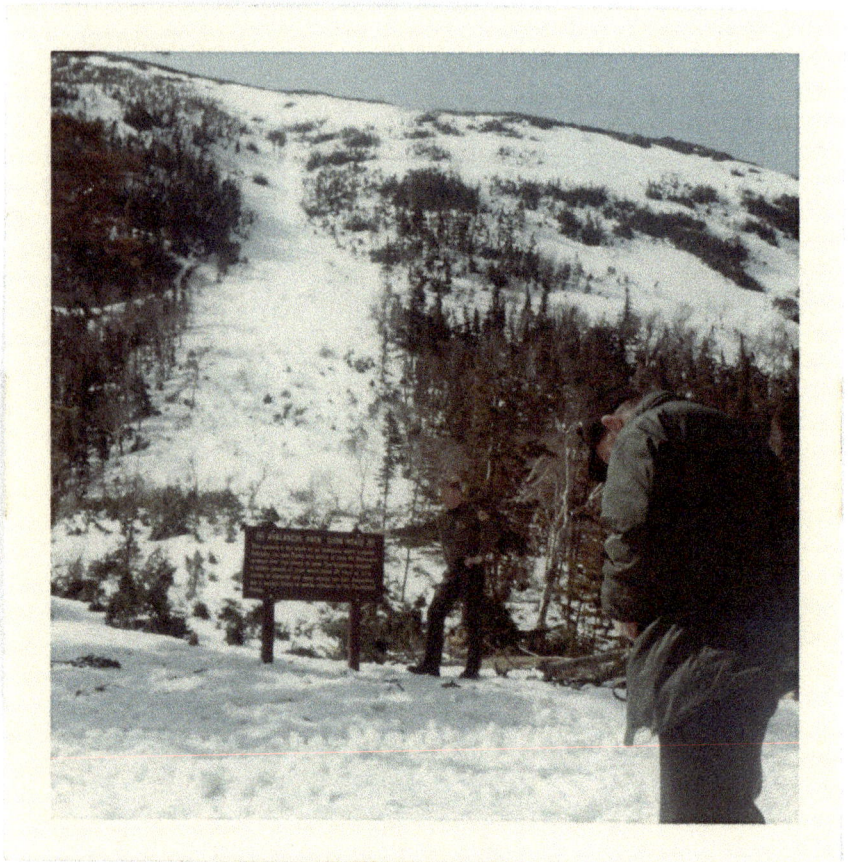

Snow Ranger Rene LaRoche standing at the base of the 1969 slide path on Lion Head (early 1970s). By 1982, the massive avalanche scar had disappeared. Text of sign below.

AVALANCHE PATH (LION HEAD)

This opening is the result of an avalanche which occurred February 26, 1969. During the winter of 1969, Mt. Washington received over 500 inches of snow. The avalanche released 5 million pounds of snow which broke off trees up to 10 inches in diameter and swept across this trail. Avalanches are a serious threat to winter climbers on the Presidential Range.

XXIV
BREAKING PATTERNS

If I cease searching, then, woe is me, I am lost.
That is how I look at it – keep going, keep going,
come what may.

—Vincent van Gogh

Mount Washington Observatory Surface Weather Observations (12:00 to 1:00 p.m.): Temperature -7°F; winds out of the west averaging 64 mph; visibility 0 miles; snow/blowing snow/fog; windchill -44.0°F; peak wind gust: 75 mph.

Ravine of Raymond Cataract (3,800 ft.)
Mount Washington
Sunday, Jan. 24, 1982
12:15 p.m.

Matt Pierce is refusing to give up. In addition to his efforts to hike into Huntington Ravine earlier to search Escape Hatch and Alpine Garden, maintain some semblance of calm among guests at Harvard Cabin, and tend to weathered searchers, he and a small group of volunteers now slog into the yet unsearched Raymond Cataract.

Sandwiched between Tuckerman and Huntington Ravines, Raymond Cataract, named after Maj. Curtis Burritt Raymond (1816-1893) who was a trail steward in the area, serves as yet another collection point for wind-raked snow, errant scree, and water draining in from Alpine Garden above.

"It would have been a difficult route for that team because they were walking up into a giant bowl," says Ryan Knapp of the Mount Washington Observatory. "There was a lot more snow depositing in there, making it even deeper than what searchers over on Lion Head were experiencing. It's basically a giant funnel, so not only did they have a strong headwind that day, but the winds would be funneling their way down toward the middle of the ravine."

Unlike its more popular neighbors to its left and right, Raymond rarely has visitors. On the rare occasion someone does venture in, it is typically by mistake. Those who've found trouble on the Alpine Garden find even more of it in the Cataract, and that is why Pierce and his companions have come.

Over time, backcountry enthusiasts under duress have established consistent patterns of behavior on the eastern aspects of Mount Washington and elsewhere in the White Mountains. By cross-referencing those patterns with a missing person's planned itinerary, the day's wind speed and direction, the visibility, and a hodgepodge of other variables, search planners can focus resources on the locations of highest probability.

"If you're coming up Pinnacle, Odell's, or South Gully, you're probably going to go left to the west when you top out," says Rick Wilcox, former president of Mountain Rescue Service. "You then have two options: descend the Escape Hatch or go across Alpine Garden to the Lion Head Trail. But over the years, many people not familiar with these descent routes have gotten into trouble. The Escape Hatch is a little bit harder to find unless you're familiar with the ravine. The gully might not have seemed that bad on the way up. But when climbers get above the gully in heavy wind, fog, and snow, they don't navigate well and can wind up somewhere between the Escape Hatch and Raymond Cataract. They will often go looking for Lion Head, but what they don't realize is that you have to go back uphill to get around the top of Raymond Cataract to get over to Lion Head. So they get sucked down into Raymond's and wind up trying to follow the brook down, which is very dangerous because if they fall in or try to cross the brook, it's all open water. It's really nasty in there, and they often spend the night in the trees not far from Harvard Cabin. There've been instances where people in there have been in voice contact with people at Harvard Cabin. We know they're alive, but they don't get out of there until the next morning. It's a common descent problem."

In addition to the obstacles that exist in Raymond all year long, the Cataract is also susceptible to avalanche hazard in winter. Westerly and northwesterly winds deposit lots of snow there, just as they do in the adjacent ravines. Joe Gill, who is leading a small team toward the rim of upper Raymond as Pierce and his team move into the ravine itself, recalls the carnage caused by an epic avalanche that occurred in

Raymond in February 1969. "Following that event, you could look far up into the ravine into the late 1980s,' he says. "The slide had gone all the way across the Huntington Ravine Fire Road, and the whole area was just knocked flat. The Forest Service put up a big sign on the Tuck Trail describing the avalanche and marking where it ran out. That was one hell of a winter; things were sliding everywhere. "

Fortunately, that event, though memorable, did not result in any fatalities. To date, the only avalanche fatality in Raymond Cataract occurred on April 11, 2019, when Nicholas Benedix, 32, was killed while backcountry skiing alone. Benedix, who was from New Hampshire, was the 15th avalanche fatality and 161st person to perish on Mount Washington.

Lion Head (5,000 ft.)
Mount Washington
12:15 p.m.

Joe Gill and his team are above treeline, but not out of the woods yet in terms of safety. Because of its exposure to high winds and snow deposition, the snowpack on upper Lion Head is notorious for its instability. "We were careful in the open section before we topped out because there was potential for a little slide there," says Gill. "The patch of snowfield right at the top could form a wind slab pretty quickly." What makes this area especially precarious in winter is the series of cliff bands and steep drops, also known as terrain traps, that lie just below these snowfields.

So far, the three have successfully made it across the small but unsettled snowfield, but their relief is short-lived. Kamman suddenly drops almost completely out of sight. He's sprung a spruce trap concealed beneath the drifting snow.

"It's the only time I've been in snow just about to my neck," Kamman says. "Those guys had to help me get out of it." With significant effort on the part of Gill and Meduski, Kamman is extracted from what could have proved fatal for him had he been alone. Undeterred, however, they continue upward, no worse for wear.

"That day I just followed Joe and did what he did because he was the most experienced of the three of us," says Meduski today. "He knew the terrain really well." Kamman, too, had full trust in Gill's leadership and experience. "I felt like part of the team. I looked to Joe to keep us out of trouble, and I felt that if I'd allowed myself to exceed my limits, Joe would have put the brakes on that. He would have kept us safe. I never felt pressure that I had to do it. I wanted to do it."

With Lion Head Rock behind them, Gill, Kamman, and Meduski reach the crest of the massif, which is essentially a ridge separating Tuckerman Ravine and Raymond Cataract. Here, the trio is hammered by the full brunt of the westerly winds. "It wasn't a whiteout, but it was unpleasant," recalls Gill.

Rather than continue up to Alpine Garden Trail, they contour over to the rim of Raymond Cataract. Contouring is when hikers follow the contour of the terrain, as your fingers do on a topographical map, and try to stay at the same elevation as they work their way across. Gill, who's utilized this technique many times before, positions his team to get a better look down into Raymond. Following this line will bring them to the southern end of Huntington Ravine, where they can begin to search the tops of the gullies.

As they do this, they'll contend with high winds prodding their left sides. Once in the shadow of Washington's summit cone, the winds will temper just enough to allow for better walking but not to improve visibility in the near whiteout. Alpine Garden is also riddled with deep and elongated sastrugi, that is, areas of wind-eroded snow, that will require them to bust through to continue forward progress. The flatter plain of the garden does not mean their day will get any easier.

Huntington Ravine (4,200 ft.)
Mount Washington
1:30 p.m.

Mount Washington Observatory Surface Weather Observations (1:00 to 2:00 p.m.): Temperature -7°F; winds out of the west averaging 60 mph; visibility 0 miles; snow/blowing snow/fog; windchill -43.2°F; peak wind gust: 74 mph.

Great Gulf: Temperature: 4°F; winds are low; visibility daylight; light snowfall.

Snow Rangers Brad Ray and Rene LaRoche stand by in the idling

USFS Thiokol on the Huntington Ravine Trail as a small team of searchers heads back into the ravine to make one last check for any sign of Hugh Herr and Jeff Batzer. The team's assignment is to check the scree field at the base of The Fan for any sign of fresh footprints.

This ground search of the scree field was not the original plan. When Team Leaders Bill Kane and Joe Lentini and the other members of MRS arrived back at Pinkham from their unsuccessful attempt to get up the Auto Road and over to Huntington, the planning team discussed sending four members of MRS back into the ravine to attempt to climb Odell Gully, the point last seen for Herr and Batzer. Kane and Lentini, along with Doug Madara and Steve Larson, were to attempt Odell in teams of two. But that didn't happen. "We didn't go into the ravine," says Lentini. "We were done at that point."

Kane explains that the risk of climbing that afternoon was just too great. "The problem was that the deposition of snow was so significant that climbing Odell was out of the question. A small team did go into Huntington to look for tracks."

MRS member Dana Seavey was part of that small team and recalls the difficult conditions searchers were facing. "Travel through the scree field was very difficult, as the larger boulders were mostly exposed. We had to do a lot of climbing up, down, and around the big boulders exposed in the talus. You really had to squeeze through."

In the end, their efforts were in vain. They found no signs of Herr and Batzer.

South Rim of Huntington Ravine (5,000 ft.)
Mount Washington
1:30 p.m.

Despite the difficulty of their forward progress, Joe Gill's team of three is managing to continue its search, "They were the ones who fought and got to the top of Lion Head and went over to the top of Huntington's, and Odell's in particular, to see if Herr and Batzer were pinned down or hung up in the gully," says Bill Kane.

"I could see The Fan below but didn't want to lean over too far," says Gill. "The wind was really blowing. After checking the top of Raymond's, we started our search at the top of Escape Hatch and then moved along the edge of Huntington's looking over the tops of the gullies to see if there were any fresh footprints coming out of them. I did see some older ones coming out of one of the gullies and heading in the direction of Lion Head. I can still see the prints like it was yesterday—nothing terribly significant about them really, but it's funny the things your brain stores with clarity and what it doesn't."

Although footprints are one of the signs they're looking for, Gill is confident that the ones he's found have been there for some time. "They had been pretty well scoured by the wind. I felt the prints were likely older than what would have been made by Herr and Batzer the day before and that they should probably be discounted."

Raymond Path/Cataract (4,300 ft.)
Mount Washington
1:45 p.m.

David Moskowitz is reveling in a splendid ski as he searches Raymond Path. He'd worked the front desk at Pinkham on Friday as Hugh Herr and Jeff Batzer made their dash up the Tuckerman Ravine Trail toward Harvard Cabin. Like many AMC employees on this Sunday, he's been assigned to search this area after conservation officers on snow machines were unable to do so because of deep snow.

"The weather wasn't terrible where I was," Moskowitz recalls. "There was just a ton of snow, and it was still snowing. I skied from Harvard Cabin to the connecting trail to check for any tracks from someone who might have descended Raymond Cataract or Lion Head. It was a beautiful, peaceful ski."

In Raymond Cataract, just above Moskowitz, Matt Pierce and his team are having a completely different search experience. "We went up the Lion Head face as far as we could via the south nose and cut over," Matt says. "The snow was deep and soft. When it got up to almost my armpits, I thought, 'This is too steep, too scary.' Even though we were in the trees, it just wasn't stable. It was time to get out of there. We were getting covered in snow, our mittens were getting wet, and the snow was working its way into our gaiters. The situation was going downhill fast, so we went back to the cabin. I was definitely concerned about avalanche where I was, even though we were in the trees, because snow that's that deep has got some buildup on the top portion of it, and the bottom was sugar snow. That's not good."

Below Alpine Garden Trail (5,000 ft.)
Mount Washington
1:50 p.m.

Battling winds that could send them plummeting down the headwall to The Fan below, Gill and his teammates search the tops of Escape Hatch, South Gully, Odell Gully, and Pinnacle as best they can. Rather than work their way back to Escape Hatch, Gill elects to take the team back across Alpine Garden to Lion Head, where they'll descend. "Given what I knew about the avalanche conditions on the way up Lion Head, it would have been a little reckless of us to exit Escape Hatch," he explains.

Alan Kamman still remembers the effect this search had on him. "To this day, I feel like that was one of the most epic things I've done in the mountains. All it was, really, was a winter hike on a shitty day, but it had a lot of consequence to it. It was kind of exciting, kind of critical. I like the responsibility of needing and wanting to find people who are in trouble. I thought we had a good chance of finding them when we were going up and moving toward Huntington Ravine. That was some of what was going through my head. I wasn't cold, or feeling like I was in over my head. I felt pretty good, though I did get a bit of nip on my face, even though I was wearing goggles."

At just before 2:00 p.m., as Gill's small team again contours Raymond over to Lion Head, he radios Pinkham to inform them of the instability he encountered earlier that day on the Winter Route. The official log reads, "Radio. Unit 24 reports slides on Lion's Head." Many decades later, Gill still recalls this message. "I reported very unstable snow. I saw no slides, but I felt it going up."

At this point, the day's searches are concluding, and Herr and Batzer are still missing somewhere on the mountain. Over the course of the day, teams have confronted significantly escalating risk, and although battered by the weather, all will be returning to Pinkham unscathed. A lot of skill and experience, combined with a little bit of luck, is allowing searchers to return home, rewarm, and rest. Some will return the following morning, when the search for Herr and

Batzer will narrow and become much more technical in nature.

XXV
GEARED UP

Getting lost along your path is a part of finding the path you are meant to be on.

—Robin Sharma, author

When Geoffrey May and David Boudreau set out from Newton, Mass., in Boudreau's 1980 CJ-7 on Saturday morning, Jan. 23, intending to do some winter hiking in the Presidential Range, they cannot imagine the role they will be called upon to play during what will become a momentous weekend in the White Mountains.

After making a brief stop at Eastern Mountain Sports in North Conway to rent snowshoes, they arrive at Pinkham Camp at 2:00 p.m. Muscling their heavy packs onto their shoulders, they head directly to the Trading Post to check the weather forecast and sign in.

"Neither of us was in great climbing shape that winter," Boudreau recalls. "Our plan was to hike across Great Gulf and up to treeline. If our legs were underneath us enough and the weather was cooperating, maybe we could climb Madison and Adams or even do a traverse. We checked *The Boston Globe* weather page before we left Newton, which included the current conditions from the Mount Washington Observatory but no forecast back then. So we knew before we left that a traverse was highly unlikely, but I was cool with a walk in the woods. We checked the forecast again on the bulletin board at Pinkham, and that's when we realized we probably wouldn't be able to advance above treeline that weekend. We had a compass and a topo map, but no means of receiving forecast updates. We were mentally prepared to turn around at treeline."

For his part, May says, "We weren't sure what to expect when we got to Pinkham. It was just wintertime in New England. We were equipped, and we were going to take it as it came. Our goals were modest, and we were going to be in the trees and protected. We were trying to put ourselves in a position to climb Madison, but we knew the timing and weather would have to be right for that. We were staying flexible."

If Boudreau and May move ahead with their planned route, it will take them over the Old Jackson Road onto the Madison Gulf Trail. At the trail junction, they'll take the Osgood Cutoff to the Osgood Trail and head up Mount Madison to treeline. The trail junction lies at the lower portion of Great Gulf. They are not intending to take the Great Gulf Trail at this junction. That route would lead them deeper into the Gulf than they want to be in this weather. The junction is where Herr and Batzer have ended up instead of reaching Central Gully.

Sherburne Ski Trail
Pinkham Notch
Sunday, Jan. 24, 1982
3:00 p.m.

As it turns out, after setting off behind Pinkham Camp, Boudreau and May never pick up the trailhead for Old Jackson Road. "Instead of taking a right, we took a left and somehow ended up on the Sherburne Ski Trail," says May. The snow depths in the area, even in the relative security of Pinkham Camp, are clearly causing navigation problems. "Usually, I can tell the difference between an old road and an old trail," Boudreau says. "It gives you an idea of what the snow depth was. We weren't even conscious of where we were."

Just after 3:00 p.m., Boudreau and May are the beneficiaries of a backcountry intervention. Misha Kirk is on his way back down to Pinkham Notch Camp (PNC) from the Tuckerman Caretaker Cabin. He is not happy about the vain efforts of the day's search and will later write in his journal, "I cat-napped listening to the radios. ... As dark approached, the search was called off until daybreak. Shortly after, I left Tucks for PNC. I was frustrated, but at least rested up."

He then writes about his encounter with Boudreau and May: "As I neared PNC, I ran into two fellows hiking up. Each had huge packs with enough equipment for at least a week. I stopped and chatted with them. ... They told me they were heading for Great Gulf and thought they were on Old Jackson Road. Boy, I thought, 'There are a lot of turkeys in the mountains today.' I told them no, not quite. Then they asked me if they still continued up, could they get over to the Osgood Ridge. I patiently showed them where they were and where they had gone wrong. We had a good laugh, but I'm sure not for equal reasons."

Boudreau vividly recalls what will not be their last meeting with Kirk. "I remember just being a little embarrassed that I wasn't up to Misha's level in terms of knowledge and so forth. But when I found out later who he was, I didn't feel as bad. He was very nice and very patient with us, and it was very respectful. I was impressed with that guy, especially after what happened when we next met."

Kirk doesn't mention the active search that is underway on this side of the mountain. He bids them goodbye and continues his walk toward Pinkham. Boudreau and May hike for about five more minutes in the dark before finding a flat space at least 200 feet off the "Sherbie," where they can camp legally. "We decided to stop right then and set up our tent," says May. "That's how bad the weather was. It was snowing, windy, and cold. Things were 'in full condition,' as they say."

May's fingers are numb from the windchill, and he struggles to thread a tent pole through the nylon housing on Boudreau's cherished North Face VE-24 expedition tent. A few expletives later, he's finally able to force the pole into compliance, but not without a minor alteration. "I remember feeling bad because I bent one of the tent poles setting it up in the blizzard," he says. But Boudreau is too focused on his own battle on the opposite side of the tent to notice.

May, 24, is home on break from graduate school at the Idaho State University where he studies geology. He and Boudreau, 23, a marketing administrator at Honeywell Information Systems in Waltham, Mass., have been friends since elementary school. They did Cub Scouts and youth sports together and attended St. Sebastian's High School in Needham, Mass., where they started backpacking, rock climbing, and winter climbing together.

Although they may not be in their best climbing shape on this day, they have built extensive resumes in these and other ranges. May has climbed Mount Rainier (14,417 ft.) in Washington State, Mount Hood (11,249 ft.) in Oregon, and the Grand Teton (13,775 ft.) in northwestern Wyoming. While in graduate school, he also took a course in Advanced Wilderness First Aid. Boudreau has completed two Presidential Traverses in summer, the Franconia Ridge Traverse, and the Bonds, and spent a month in the Canadian Rockies climbing glaciers. In February 1981, Boudreau and another hiking partner summited Washington via Boott Spur and overnighted on a snowdrift before descending Lion Head the next morning. The two friends have climbed Washington together and separately a half-dozen times.

With the tent set up and rocking back and forth as the unrelenting wind and snow race through Pinkham Notch, May and Boudreau get their packs inside and settle themselves into their night's shelter. They have not packed for a light and fast trip. Quite the contrary. "We were very conservative with our packing," Boudreau says. "This was prior to the ultralight backpacking days and in the dead of winter. We were prepared to stay out for a week, so we took a couple of extra days' worth of food in case we had to ride out any weather events."

May, too, recalls how thoroughly they had prepared for the backcountry on those early outings. "Our packs were heavy—easily 70 pounds each—but we were young." They each packed or carried enough gear to fill a small outfitter's shop:

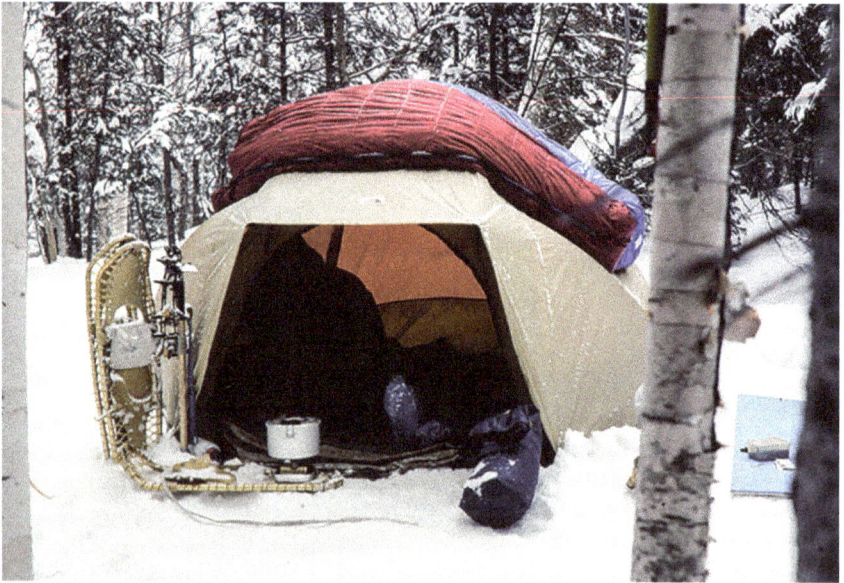

Campsite of Geoffrey May and David Boudreau during calmer conditions.

Zero-rated sleeping bag

Polypropylene long underwear

Multiple pairs of Dachstein wool socks with sock liners

Wool knickers

Fleece pants

First-generation Gore-Tex shell pants and jacket

Wool sweaters: light and heavyweight

Expedition down parka as "an emergency stopgap"

Balaclava wool hat/face mask

Dachstein mittens and Gore-Tex overmitts

Cookstove with white fuel

Sleeping pad

Crampons "in the event we could get up on the ridge"

Walking-length mountaineering axe

Chippewa leather boots lined with sheepskin (May)

EMS technical boots with felt insulation (Boudreau)

Knee-high overboots

Down booties

Flares (May)

Nylon rope (May)

Paracord (Boudreau)

Snow shovel

North Face VE-24 tent with snow pegs and ice screws

First-aid kit (both)

Blistex

Sunscreen

Map and compass

Snowshoes

Glacier glasses

Mess kit and silverware

Insulating mug

Several days' worth of food, including freeze-dried meals

Small tubes of marzipan (almond paste) for emergency energy

Headlamps with 4 D-cell batteries and "very limited battery life"

Candle lantern to limit headlamp use in tent

The two fire up the cookstove and prepare two freeze-dried meals. Despite Mother Nature's active protest outside, they settle into their down sleeping bags and rejoice in the official launch of their multi-day adventure.

"Looking back, it's a little ironic that we were up there then," says Boudreau. "We'd tried for three or four straight years to do a winter traverse of the Presidentials, but because of the bad weather, we usually ended up getting one peak in or only going to treeline. One year, we got to treeline and had to camp out for three days waiting for the weather to clear and then never got anywhere. It was always just blowin' and snowin' up above treeline."

The following morning, Boudreau and May plan to regain their bearings and link up with Old Jackson Road, which will take them north along the eastern flank of Mount Washington and, they hope, to points beyond if the weather improves. "Going into Great Gulf for that trip was Geoff's idea," says Boudreau today. "I'd seen the Gulf from Star Lake in Madison Col but had never actually been through it before. It just sounded like a good idea to me. If we got up to treeline at Madison or Adams and confirmed that we weren't in good enough physical condition to continue onto the ridge, we'd just have a nice snowshoe in the woods for a few days."

At about 6:30 p.m., Boudreau will extinguish the candle lantern and they will call it a night. Encased in their warm sleeping bags, they have no concept of how important their presence on the mountain will be or how critical what they've brought with them will become.

XXVI
FRUSTRATION

It's the terror of knowing what this world is about. Watching some good friends screaming,
"Let me out!" Pray tomorrow gets me higher, higher, high.
—David Bowie and Queen, *"Under Pressure"* (Billboard Hot 100 January 1982)

Pinkham Camp
Pinkham Notch
Sunday, Jan. 24, 1982
4:00 p.m.

Conditions above treeline continue to worsen, as the last remaining vestiges of daylight slide westward and the search for the two missing climbers is suspended for the day.

Mount Washington, always fraught with risk in winter, seems to be fortifying itself for another round with rescuers when they regroup and return in the morning. The ambient air temperature is flirting with double digits below zero and continues to backslide, along with dangerous windchill factors. Tropical-force wind speeds are expected to reach 100 mph the following day. Day two of the search for Hugh Herr and Jeff Batzer promises to be the mountain's version of a Category 2 hurricane in January, and venturing outside will be hazardous for anyone unable to stay in constant motion.

Weary searchers intermittently file into the Trading Post. They make quick work of the late lunch prepared for them by the AMC kitchen crew. Thousands of calories spent during their exertion in the cold are replenished.

MRS Team Leader Bill Kane tells them, "We're going home until tomorrow morning," expressing the consensus reached by fellow team leaders and other planners. The official report reflects their thoughts at the time: "The first day's search exhausted a number of possibilities outside of Odell Gully, but [searchers] couldn't thoroughly search the Gully itself because of weather conditions. Plans were made to reunite forces in the morning and continue with the search attempt."

Not everyone is happy with that decision. "We're just leaving them up there to die?" MRS member Steve Larson asks Kane. It is more a statement than a question. "We're the only ones that can get them," he urges. Kane recalls the exchange with his teammate and a few others who wished to go back outside and up. "But I told them it was just too dangerous, and that we'd go back up there the next morning."

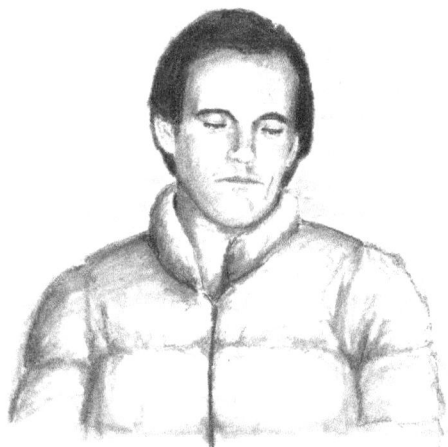

Bill Kane

The frustration some are feeling that evening is indicative of the drive and commitment searchers bring to every outing. "Basically, you have a sense of purpose," says Larson today. "You have a desire to help, and you're just getting shut down. I'm just a soldier, and I want to go out there to try to help. You feel like you have more time in the day and that time is of the essence, because you worry people won't survive the night."

Now having served on MRS for over four decades, Larson has grown more sensitive to the heavy weight team leaders carry when out on a mission. "I was not in a leadership position at the time," he acknowledges. "The pressure of being responsible for all of these people is immense. You have to think first about the safety of your rescue teams."

Plans for day two of the search are not yet fully formed when searchers are sent home Sunday night. "We had a rough idea of what we were going to do, because at that point people had only searched the bottom of the gullies," says MRS Team Leader Joe Lentini. "It was pretty much assumed that the next day, if we went out, we'd be up in the gullies."

Over the course of the afternoon, having made their own selfless contributions to the search for their young cabinmates, Harvard Cabin guests Jim Frati, Hank Butler, Bob MacEntee, Paul Geissler, Kacy St. Clair, and Layne Tyrrell collect their gear and head homeward.

With the cabin empty of guests, Matt Pierce prepares to descend to Pinkham carrying his wet gear. He'll grab some food at the cafeteria, dry out his gear, stay the night, and head back up in the morning following breakfast. But before shutting the rustic cabin's heavy wooden door behind him, he makes one last entry in the log:

> Two climbers missing since yesterday. The AMC, Forest Service, Fish & Game, and the MRS were all involved to no avail. The climbers, Hugh & Jeff, were last seen heading up Odell's 9:00 AM Sat. We've found the pack of one of them but nothing else. Tomorrow the search will continue...
> —The Caretaker

XXVII
INTERSECTIONS

The terrible 'Ifs' accumulate.
—Winston Churchill

Great Gulf: Temperature: 3°F; winds are low; visibility: dusk; light snowfall.

Old Jackson Road/Mount Washington Auto Road (2,600 ft.)
Sunday, Jan. 24, 1982
4:00 p.m.

At this late hour, when most of the rescuers have been called back, one team still remains on the search. After teaching a winter camping workshop on Sunday morning, Jeff Tirey and AMC crew member Jack Corbin were recruited to form a small team, along with AMC crew member Mike Waddell, to look for signs that Hugh Herr and Jeff Batzer might have used the Mount Washington Auto Road as a bailout route. They set off from Pinkham at 1:30 p.m. and hiked north on Old Jackson Road (OJR) on their way to the point where it meets the Auto Road just above the two-mile mark.

Directly across the Auto Road, OJR intersects with Madison Gulf Trail, which leads into Great Gulf Wilderness. Great Gulf is not part of the searchers' equation because Herr and Batzer had been ice-climbing in Huntington Ravine, and it was highly unlikely they would end up there. But in fact, Great Gulf is exactly where the two remain lost and trapped.

Old Jackson Road leaves Pinkham Camp and climbs steadily, and sometimes steeply, for 1.8 miles until it reaches the Auto Road. The route is positioned well below treeline, which is why this assignment is allowed to continue into the evening.

"OJR wasn't that bad," recalls Jeff Tirey today. "It was just a lot of breaking trail, so we did rotations to share the work. It was a great snow year in 1982. You had to use snowshoes, because if you didn't, you were in deep, deep trouble."

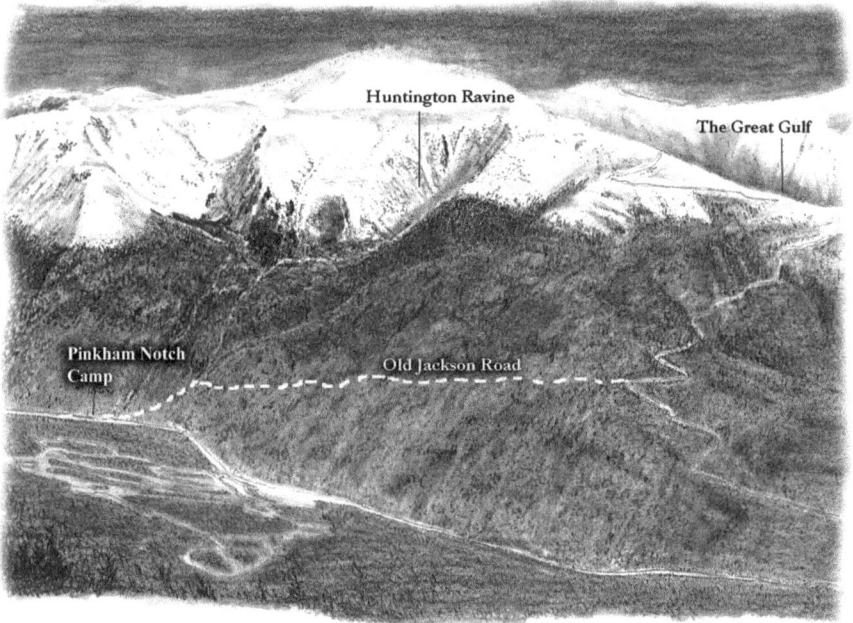

Old Jackson Road from Pinkham Notch to the Mount Washington Auto Road.

As they arrive at the intersection of OJR and the Auto Road in late afternoon, they find the surroundings eerily peaceful. The occasional drone of heavy trucks moving across Route 16 down below and the distant, crashing sound of the westerly winds moving over exposed terrain higher up do not compare with the extreme conditions other teams have been reporting.

The three stand in a horizontal line from one side of the Auto Road to the other and methodically scan it for boot prints, discarded gear, or other signs of the missing climbers. Sunset is still 43 minutes away, but darkness has already settled in. Toward day's end in January, the ambient light is smothered by the steep walls of the Northern Presidential Range. So the three searchers switch on their clunky D-cell headlamps and continue walking upward in unison. As the narrow beams of light sweep back and forth on the road, the only signs of human activity are the bulldozer tracks carved in the snow by the sharp cleats of the Observatory's Thiokol, which shuttled a team from Mountain Rescue Service up the mountain earlier in the day.

Tirey, who previously worked for the Randolph Mountain Club and the Mount Washington Observatory, has taken the week off from his engineering job in Winchester, Mass., to complete a multi-day Mahoosuc Traverse with friends. But that trip will be delayed by at least a day. As Tirey and his two companions round the corner near Two-Mile Spring, the thought of a winter excursion for pleasure is the furthest thing from his mind. For one thing, he's not optimistic that Herr and Batzer are still alive as their confounding disappearance enters its second frigid night. But his selfless involvement in the search for them is also serving as a trigger, forcing him to contend with the haunting memory of his own brush with death two years earlier on this very mountain range.

On the morning of Easter Sunday, April 6, 1980, Tirey and Richard Morse set out from Gray Knob Cabin on Mount Adams to do some ice climbing in King Ravine. Their plan was to descend Great Gully to the floor of the ravine and climb a frozen waterfall located at the bottom. After the technical climb, they would reascend Great Gully and return to the cabin, where Tirey was the caretaker and Morse was staying with four companions.

"We reached the top of Great Gully at 7:30 a.m. to descend to the frozen waterfall," says Tirey. "But before we glissaded down, I tried to trigger an avalanche to see if we were at risk. We'd gotten only six inches of snow the night before, so it didn't seem like it was super high-risk."

With Morse standing a short distance away, Tirey stomped on the snow trying to force its release. "I was doing what I could to get a slough to go, and I was doing it at the point of convexity of the head of the gully because that's where most of the stresses are in the snow."

At that point, Tirey wasn't able to trigger a slide. But he realized later that he had made a tactical error. "It was early April, and I wasn't thinking about the fact that the temperature can change 20 to 30 degrees from early morning to mid/late morning," he says today. "That difference can result in snow melt that creates a slide plane for loose snow." As it turned out, there were stresses, but they did not create a snow slide until a few hours later when the two were on their way back up the gully at about 8:30 a.m.

Tirey and Morse were not roped together as they ascended. To some, this may seem like a reckless decision, but for climbers it's about weighing the risks and mitigating them. "It was a conscious decision not to rope up," says Tirey. "When roped, you are inextricably tied together so, for better or worse, if one falls you might both fall. It seemed safer to climb without the rope because once we were off the ice, we were just traveling on snow."

Between 9:30 and 10:00 a.m., the two were almost at the top. Morse was off to the side, and Tirey recalls being right in the center of the gully. "All of a sudden, [Morse] said, 'Hey, what's that crack there?' I looked up and ahead four to five feet, and there was a crack in the snow on the slope that ran across the entire width of the gully. I knew what that meant. I was like, 'Oh shit, this could go.'"

They immediately stopped their ascent for fear of setting off the slope. A pillowy wind slab at the top of the gully had weakened as the temperature rose that morning. They each needed an anchor in the snow to hold them in place if things did let loose. "I was going to plunge my ice axe into the snow so that if it did let go, I'd hopefully have some type of belay going for myself," says Tirey. "I lifted my arm to plunge my axe in, and the whole thing let loose. The motion of my body was enough to kick it off. So I was the one that triggered that avalanche, and it was just a hell of a long ride."

Both climbers were pulled from their stances as gravity assumed control of the 4-to-6-inch-thick slab. Interestingly, this was not the first time Tirey found himself in an avalanche. While attending college, he was climbing Maine's Katahdin when he was caught in one, so he had a sense of what he needed to do if he hoped to survive. "Because of my experience on Katahdin, I knew to try and keep my feet pointed downhill and to swim with it," he says. "I couldn't do much about the fact that I had crampons on, so I knew that was going to be an issue. As I started sliding, the heel of one of my crampons caught and spun me around so that my back was facing downhill. I didn't want to be going downhill backwards, so I managed to free my foot and turn back around. I was still trying to self-arrest, but I was riding on top of all of the snow that was sliding, so I couldn't plant the point of my axe."

Tirey and Morse ended up plummeting hundreds of feet with such speed that they were unable to use their axes to stop or even slow their fall. Then, toward the bottom of the gully, this potentially catastrophic event delivered its knockout punch. "We rode the way down, and all of a sudden, I found myself floating," Tirey recalls. "Then I realized where I was. We had shot off the top of the frozen waterfall we'd climbed earlier, and I realized I was going to drop a couple hundred feet to the ground below. At that point, my body told my mind to just shut down. So everything from the moment I went airborne until I came to a stop at the base of the frozen waterfall is all blank. I have no recollection of it at all."

Tirey estimates he and Morse fell 1,500 to 2,000 feet. Although badly injured, neither was buried. "Luckily, there wasn't enough snow to form a deep deposition," says Tirey. "We were on top of the snow when it stopped."

They were rescued after hikers heard Tirey screaming for help at approximately 10:00 a.m. One of the good Samaritans, Justin Whitney from Winthrop, Maine, bushwhacked through deep snow and a boulder field and reached them at noon. After treating them with guidance from the injured Tirey, Whitney hiked out at 2:00 p.m. to notify authorities. At 4:00 p.m., some six and a half hours after the avalanche, Whitney was able to reach Pinkham Camp by phone.

Misha Kirk and Pinkham Notch hutmaster Jon Martinson arrived on the scene at 9:00 p.m. By 10:00 p.m., 40 rescuers—from New Hampshire Fish and Game, the U.S. Forest Service, the AMC, and Mountain Rescue Service—were also there. Among the 18 members of Mountain Rescue Service who responded were Albert Dow, Michael Hartrich, Joe Lentini, and Bill Kane.

After four and a half hours of carrying two litters through deep snow, the rescuers arrived with Tirey and Morse at the trailhead on Route 2 at 2:30 a.m. Morse, who was knocked unconscious by the fall, suffered a concussion, fractured ribs, and fractured vertebrae. Tirey fractured both ankles, a breastbone, and two vertebrae. Both suffered frostbitten feet.

Today, Tirey offers an objective assessment of his decision-making on that Sunday in 1980. "Hindsight being 20/20 and having about 45 years to reflect on that incident, there's a lot of things I would have done differently," he admits. "I didn't pay close enough attention. Like many climbers who are young and dumb, I ignored some signs. I did test for signs of avalanche, but conditions change over the course of hours, and I didn't take that into consideration."

The avalanche in King Ravine could have easily caused Tirey to hang up his climbing gear and walk away from the mountains altogether. Instead, he leaned in. He would not only return to climbing, he would fully engage himself in volunteer search and rescue missions. He would go on to become one of the founding members of the Androscoggin Valley Search and Rescue Team (AVSAR) when it was organized in 1988.

Like all backcountry search and rescue personnel in New Hampshire, Tirey was drawn to the work by a deep sense of purpose and recognition that the line separating them from the people they're helping is razor thin. "When you've been on the inside of a litter, it is much easier to understand what the person is going through and the relief they can feel being removed from danger. You can't change their circumstances, but you can give them some reassurance that things should get better. Not always, but usually. For me, this was payback for the generosity of time and expertise that others had given me. I feel extremely lucky to have survived my own accident when I was sure I wouldn't. It completely changed my perspective on the notion of community service and my own participation in that effort. … I have come to believe that when you have various skill sets, you should use them when you can to help other people. That's just being part of humanity."

Though some thoughts of his earlier traumatic experience are creeping into Tirey's consciousness as he and his teammates scour the Auto Road, all three are focusing on the task at hand. With no indication that Herr and Batzer have been here, they move back in the direction of the OJR trailhead. The creak and snap of their cold wooden snowshoes on hardpacked snow is replaced by a wispy "whoomp" as they step into the heavy powder blanketing the trail. Their backs now to the Auto Road and the entrance to Madison Gulf Trail, they hike back toward Pinkham.

Unbeknownst to them, they are the closest any searchers have come to Herr and Batzer since the search began 12 hours earlier.

Great Gulf/Madison Gulf Trail Junction (2,247 ft.)
4:00 p.m.

Hugh Herr and Jeff Batzer stand atop deep snow reaching the

handrails of the wooden footbridge that spans the West Branch of the Peabody River. When they first crossed the bridge at 8:30 a.m., they felt a sense of progress, believing it was their gateway to Madison Hut and self-rescue. Both are famished, dehydrated, and exhausted. They're dejected by the realization that their expended effort has led them on yet another path to nowhere. For the subdued Herr, it is further confirmation that death is imminent.

Neither is aware that searchers are two miles away from them on the Auto Road. And even if they were, in their present state, two miles might as well be 10,000. No one is coming for them.

"It was 2 or 3 in the afternoon, and we couldn't understand why we weren't at the hut," Batzer says. "So we turned around and headed back down, which was a lot easier than climbing up. We got back to where we'd started out that morning, where there's this modern bridge in the middle of the woods, but we still couldn't get anywhere. It was discouraging."

In fact, Herr and Batzer have covered only 1.7 miles in seven and a half hours, having set off at 8:30 a.m. toward Madison Hut from the trail junction only to return to their starting point.

Unsteady on their feet because of the onset of muscle failure, the two are careful to avoid falling off the narrow wall of snow and down onto the ice-covered river. Darkness is taking hold in this deep glacial cirque, as is the stark reality of a second night out in the wilderness. Each scans the riverbanks hoping to find shelter for the night.

On the opposite side of the river, some 100 feet away from them, is a large boulder. Having survived the previous night under one of these, they cross the footbridge, link back up with the Great Gulf Trail, and move in the direction of the 10-by-10-foot glacial erratic. Once parallel to it, they descend a steep 20-foot embankment carved over time by raging waters from thousands of spring snowmelts.

"The strange thing is we were able to see the bridge from the boulder," says Batzer. "It seemed like such a strange place to potentially die, right next to a bridge that would've had so many people there at one point building it."

They waste no time preparing the shelter for another round with the cold. "We started with same approach as the night before, with branches," says Batzer. "There weren't as many as there were farther back in the gulf, and it was harder to collect them because we were so weak. We had to work hard."

They lay a bed of spruce and fir branches in an empty space between the boulder and the ground. The space is neither flat nor deep enough for them to get fully inside.

Then, without warning, Herr collapses onto the snow. With Batzer's help, he regains his feet only to drop to the ground again.

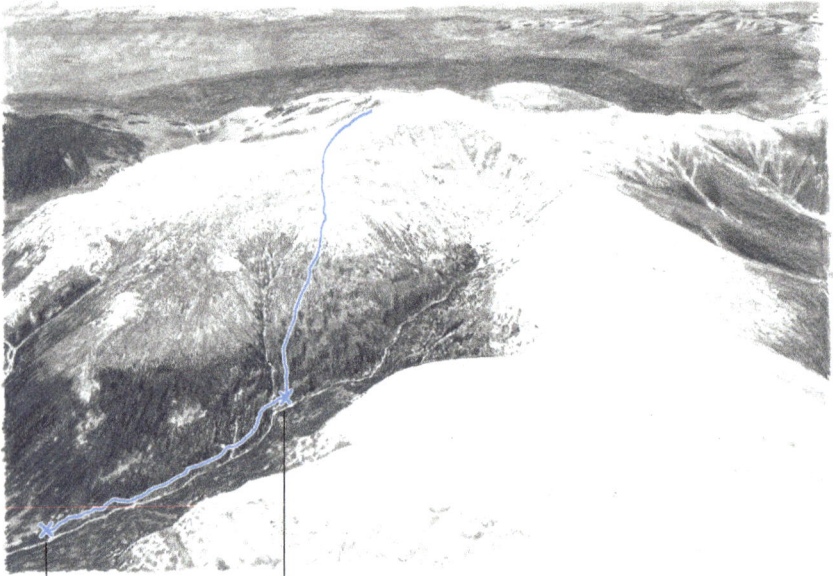

Hugh Herr and Jeff Batzer's bivouac on the night of the 23rd

Bivouac on the night of the 24th

"My feet were numb, and I couldn't balance," says Herr. "It wasn't even a thought at the time. Out there, I didn't think I was going to live, so I wasn't even thinking about my body parts. I didn't care."

"He probably collapsed because he was so cold and exhausted," says cold-weather injury expert Dr. Gordon Giesbrecht. "People can walk long distances on frozen feet, and you don't feel it, but it can still be tough to maintain balance."

Herr slides himself onto the thin layer of branches lining the floor of the empty space where he's joined by Batzer. As they sit next to one another, they unlace their stiff leather boots and in unison begin to pry them off. But neither can remove them because the tips of their socks are frozen to the boots' interior. Using the blades of their ice axes, they slide them down in between their feet and the boots and saw off the tips of the socks.

As they did the previous night, they leave their boots off, jamming them down into the bottom of the void. "We were still concerned about frostbite damage," says Batzer. "What we should have done was to keep our boots on and wrap our feet up. Then we'd be ready to go when we got our strength back and just take the frostbite damage. At that point, our concern should have been on maintaining our core temperature, but we were so concerned about frostbite that I took my 60/40 parka off and wrapped it around our legs."

They are feet in, but because the cave is so shallow, they can only get hip deep, leaving most of their upper torsos exposed. Herr, 5-foot-9 and 130 pounds, and Batzer 5-foot-7 and 120 pounds, cover themselves with the remaining boughs. They face one another and hug as they did the night before to preserve the waning vestiges of body heat. "We had a ton of branches under and over us on the first night, but on the second night there were far fewer."

As they lie in their rudimentary emergency bivouac and brace themselves for the long night ahead, Sgt. Carl Carlson of New Hampshire Fish and Game notifies their families by phone that the pair is missing.

"My mom and dad and my oldest brother and his wife had gathered at my parents' house for the Super Bowl," recalls Batzer. "They were just about ready to sit down to eat lasagna when Fish and Game called. They told my mom there were 30 to 40 people searching for us and to wait there because there was going to be an early morning search for us on Monday. At that point nobody was able to eat, and my parents and brother were quickly making plans about how they all were going to be able get to Mount Washington by the next day."

In her book *Second Ascent: The Story of Hugh Herr*, author Alison Osius relates that when Herr's parents were informed by a phone call from their son Tony that his youngest brother and Batzer were missing, their mother Martha's initial response was consistent with the independence and self-reliance she and husband John had instilled in their children. "Knowing Hugh…," she began. "He's always inclined to make the most of any climbing trip, to squeeze in one last climb." But Tony, who was very concerned, called his mother a second time to talk about the situation. "You know how those boys are," she said again, gently. "They're probably just getting in now. Let's just see what the morning brings."

The morning would not bring relief, however, Since leaving Harvard Cabin Saturday morning, Herr and Batzer have traveled through some of the most difficult terrain anywhere, with no food or water. They are in such a caloric deficit that their bodies are now consuming themselves for energy.

"We were not giving up, though," says Batzer. "I can remember crying out to God for help that night. We were encouraging each other, not undercutting or criticizing the other. We were always fighting for the other person."

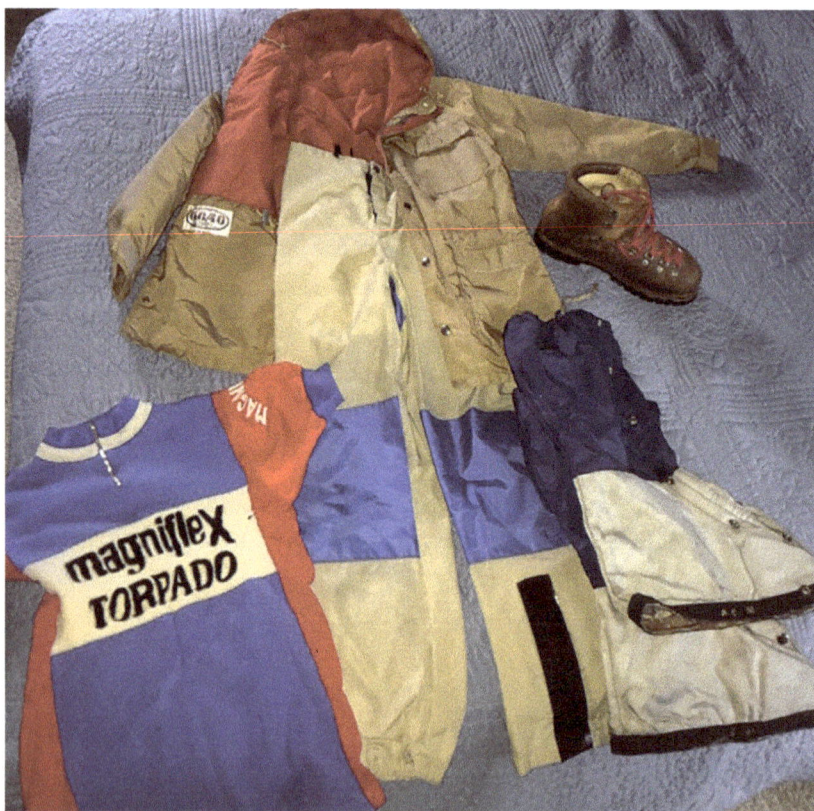

The clothing Jeff Batzer was wearing during his ordeal in Great Gulf.

XXVIII
PRIMED

Darkness crept back into the forests of the world.
Rumor grew of a shadow in the East, whispers of a nameless fear...
—Galadriel, *Lord of the Rings*

Mount Washington Observatory Surface Weather Observations (6:00 p.m. Sunday, Jan. 24, to 5:00 a.m. Monday, Jan. 25): Lowest temperature -24°F; winds out of the west averaging 72 mph; visibility 0 miles; snow/blowing snow/ fog; lowest windchill -71.0°F; peak wind gust: 85 mph.

Cutler River Drainage
Mount Washington
Monday, Jan. 25, 1982
Early morning

Dawn arrives to find Mother Nature still laying siege to Mount Washington. It's been more than 30 hours since winds shifted west and launched their unrelenting snow assault on the eastern side of the mountain. Banner after banner of wind-driven snow jettisons from the rims, ridges, and ledges of Cutler River Drainage. Tuckerman, Raymond, and Huntington Ravines—and every slope in between— are suffocating. A close look at the weather patterns leading up to this day reveals the risks being assumed by anyone venturing into the high country, as dozens of rescuers are about to do.

Winter on Mount Washington is like a giant canvas with precipitation the medium, temperature the brush, and wind the artist. High- and low-pressure weather systems that arrive on one of three storm tracks drive erratic fluctuations in air temperature, precipitation type, and wind direction, creating unpredictable weaknesses in the snowpack. Snowfall that is heavy and wet (high density), light and fluffy (low density), rain, sleet, or any combination of these can set up hazards.

During the month of December 1981, 54 inches of snow fell on the mountain. Every nook and cranny beneath alpine vegetation or between rocks and boulders was now chock full. Winds then polished the snow down to a flat, firm surface. This allowed winds of varying strength to transport snow across the terrain and into the lee areas of the mountain. The average wind speed in winter is 45 mph. From October to May, the windiest months on Washington, the summit experiences hurricane-force winds 15 days per month and winds of 100 mph or more seven to eight days per month.

The first four days of the new year brought 15 inches of heavy, wet snow. Above-freezing temperatures and about an hour of light rainfall on Jan. 4 added water and weight to an already heavy snowpack.

One day later, on Jan. 5, the first of three critical changes in the snowpack occurred. Temperatures dropped sharply below freezing and never looked back. From Jan. 10 through 12, the ambient air temperature ranged from -18°F to -31°F. So the heavy, wet snow that had fallen the week before froze solid, creating a thick layer of crust. Known as a "melt-freeze crust," this layer can become a slick bed for future snow to slide on.

Throughout January, there was periodic snowfall, and because temperatures were so cold, it remained light and fluffy. From Jan. 17 through 19, temperatures plummeted to between -13°F and -39°F. The crystals within the plate-shaped snowflakes that were resting on the terrain or freshly falling were so weakened by the arctic air that they were slow to bind together and consolidate. Extremely strong, sustained westerly winds on Jan. 17 and 18, reaching 114 miles per hour at their peak, removed any of the new snow still sitting on open slopes.

Between the hours of 1:00 a.m. and 2:00 p.m. on Jan. 20, the summit of Washington received 2.1 inches of low-density snow. Another round of strong, sustained westerly winds, with gusts approaching 140 mph, again scoured newly-fallen snow from exposed open areas and deposited it into lower elevations on the eastern aspects of the mountain, where it accumulated in areas protected by terrain features or areas with dense trees.

More moderate wind speeds, ranging from 15 to 40 mph, are ideal for building slabs on the mountain's major avalanche paths. At these lower speeds, cold, dry snow will gradually form slabs, often taking 24 hours or more to form a large one. They tend to do so higher up, in established avalanche paths. But because of the mountain's topography, westerly winds like the ones blowing during this rescue attempt are particularly effective at building slabs in lee terrain.

When winds exceed 60 mph, they will move copious amounts of snow very quickly. Low-density snow, the kind that fell from Jan. 23 to 25, is easily transported. Under the right conditions, an inch of snow that falls on Alpine Garden can become a 10-inch-thick wind slab somewhere else. Winds at this speed strip snow off the surface of exposed areas and send it into the air, a process known as "turbulent suspension." Such winds will push snow over cliffs or ravines, where the air then becomes turbulent, slows down, and deposits the snow onto lower terrain.

On Saturday, Jan. 23, when Hugh Herr and Jeff Batzer went missing, seven inches of light, fluffy snow fell on the mountain. Early in the day, southerly winds were moving it north and depositing significant amounts of snow into northern ravines like Great Gulf, where Herr and Batzer have become lost. Late in the evening, the southerly winds shifted to the west, and wind speeds decreased to around 30 mph forming softer, weaker slabs on east-facing aspects such as the Cutler River Drainage. This was likely the start of the development of the weak, soft layer of snow sitting on top of the hard, melt-freeze crust, and represents the second critical change in the snowpack.

The relentless west wind overnight and into Sunday, ranging from 50 to 55 mph, coupled with additional snowfall and rising temperatures, increased the size of these east-facing soft slabs. Then stronger wind speeds and warmer temperatures created a slightly denser layer on top of the softer layer below it. This softer layer, sandwiched between the Jan. 5 melt-freeze crust and the more dense snow on top of it, acted as a weak layer, creating a strong-over-weak unstable snow structure. This was the beginning of the third and final critical change in the snowpack.

Now on Monday morning, the winds are still moving walls of snow to the east, loading the ravines. It is likely that avalanches triggered by natural forces occurred somewhere on the mountain the previous day but were not witnessed because of the extreme weather conditions limiting visibility.

A broad area of low pressure out toward Quebec is traversing the region and pulling cold air down from the Canadian plains. As this arctic air mass sweeps across the Great Lakes, it will move into the area. Winds coming from the west will get even stronger, sustaining the transport of snow.

Four components must be present for a slab avalanche to occur: a steep slope of 30 degrees or more, snow cover with a weak layer beneath it, and someone or something to set it off. At this early hour, the eastern side of Mount Washington is primed. As searchers roll out of bed and prepare to depart for Pinkham, they face a mountain where localized instability in the snowpack could pose significant risks, underscoring the need for caution. The mountain's hammer is cocked, and they will need to keep their guard up so as not to pull the trigger.

XXIX
PERSEVERANCE

Starting to race through the final chapters of the [Lord of the Rings]
trilogy…honestly sorry to see it drawing to an end, which is ironic because it is
now so exciting and full of suspense that I do not want to put it down
(it is a sad race to the end!).
—Albert Dow, in a letter to his family Jan. 23, 1981

Great Gulf: Temperature: -14°F; windy; visibility darkness; light snowfall.

Emergency Bivouac Site (2,247 ft.)
Great Gulf Trail Junction
Monday, Jan. 25, 1982
5:30 a.m.

Jeff Batzer winces as he gently palpates the middle finger of his
left hand. It was just after midnight when the realization hit him that
he'd lost his ability to keep both hands warm. It seemed inconsequential
two days earlier when one of his Gore-Tex overmitts skidded down
the ice in Odell Gully. Batzer's brain, sensing alarm, immediately
activated his ego, which underplayed the mistake, allowing him to
dismiss the lost piece of gear as a minor inconvenience. Nothing to
see here; I'll be fine. Just keep climbing! But after two days and nights
in extreme conditions, Batzer's left hand is now freezing from the
absence of blood flow. Unfortunately, it isn't yet numb enough to
deaden the feeling of a sharp pencil point being driven into the tip of
his nearly frozen middle finger.

Winds, which had remained calm once Herr and Batzer reached
the floor of Great Gulf on Saturday afternoon and seemed to be the
only thing going right for them, are now pounding the lower portion
of the Gulf where the pair are hunkered down. The ambient
temperature, which had been holding steady at or just above zero, has
also begun a steep slide made worse by the windchill. Sunrise is 90
minutes away and will only serve to make their dire circumstances
more visible to them. Restorative sleep remains as elusive as the way

out of the Gulf.

"I was never able to sleep during the entire ordeal," says Batzer today. "I was just so miserable and wide awake the whole time even though I was exhausted."

As they rest beneath the layer of spruce and fir boughs blanketing them, Herr and Batzer are readying themselves for a final self-rescue attempt. They're remaining as still as possible to preserve their energy, embracing to retain warmth, and offering each other positive encouragement. "There was still no tension between us," says Batzer. "Hugh was fighting for me as much as I was fighting for him. It was maybe 1:00 or 2:00 a.m., and we told each other we'd have to preserve our energy in order to get out that morning. We were facing exhaustion, we were extremely thirsty and cold, but we felt like we had enough strength for one final attack. We knew we weren't going to be able to keep doing it. It was definitely starting to get the best of us."

Perhaps because of his two immersions in the icy river, Herr's physical condition is worse than Batzer's. He is freezing to death from the feet up. Batzer is holding on, but his ability to do so is tenuous.

"Hugh was definitely in worse shape," acknowledges Batzer. "I realized he was not going to be good for an attempt out. He was delirious, not talking much, and not very responsive to my encouragement to move out. I kept telling him we had to make one last attempt. He was very calm, almost deadpan, but totally without energy. He had always been the leader on our climbs. When I was really fearful, he'd say, 'Hold it together Jeff, don't panic. We're going to figure it out. We'll be all right.' But on that Monday morning, the roles were reversed."

Batzer's 60/40 winter parka they've used to wrap around their legs for warmth during their two overnights is now frozen and useless. The contorted and rigid garment relinquished all insulating properties after Batzer perspired heavily in it on their failed attempt to reach Madison Hut the day before.

"This was a huge epic for these guys," says Dr. Gordon Giesbrecht. "They had three things going on: They were completely dehydrated, malnourished, and suffering from frostbite. Their extremities froze because there was no blood flow. There were ice crystals forming in the tissues. Tissue is composed of 70 percent water, so when it freezes, the ice crystals themselves can do damage. We tell people to never rub frostbite because you're moving ice crystals in there. Then once the area eventually thaws, there will be a lot of blood there that will re-profuse throughout the body. Capillaries and tissue will be damaged or destroyed, sending toxins into the kidneys and bloodstream."

The next phase in their preparation to extract themselves from Great Gulf requires an enormous investment of energy—and they have very little of that left. They need to don their alpine boots, which are frozen and as solid as the boulder that partially shelters them. "We needed to try to get our boots on," Batzer recalls. "We had to get ready even though everything was frozen and make an attack in the dark. We knew we needed to get moving because if we stayed there, we were going to die."

Eastern Mountain Sports
North Conway, N.H.
5:50 a.m.

Albert Dow laughs as he shivers. From the passenger seat of friend and Mountain Rescue Service teammate Dana Seavey's car, he rocks back and forth rubbing his gloved hands together.

"Albert and I drove up to Pinkham together in my old Ford Maverick that had no heat in it," recalls Seavey. "I know it sounds strange today, but I recall joking with Albert in the car, and I remember—at the first steep switchback on Route 16 just before Pinkham—thinking to myself how much fun I was having."

Like Dow, Seavey works as an instructor/guide for MRS Team Leader Joe Lentini at the Eastern Mountain Sports (EMS) Climbing School. As was customary back then, MRS members often met at EMS, or across the street at International Mountain Equipment (IME), to carpool for callouts.

Two years earlier Seavey, like many of his teammates, moved to North Conway to pursue his passion for climbing. At the time he knew no one, and it was Dow who went out of his way to make the newcomer feel welcome.

"When I moved to North Conway by myself to become a climber

in 1980, it was initially a bit intimidating," says Seavey. "I was on the fast track, but I still felt like a Gumby in the elite North Conway climbing scene. Becoming friends and guiding and climbing with someone like Albert allowed me to feel like I finally belonged. We climbed a lot together on mixed rock and ice on Mount Willard in Crawford Notch. He would use rock climbing protection instead of ice screws and would just cruise up the gullies. I really looked up to Albert. In fact, I idolized him a bit. He was super fun to be with. He had no ego and was such a gifted athlete and climber."

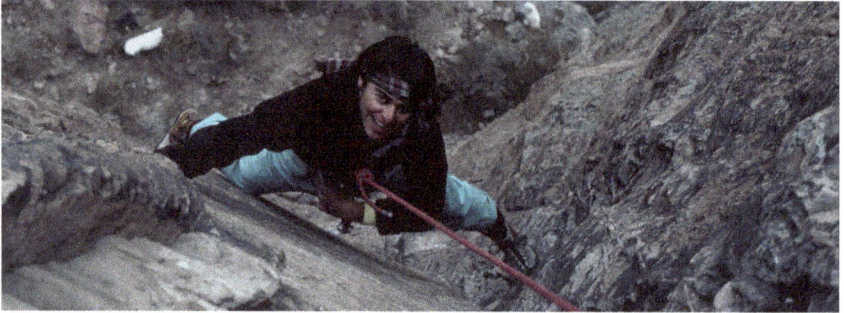

Albert Dow finding complete joy in Albuquerque, N.M.

Dow, Seavey, and other members of MRS who are en route to Pinkham know it is likely that some of them will be assigned to searching gullies in Huntington Ravine. Today, Seavey reflects on Dow's mindset as they approached Pinkham. "Albert wasn't all that thrilled about the possibility of climbing that day. In no way was he saying he was afraid or concerned about safety; he just did not enjoy basic ice climbing as much as he did rock."

Dow's younger sister, Caryl, would learn later that her brother was wary of the conditions, but that his wariness was overpowered by his sense of service. "That morning, Albert shared with someone close to him that he was concerned that the snowpack conditions were horrific," she says. "But he said, 'I have to go.' Like the rest of his teammates, my brother went out not because he was forced to go, but because someone needed help."

As Seavey pulls into the freshly plowed parking lot of Pinkham Camp, he is surprised by the number of vehicles already there given the extreme weather. "We spent five minutes or so sorting through gear," says Seavey. "Albert definitely liked to climb light, and I remember him putting the gear he didn't need in the back seat of my car: an extra parka, gloves, and some other gear. He said, 'I'm not going to need my rock gear, so I'm going to thin my pack down.' Then we headed inside to get breakfast."

"During that ride up with Albert," Seavey adds, "I was saying to myself, 'Look at you, Dana! You're driving to a big rescue with Albert Dow!' Life was just so good at that moment, until it wasn't, only hours later."

Once planning for the day is complete and teams are dispatched to their assignments, a critical and increasingly dangerous phase in the search for Hugh Herr and Jeff Batzer will begin. For Dow, Seavey, and their fellow searchers, it is a race against time … and time is winning.

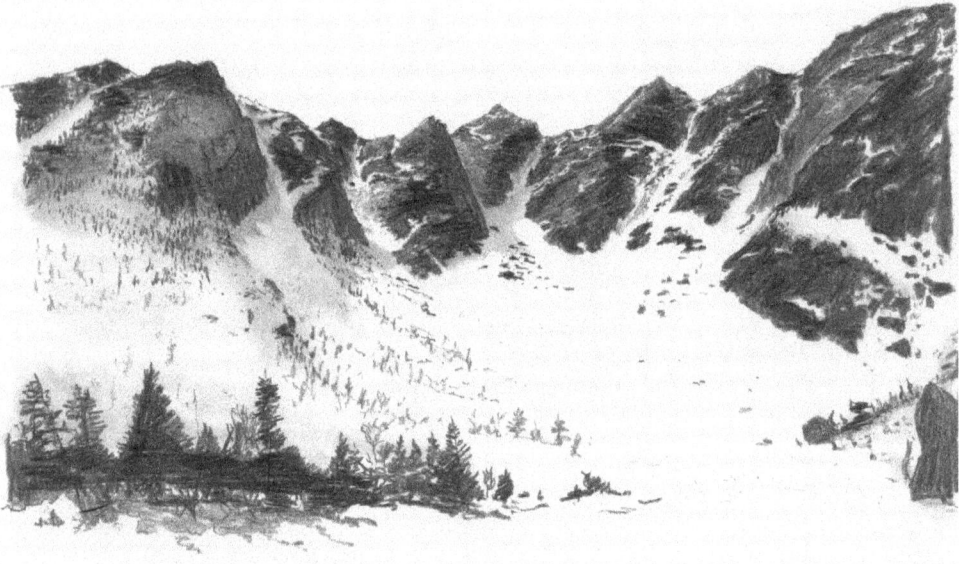

Huntington Ravine

XXX
TREADING LIGHTLY

It does not do to leave a live dragon out of your calculations,
if you live near him.
—J.R.R. Tolkien, *The Hobbit*

Mount Washington Observatory Surface Weather Observations (7:00 to 8:00 a.m.): Temperature -26°F; winds out of the west averaging 84 mph; visibility 0 miles; snow/blowing snow/fog; windchill -75.6°F; peak wind gust: 92 mph.

Pinkham Notch
Monday, Jan. 25, 1982
6:45 a.m.

The comforting aroma of freshly-cooked bacon and coffee wafts through the expansive dining room at AMC's Pinkham Camp. The complex is filled with guests of the Joe Dodge Lodge, who have decided to stay out of the day's brutal weather, and searchers readying themselves for their unavoidable confrontation with it.

Conversations among both are filled with worry and conjecture about the two missing climbers. "There was this dark mood over the whole camp, and it was really all-consuming," says AMC crew member Alan Kamman, who had been searching on Lion Head the day before. "No one at camp had slept well because we knew Hugh and Jeff were out there. Everyone knew the consequences were really grave, and it just permeated everything."

Huddled at a table in the back corner are members of the planning team, who are carefully plotting a strategy for the day's search. All agree that the focus will be technical in nature, and that small teams from the all-volunteer Mountain Rescue Service will do the heavy lifting. "The plan was to go into Huntington Ravine and climb the gullies," says MRS co-Team Leader Joe Lentini. "Herr and Batzer had supposedly done Odell's, so we would search there, and also the gullies to the left of it in case that's where they descended."

At this point, approximately 600 feet of Odell Gully remains unsearched, and planners have to consider the possibility that Herr and Batzer might still be in there.

Bill Kane, Lentini's co-team leader, recalls the glimmer of optimism he still held on to that morning. "I thought if the two were in a place where they'd have a level of shelter, they could still be alive. A few years before, we'd rescued guys who'd been on the mountain for a day and a half. So we asked ourselves how they'd have gotten back down, because they weren't in the obvious places where we thought they'd be. Everybody was on edge, everybody was worried, because we had two kids up there. We knew we were in a dangerous situation."

As planners continue their work, word spreads among some of the searchers that Hugh Herr is a well-known and exceptional climber. One of Herr's idols, Henry Barber, had been alerted about the search for Herr and Batzer by a mutual acquaintance and called to relay this information to a member of the search team by phone. "I had a view of Huntington Ravine from my living room window and was at my house when Hugh and Jeff were lost," Barber recalls today. "All I could see was the shrouded mountain and plumes of snow blowing off the peaks. It was westerly, so the clouds were boiling in over Monroe and the Southern Presidentials, and every once in a while, there was enough visibility that I could see the wind blowing off Jefferson, Madison, and Adams. I said something to the searchers based on what I knew about Hugh. All I could do was let them know that."

Dana Seavey, who had driven to Pinkham with teammate Albert Dow, remembers hearing the buzz about Herr that morning. "We were told Hugh was a world-class climber. We knew these guys were fit and tough, but being able to climb 5.8 doesn't necessarily equate to navigating a whiteout."

Michael Hartrich also recalls hearing the talk about Herr. "It turns out that Hugh was a budding superstar," he says. "So to me, he wasn't just blunting around up there. Even though he wasn't an experienced ice climber, ice climbing has always been looked upon as something that anybody can pick up. Rock climbing takes technique and skill, but ice climbing is a pretty simple thing. So the idea was that these guys might have been fully capable of this. But where were they?"

Lentini says today that Herr's reported skills did not matter in the moment. "They'd left gear behind because they were going to come back, so no matter how skilled they were, they were still missing, and we had no idea where they were."

Every planner and search team member is highly aware of the ongoing avalanche hazard that this day presents. But it is important to note that in 1982 avalanche awareness, education, forecasting, and knowledge of how avalanche terrain should be navigated was markedly different from what it is today. The focus back then was on already established slide paths in Huntington and Tuckerman Ravines, with most avalanches occurring on the Tuckerman headwall itself.

"Back then, the ravines were either open or closed," says Rene LaRoche, then a snow ranger and member of the planning team. "We'd go out in the morning and check Huntington and then Tuckerman's. If we saw avalanche danger, we'd hike up each side of it and try to come down and start a slide. If it wasn't that dangerous, we'd tie together and come down on top of it with a spotter. We didn't have avalanche beacons or anything. In the springtime, we'd use rifles to shoot at ice above the headwall to make it fall onto the snowpack below. We'd shoot off a car-sized chunk to start the slide and then open the ravine to skiing. If we still couldn't get it to slide, we'd shut the ravine down."

With over two decades of experience in Cutler River Drainage and training in avalanche hazards, LaRoche and Brad Ray are important members of the planning team. "The discussion that morning was about being aware of the snow conditions, so everybody was well aware of the medium-to-high avalanche danger," says Lentini. We're there with Brad and Rene, the avalanche forecasters. We all knew that avalanche conditions had gone up overnight, so we were being really careful of where we were going to travel."

The difficulty in planning for a situation that is so chaotic, a situation that will actively resist detailed plans because the system itself is so unpredictable, highlights the enormity of the task the planners and searchers have taken on. Despite careful advance planning, decisions will be made by individual search teams in real time and based on circumstances as they arise. "We didn't discuss what we'd do if we went up above the gullies on Alpine Garden, and there wasn't a specific plan for descent. It was up to each individual climbing team to decide how they'd get back down," says Lentini.

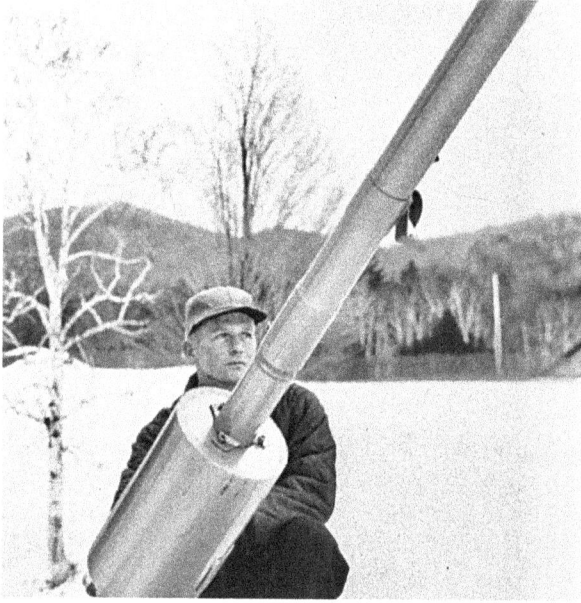

Young Snow Ranger Brad Ray pictured with an avalauncher. Used as an avalanche mitigation tool, the avalauncher can deliver a kilogram of high explosives up to 2,000 meters away. In April 1966, two snow rangers and a bystander were injured when a pre-detonation occurred during use in Tuckerman Ravine.

Steve Larson, who will be one of those climbing the gullies, recalls that the planners left a lot up to the MRS members themselves, given the unpredictability of the circumstances, weather, and terrain, "The plan was for us to search the gullies and make decisions based on what we found," he says.

Although the parking lot at Pinkham is already full, and foot traffic is high at this early hour, the New Hampshire press has yet to pick up on the extent of the search. Throughout New England, attention remains on World Airways Flight 30, which skidded off the end of the runway at Logan Airport on Saturday night, the same day Herr and Batzer went missing But very soon, attention will turn to Mount Washington and Pinkham Notch.

XXXI
INTO THE BREACH

There are memories that time does not erase. ...
Forever does not make loss forgettable, only bearable.
——Cassandra Clare, American writer

Mount Washington Observatory Surface Weather Observations (7:00 to 8:00 a.m.): Temperature -26°F; winds out of the west averaging 84 mph; visibility 0 miles; snow/blowing snow/fog; windchill -75.6°F; peak wind gust: 92 mph.

Dining Room at Pinkham Notch
Monday, Jan. 25, 1982
7:30 a.m.

Harvard Cabin caretaker Matt Pierce doesn't quite know what to do with himself. As he sits among guests of Joe Dodge Lodge, AMC staff, and searchers, he is confronted by many more menu options and much warmer temperatures than he's used to in his usual haunt. But amid the loud hum of caffeine-infused conversations, one memory from that morning still resonates more than four decades later.

"Everyone that was involved in the search was there to be fed well and get a briefing," says Pierce. "I remember that Albert [Dow] sat down next to me at my table. I knew who he was, but it was the first time I'd ever met him. I can remember watching as the young women sitting at the table with me all smiled as soon as he sat down. He was just one of those people who was really personable and had a great smile. I immediately wanted to talk with him because he seemed like a really nice guy, a laid-back and quietly confident person. We talked about the two missing climbers, the weather conditions, and the fact that none of us really knew where we were going yet at that point."

It is just before 8:00 a.m. when the planning team calls Pierce, Dow, and others involved in the day's search out of the noisy dining room and into a quieter part of the building. Whether climbing or not, everyone present is briefed on the medium-to-high avalanche hazard and given their specific assignments.

Unit 1: Steve Larson and Doug Madara will climb the left side of Odell Gully.

Unit 2: Joe Lentini and Tiger Burns will climb South Gully.

There is no Unit 3 designated.

Unit 4: Michael Hartrich and Albert Dow will climb the right side of Odell Gully.

Unit 5: Bill Kane (team leader), Paul Ross, Frank Hubbell, Rob Walker, and Todd Swain will coordinate from the left buttress of Odell and The Fan.

(Note: The official report indicates that Unit 1 will climb Odell Right, and Unit 4 Odell Left. Members of both teams indicate this is not accurate and agree that they climbed the routes indicated above.)

At the conclusion of the briefing, everyone proceeds to the Pack Room located on the lower floor to retrieve their gear. From there, the units head to the idling Forest Service Thiokol, where they'll be transported into Huntington by Snow Rangers Brad Ray and Rene LaRoche. After dropping off the climbing teams, the Thiokol will return to Pinkham and shuttle the second wave of searchers into Huntington, where they'll search the ravine floor and be on standby in the event trouble emerges in one of the gullies.

"I remember talking with Albert [Dow] and Joe [Lentini] near the Tuckerman Trailhead before they left for Huntington," says MRS teammate Dana Seavey, who'll be part of the second wave heading into Huntington. "Joe was talking to Albert and me about what gear we should bring, because he always packed extra gear. But Albert liked to travel really light, and Michael [Hartrich], who was heading up with them, always had the smallest and shittiest looking rack but would climb circles around most of us. Me being the follower, I adopted the same approach. I'm not sure who was right, but the 'less is more' approach was certainly satisfying at the time. Albert admired Michael and considered him his mentor, and Albert was mine."

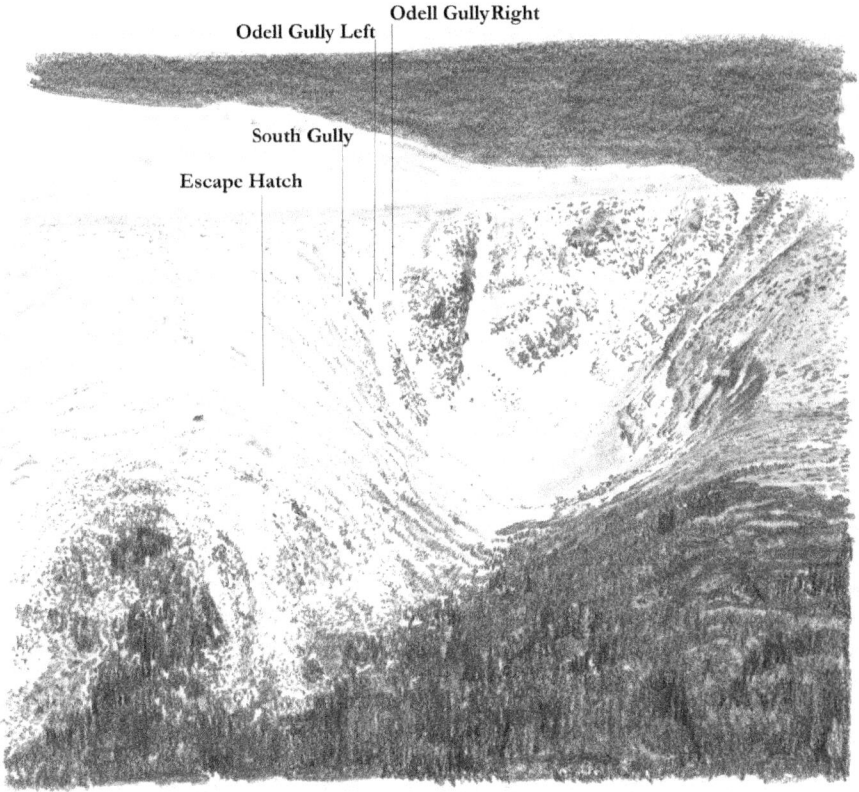

Odell Gully Right

Odell Gully Left

South Gully

Escape Hatch

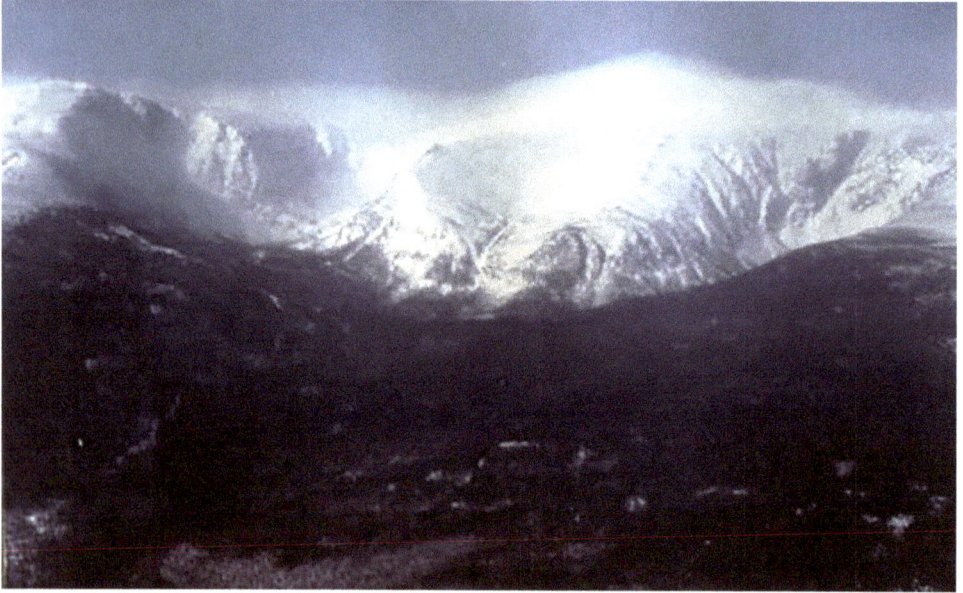

High winds and blowing snow on Mount Washington during the search for Hugh Herr and Jeff Batzer.

XXXII
BROTHERHOOD

You never know how strong you are until being strong is your
only choice.

—Bob Marley

Mount Washington Observatory Surface Weather Observations (8:00 to 9:00
a.m.): Temperature -25°F; winds out of the west averaging 78 mph; visibility 0
miles; blowing snow/fog; windchill -73.0°F; peak wind gust: 88 mph.

Fire Road (3,700 ft.)
Huntington Ravine
Monday, Jan. 25, 1982
8:30 a.m.

Snow Ranger Brad Ray repositions himself on the bench seat of the Forest Service Thiokol he's finessing up the snow-clogged Fire Road toward Huntington Ravine. To his right, Rene LaRoche has the "Oh shit" handle of the passenger door in a death grip as he tries to maintain contact with the seat. Behind them in the fully exposed flatbed are 11 members of Mountain Rescue Service, all of whom are working to maintain a low center of gravity so as to avoid being tossed out.

Sitting between Ray and LaRoche, and taking the jostling in stride, is Tuckerman, a husky/shepherd mix owned by Ray. It is not uncommon for Tuckerman to spend as much time in the Cutler River Drainage as his human companion, and the bond between them runs deep. "Tuckerman was an independent spirit who was famous for leaving the snow ranger cabin at Hermit Lake one afternoon and walking back to the house where he and Ray lived at the time in Gorham," says Rebecca Oreskes, Ray's widow.

The Thiokol passes by the Huntington Cache, a rugged structure built with two-by-fours, live-edge plank siding, and a peaked roof

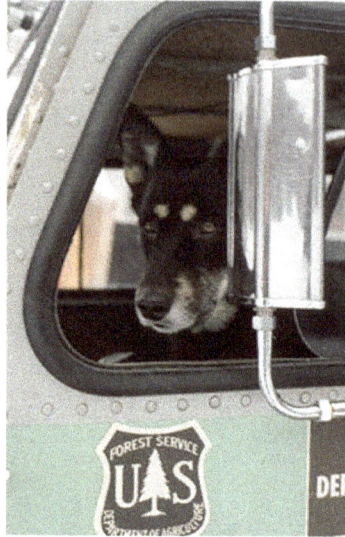

Tuckerman waits patiently for his human companion, Brad Ray, during the search for Hugh Herr and Jeff Batzer.

with cedar shingles. Inside the cache are basic first-aid supplies, Stokes litters and/or toboggans, blankets, shovels, and avalanche probes. The Huntington Cache is one of several strategically positioned in the Cutler River Drainage to provide ready access to rescue equipment in the event it's needed somewhere on this side of the mountain.

For the first time in 48 hours, it has stopped snowing on Mount Washington, but high winds continue limiting visibility and lowering the air temperature. As the trail levels off, Ray and LaRoche put eyes on the massive wall of rock, snow, and ice runnels jutting from the floor of the ravine. In a good snow year like this one, Ray will be able to drive the Thiokol up onto the lower portion of The Fan because the steep boulder field is now completely covered by wind-deposited snow.

Vivid memories of previous visits to the ravine are colliding with the MRS team members' unsettled thoughts about the challenging climbing routes they will soon be facing. In January 1980, for example, Bill Kane, Michael Hartrich, Albert Dow, Steve Larson, Misha Kirk, and six other members of MRS were shuttled into the ravine by Ray and LaRoche to help an ice climber who'd fallen 250 feet down Odell

Gully and onto the exposed scree of The Fan. Although he suffered significant trauma, he would survive the fall.

Bill Kane, who will coordinate this morning's search with Paul Ross, played a key role in that 1980 rescue, along with Todd Swain, Rob Walker, and Frank Hubbell. Kane, an emergency medical technician, had warm packs in his medical kit. Because the victim was showing signs of hypothermia, Kane and Kirk applied the packs to parts of his body where heat loss is more significant. The effectiveness of this warming technique had a strong effect on Kirk, as noted in his report: "I feel hot packs are more than worth their weight and cost and should be on any winter rescue in the future." Unbeknownst to Kirk at the time, the decision to add warm packs to his med kit will play an important role in the events that will transpire in the search for Hugh Herr and Jeff Batzer.

As the Thiokol reaches the base of The Fan, where the team from MRS will disembark and hike up to their assigned routes, it is important to note where the team was in its evolution in January 1982, when the organization was much more loosely structured than it is today. At that time, team members were called upon, completed their task, and returned to their day-to-day existence. "There wasn't much training in the 1970s and '80s," says then MRS President Rick Wilcox, who at the time of the search for Herr and Batzer was guiding clients on Aconcagua. "We were just guys on the street who were decent climbers, and if you could climb, you just signed up for MRS. We knew who was competent and who wasn't. We were probably most concerned with whether members of the team got along well with each other. We were definitely competent, but not trained to the level we are today."

Steve Larson, who along with Doug Madara is assigned to climb Odell Gully, has high praise for the way Wilcox cultivated the team back then. "Rick created a culture where the best climbers served, and I think history has shown that it's easier to teach a climber to rescue than to teach a rescuer to climb. But in 1982, we all trained informally; there was no system."

Despite the absence of formalized structure, MRS was a vital presence in the climbing community, even in its earliest days. Joe Lentini, who will climb South Gully with Tiger Burns, warmly recalls the close ties MRS team members shared back then, and still share today. "Those were some of the toughest people on the crew back then—and I'm not saying it in a macho way. They could deal with tremendously bad conditions and nobody would complain about it. Climbers taking care of other climbers. I still can't believe we actually did some of these things together."

The team's high level of technical climbing expertise, experience operating in difficult terrain and extreme weather, and the fact that they were constantly looking out for one another are all reflected in the fact that prior to January 1982 no member of MRS had been seriously injured during a callout.

But that will change on this day, and the effects of the day's events will have a permanent impact on MRS and on the climbing community in the White Mountains. The evolution that MRS has undergone in the intervening years, including a more formalized structure, systematized training, and an increasing array of rescue strategies, is in large part the result of the increased awareness generated by the experience these 11 team members will have as they move toward their assigned routes.

XXXIII
KNOWN UNKNOWNS

Bravery is not the absence of fear. Bravery is feeling the fear,
the doubt, the insecurity, and deciding something else is more important.
—Mark Manson, American author

Mount Washington Observatory Surface Weather Observations (9:00 to 10:00
a.m.): Temperature -23°F; winds out of the west averaging 77 mph; visibility 0
miles; blowing snow/fog; windchill -69.9°F; peak wind gust: 86 mph.

The Fan
Huntington Ravine
Monday, Jan. 25, 1982
9:00 a.m.

The air is so viciously cold in Huntington Ravine that if boiling water is thrown into the air, it will freeze before it hits the ground. The wind has deposited so much snow beneath the searchers' boots that it covers most of the gnarly scree and boulders that would normally require extra time and effort to travel over. Today, the firm snowpack offers a straightforward ascent of The Fan. It is not long before the 11 members of MRS get above the small trees made invisible by the epic snow depths and reach a height where the gullies of Huntington begin.

Gusts of wind taunt them as blowing snow peppers the portions of their faces that their wool face masks can't shield. If Hugh Herr and Jeff Batzer are still in Odell Gully, they are most certainly dead and frozen by now, unless they've been able to dig a snow cave. But the team members don't know that the two are really about 2.4 miles north of the ravine as the crow flies, having been swallowed by Great Gulf Wilderness.

Few words are spoken. Each man knows what's in store and

what's at stake. Plus, it's just too damn cold to stand idle and chat. They're ready to get on with it. Joe Lentini and Tiger Burns (Unit 2) find the ends of the climbing rope they'll share as they traverse over to South Gully, and each ties a figure-eight knot to his nylon climbing harness, which connects them to each other. Steve Larson, Doug Madara, Michael Hartrich, and Albert Dow, all of whom will climb Odell, follow suit.

Bill Kane, Paul Ross, and Todd Swain (Unit 5) climb unroped up firm snow in Odell. They will ascend the 60-degree snow slope to a small perch on a buttress 100 feet above them. There, Kane and Ross will coordinate the search of the gullies and floor of Huntington Ravine, and the three of them will monitor the progress of Larson and Madara (Unit 1) and Hartrich and Dow (Unit 4) as the two sets of partners assault the gullies. Today, the ravine will experience the basketball equivalent of a full-court press. MRS wants to finish this,

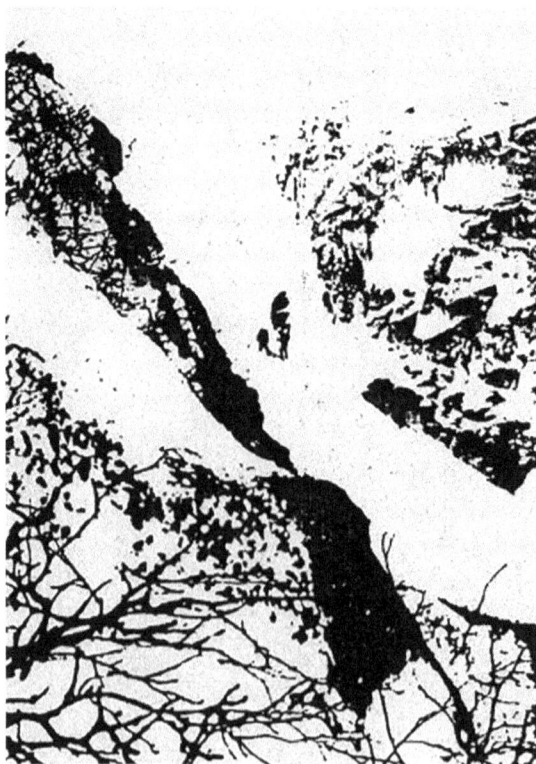

Doug Madara and Steve Larson in Odell Gully on Jan. 25.
It is so cold that the film in Paul Ross's camera will freeze.

regardless of how it ends.

Larson and Dow pull in the remaining slack in their ropes and coil them on the snow. Larson will belay Madara, and Dow will belay Hartrich. The four watch as Kane, Ross, and Swain approach the buttress. Their eyes then track beyond the buttress as they visualize their respective routes up the gully from its base, until blowing snow renders the higher reaches unseeable.

Because the four climbers cannot see their entire route, they won't see any potential avalanche hazard lying in wait until they're up there. Bill Kane remembers the specific concern he had for the four members ascending Odell. "Going up Odell, there's sometimes a cornice that forms off to the right when you're going up, and it can be really scary. I was worried about that. They weren't that heavy, but they were freaking terrifying."

Kane's concern that day reflects the uncertainty and unpredictability MRS often contended with back then when operating in winter in hazardous terrain. They all acknowledge today that their ability to predict and navigate avalanche hazard was not yet well developed. "There was no Level 1, 2 or 3 avalanche training as there is today," says Wilcox. "It was pretty minimal back then. We were not running around with avalanche transponders on, or carrying shovels or probes with us like the team does today. We didn't have transceivers to detect someone beneath the snow if they happened to be wearing a transponder. So, it was just luck if we found somebody in an avalanche. There weren't a lot of callouts for avalanche rescue going on back then anyway."

Joe Lentini, who along with Tiger Burns is nearing South Gully, says, "Back then we were starting to become aware of avalanches because we'd work with Brad [Ray] and Rene [LaRoche] on callouts, and we'd do some informal trainings with them. But the equipment was archaic. We had gotten to a point where we had used avalanche probes, so we knew about those. But the science was still pretty young. I knew a little bit, and I'd read a little bit about it. I like to say I knew 5 percent of what I needed to know back then. But snow slab did make me uncomfortable."

When considering risk and how to identify and manage it, measuring the frequency and severity of incidents is an important factor. The first recorded avalanche fatality on Mount Washington occurred in 1954 in Tuckerman Ravine, and another was recorded in 1965, when two climbers were swept out of Odell Gully. Between 1972, when MRS was formed, and January 1982, there were six avalanche incidents involving people who were reported to the National Forest Service, but none of these was fatal. Some of the incidents were fairly minor and didn't require a response. This relatively low frequency and severity of incidents helps explain the absence of urgent education and training at the time.

"Back then, avalanches were a rare entity in the Northeast," says wilderness medical response expert Dr. Frank Hubbell, who was in the ravine that morning. "We were aware of them, but they were few and far between."

At the time, the most recent avalanche to involve significant injury occurred in April 1980, when Jeff Tirey and Richard Morse were caught in one in Great Gully in King Ravine. Kane, Lentini, Dow, and Hartrich responded to that event. But despite that recent experience, most of the searchers still considered a serious avalanche to be a low risk for them.

"I think we all suffered from what I call 'testosterone poisoning' back then," says Hubbell today. "We'd all been in the outdoors, we'd all been to altitude and done expeditions. It didn't matter what Mother Nature threw at us; we believed we could work our way through it. The attitude was, 'We're going in to save lives, so the angels are going to take care of us and protect us.' We now know that's not true. When you do these things, you're putting your life on the line. We're much more conscious today about rescuer safety, and it was situations like this one that drove that lesson home."

XXXIV
LAST STAND

Optimism is true moral courage.
—Sir Ernest Shackleton

Great Gulf: Temperature: -13°F; windy; visibility daylight.

Emergency Bivouac Site (2,247 ft.)
Great Gulf Trail Junction
Monday, Jan. 25, 1982
9:15 a.m.

Hugh Herr and Jeff Batzer are encountering enormous hurdles that must be overcome if they have any chance of survival. Since rising almost four hours earlier, the pair has struggled to complete the simplest of tasks. They are cold, stiff, and grossly depleted, limiting their ability to ambulate. Herr is much worse off than Batzer and spends most of his time sitting on the bed of pine boughs they slept in overnight.

For a couple of hours, they have been in a ground fight with their frozen alpine boots. Because their socks fused themselves to the front interior of their boots, they were forced to insert the spike end of an ice axe inside the boot to cut away the frozen socks so they could pull their feet out the night before. Now they are finding it impossible to get their feet back inside.

"There were frozen clumps of sock inside the boots," says Batzer. "I had cut through three layers of high-priced, top-level wool socks and vapor barrier socks to get them off the night before, and Hugh had the same kind of scenario. As we tried to get our feet back in the boots that Monday morning, they were frozen, and the clumps of socks were blocking our ability to get our feet back in. So, once again we had to take the point of the shaft of my ice axe and try to cut the socks out of our frozen boots."

Batzer is finally able to scrape enough of the clumps of destroyed wool out of one boot to don it, but after two more hours of effort, it becomes clear that one boot is the best they're going to get. "We were able to pop the socks out of my right boot, but in the end, we couldn't get the others out," he says. "It took both of us, with all four arms pulling with full force, to put the boot on my right foot and zipper up my supergaiter. We worked on the other three boots for a couple of hours with great frustration, but we just couldn't get the socks out of them or get them back on our feet, and that of course was just devastating."

Though Herr is in dire straits, he is coherent enough to know what his friend must do to save himself. "Hugh was still hopeful first thing that morning," says Batzer. "But things were getting really bad for him, and he told me, 'It's time for you to go, Jeff. I can't follow you, and you need to get out of here. Whatever the cost, you need to get out and save yourself.'"

Batzer vehemently resists the thought of abandoning him, but Herr is insistent that he must try to self-rescue. They ultimately agree that Batzer will try to reach Pinkham Notch, where their ordeal began. "We decided to take my one remaining Gore-Tex mitten and use it as my left boot, and I was going to try to go in the direction of Pinkham Notch, which was 4.5 miles away," says Batzer. "Once I got there, I would send help back to Hugh."

His right boot now on, Batzer pulls the mitten over his deadened left foot. He will not remove either of them again. With his left hand now exposed, he is alarmed by the carnage he sees. "I noticed my middle finger had broken through the barrier glove. I touched it with my tongue, and it was like licking a pearl, and it was as white as a pearl too." The finger is frozen solid.

Herr drifts between moments of clarity and complete detachment. His deteriorating condition pulls him further away from Batzer, and closer to his own mortality. Batzer can no longer stay put. He knows time is fleeting fast for his companion.

The trees above and around them pop and sway as strong winds work over the lower portion of Great Gulf. It isn't snowing, but winds are scuffing the fallen snow from the ground, creating ground-blizzard conditions in the forest. Once on route, Batzer will not only have to spend his entire time post-holing through deep snow wearing only one boot, he'll also be doing it without the benefit of a jacket. "My parka didn't breathe enough and froze solid from the inside out," he says. "I couldn't wear it anymore. It was hard as a rock and totally useless."

Batzer kneels next to his subdued friend and hugs him. He assures Herr that he'll send rescuers for him. Then he stands, walks to the embankment behind the large boulder that shelters them, and climbs toward the Great Gulf Trail.

"When I was on my way out alone, I was confronted with the thought that Hugh might die," recalls Batzer. "I was trying to make my way out to safety and get help for him, but there was a strong impression in my mind that Hugh might be gone before anyone could get back to him. I really didn't think about too much beyond that, but I knew it would be devastating if I was able to get help and Hugh still didn't make it."

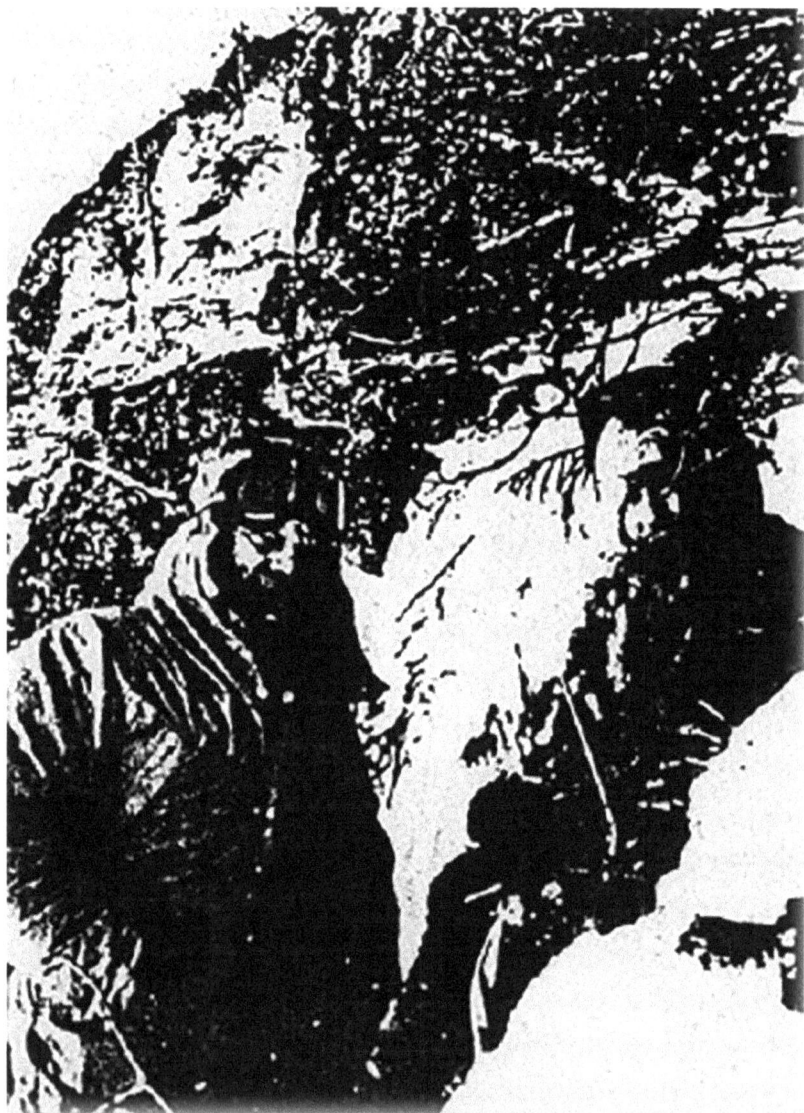

Paul Ross (left) and Todd Swain on a perch with Bill Kane (not pictured) approximately 300 feet up Odell Gully. The grainy nature of the image is the result of the frozen film.

XXXV
YOUNG LIONS

Courage will now be your best defence against the storm that is at hand
—that and such hope as I bring.
—Gandalf, *The Lord of the Rings: The Return of the King*

Mount Washington Observatory Surface Weather Observations (9:00 to 10:00 a.m.): Temperature -23°F; winds out of the west averaging 77 mph; visibility 0 miles; blowing snow/fog; windchill -69.9°F; peak wind gust: 86 mph.

Unit 5
Odell Gully Left Buttress (4,500 ft.)
Huntington Ravine
Monday, Jan. 25, 1982
9:30 a.m.

Bill Kane takes in what Mother Nature reveals of the expansive ravine. On a better day, Kane would be able to see the fine detail of the northern wall of the ravine with its water-blue ice runnels snaking their way up the rugged terrain, and the gullies of Yale, Damnation, and North, with the majesty of the Northern Presidential Range as the remote backdrop. But on this day, Kane and his two companions see only the waves of loose snow funneled upward from the ground by the raging winds. Huntington is a massive snow globe this morning. The arctic air mass, which originated in the Canadian Plains and moved across the Great Lakes, has arrived and is spawning a giant ground blizzard on Mount Washington. Off in the distance, the lower portions of the ski runs at Wildcat and Route 16 offer Kane a reassuring sense of proximity to civilization.

Along with teammates Paul Ross and Todd Swain, Kane stands 300 feet above the floor of the ravine on an approximately 9-by-5-foot perch. Just above them and still within view are Doug Madara, Steve

Larson (Unit 1) and Michael Hartrich and Albert Dow (Unit 4), who are in the midst of a methodical search of Odell Gully.

"We kick-stepped up a 60-degree slope as high as we could and stamped out a small flat spot on the buttress left of Odell Gully where it was safe enough that the slope above wasn't going to release on us if it let go," says Kane. "That allowed us to look up toward the top, where the snow cornice sometimes forms, and down below, where we could see all four of the climbers as they moved up. We did not use a rope to go up or down, but we had one just in case. There was a rock wall above us, and we had eyes on them most of the time. We were already a good 150 feet above them when they actually started on the ice. I can remember the wind almost blowing Paul off the ledge."

The ambient air temperature in the ravine is at or near -20°F. On occasion, when the westerly winds find their way from Alpine Garden down into the cirque, the windchill dips much lower. MRS member Todd Swain, a guide for International Mountain Climbing School who had also worked as a climbing ranger in the Shawangunk Mountains in New York and knew Hugh Herr, says today that standing idle in the ravine that day and watching fellow MRS members in Odell was a tough thing to do. "It was incredibly cold and windy, just brutal," he recalls.

Paul Ross, who is coordinating the search with Kane, remembers the cold but adds, "Of course, I expected it in that area of the hill in winter. I was concerned with the condition of the team and wanted them out of there as soon as possible."

"We didn't realize how much snow there was there until we got there," says Dr. Frank Hubbell, who along with Rob Walker and others is positioned below Odell Gully. "We were in the base of the ravine as they were climbing. It was pretty dramatic. We couldn't see both teams, but for a time we could see Doug [Madara] and Steve [Larson]. Steve was climbing, and Doug was belaying him from his stance above. There were times when the wind would suddenly hit Doug, and he'd blow off his belay stance to the tension of his rope. He'd be four feet off the ice, and he'd drop back onto it. We were just watching those guys with the swirling winds thinking that it was amazing they had the strength and the skills. to do what they were doing."

Meanwhile, some 100 feet below the two climbing teams, the members of MRS on standby are literally digging in for a long day of watching and waiting in case trouble strikes the climbing teams or Herr and Batzer are found.

"A group of us dug out snow caves and crawled inside so we were out of the wind," says Hubbell. "Three of us were together sitting on a bench of snow we created. I'd brought an InsuLite sleeping bag. It wasn't long before I had two folks whose feet were cold, so we wrapped our feet up in the bag to keep them warm while we waited. As we dug in, we realized that treetops were sticking up out of the snow. We were actually sitting in a snow cave on top of the trees. We were in there for a couple of hours. We eventually lost sight of the climbers, but we remained in radio contact."

While all this is happening, Harvard Cabin caretaker Matt Pierce has been conducting his own search. "After breakfast I headed back into Huntington looking in places where I thought people might not have looked," he says. "I went back to where Hugh and Jeff left their gear and was looking around the boulders there." Pierce watches as MRS team members ascend the same route Herr and Batzer had taken on Saturday. "I could see the climbers. They started up and were out of sight very quickly because it was another awful day and there was a lot of wind." Finding nothing, Pierce returns to Harvard Cabin to keep coffee on and the woodstove going in the event searchers seek respite.

Units 1 and 4
Odell Gully (4,600+ ft.)
Huntington Ravine
9:45 a.m.

Steve Larson squints as he looks up and through the ice-encrusted lenses of his glasses to where partner Doug Madara is climbing. Higher up and to the right of Madara, Albert Dow maintains a belay stance as Michael Hartrich moves over the large ice flow.

"The basic idea was to cover the entire gully," says Larson. "Because Odell is so wide, it was decided to use two teams to inspect the width and length of the flow. It's a wide flow at the bottom, and the right side leads up to the gully and eventually to the Alpine Garden. Doug and I were on the left, and Michael and Albert were on the right."

Odell typically offers climbers some shelter from the winds. Today, however, gusts spill over the rim and into the chutes of the gullies. At about 9:30 a.m., Madara, who's carrying the radio, notifies team members and Pinkham that "severe wind conditions are impeding progress." The winds are so loud and so strong that Madara doesn't notice when the radio falls out of his jacket pocket. It will be found by Larson on a snow pitch later in the day.

"Steve and I were trying to look on both sides of the gully," says Madara. "It was very windy, with bad visibility. We were taking the line of least resistance and trying to keep an eye on the snowy areas of the gully for signs that climbers might have passed through or been buried. The open, steeper ice seemed an unlikely spot to find them."

For Madara, who had climbed on high walls and in bad weather in other parts of the country, his experience on this day still ranks at the top. "I've probably been in situations that were more dangerous, just bad weather in more remote places," he says. "But this was the coldest, which was a reason to be a little conservative. I remember being worried about possible snow sliding. There are spots on Odell where people had slid out. I was seeing things I wasn't comfortable with, but you move on, you try to minimize the risk, you stay to the side, you weave your way through. It's what you do up there."

Larson feeds the rope through his belay device so Madara can continue upward. As he looks down at the rope, he notices the effect the blowing snow and brutally cold temperatures are having on his gear. "I was wearing Woolrich heavy wool knickers, and as soon as they were wet, they froze. They were rime-encrusted and bulletproof—it was like wearing armor."

Most of Larson's MRS team members are wearing the same kind of gear as he is. It is a far cry from what today's winter climbers have access to, but it worked at the time, and he was not concerned.

"In addition to the wool pants, I had on Makalus by Galibier, which were a fuzzy inner boot made of wool and leather that you'd slide into a big outer boot," he says. "I also had on Dachstein mittens made of boiled wool, long wool underwear, prescription eyeglasses, and wind pants. I had a bunch of wool on top: a Gore-Tex anorak, a balaclava with a pompom at the top that I normally wore as a hat. I always brought an extra piece of clothing in case I needed it for my upper body and one piece for the victim. I chose to wear glasses rather than goggles. Back then, we were always trying to figure out how to best cover our faces, manage our breath, and not fog our goggles because once they're frozen, it's curtains. Goggles really don't work, in my experience. The more you need them, the worse they are."

Larson and the other climbers wear helmets for protection from falls and falling ice and carry technical gear to aid in climbing the ice and snow. He vividly recalls that a critical piece of his gear failed early in the day. "After we started climbing, my crampons broke pretty quickly. I had these old-school Chouinard crampons, which can get brittle in the extreme cold. As I started up the ice bulge, the first one broke. I cursed at it and hobbled along. Then the second one promptly broke in the same place as the other one. I was able to get myself up the bulge and onto the snow. I got up to Doug at the point where there's a buttress and then the gully forks."

How Larson was able to get up the large ice is a testament to the skill MRS members brought to every eventuality they faced. "I flicked the front points of the crampons onto the ice, and then stomped on them. I was focused on putting pressure on my crampons. My heels were on the ice, and I did this all the way up the ice bulge."

A decade earlier, the thought of climbing an ice bulge in Huntington would not have been part of a climber's calculation. Advancements in technical climbing gear created what is remembered as an "ice revolution" in the Mount Washington Valley. "Chouinard crampons and shorter ice axes are what kicked it off," recalls Larson. "You had a talent pool here, and it didn't take long for them to take hold. It was kind of mind-boggling. I think it's reasonable to say that before Yvon Chouinard's visit to the Mount Washington Valley, water ice was not climbed; it was avoided. The terrain here generally allowed us to climb around ice bulges rather than take them on directly. Before the Chouinard tools, winter climbing in the Whites was practice for the 'big' mountains, and the attitude was to take the line of least resistance. With the advent of the new tools, ice climbing became a sport unto itself."

Through the 1970s and early 1980s, the equipment got better, the climbers got better, and the routes got steeper. "Back then climbing was bold," says Larson. "It's not considered bold any longer. They gave us the tools, and we went out and learned how to use them."

Larson says that as he and Madara advanced upward, they would climb a pitch of ice followed by a pitch of snow. "Doug ran out the pitch without any protection and belayed at the top off two ice screws. We had Salewa ice screws back then. Compared to today's gear, they were really primitive, having only two teeth, and they were much harder to place. We had short alpine hammers with a pic, and you stuck the pic through the eye of the screw and torqued it into the ice. The new ice screws of today you can put in by hand."

Larson still recalls the exuberance of the climbing that day, something he and his teammates shared. "We were really just a bunch of young kids, young 20-year-olds, and even the 'elders' were pretty young."

Unit 4
Odell Gully Right (4,630+ ft.)
Huntington Ravine
9:45 a.m.

Michael Hartrich makes a perfect bomber placement on the steep pitch with his ice axe. Thunk. That sound and the kinetic reaction he feels as he grips the pic end of the axe never gets old for him.

Hartrich and Albert Dow are climbing fat ice on the right side of Odell Gully and moving upward toward the top of Pinnacle Buttress and Alpine Garden beyond it. It is the same route Hugh Herr and Jeff Batzer followed two days earlier. Because Steve Larson experienced technical difficulties with both crampons lower down, Hartrich and Dow are now higher up on the route. "Michael was a man ahead of his time," says Larson. "He was an extraordinary climber."

Hartrich has been on Odell many times before, but one early experience here might have caused a less passionate climber to choose never to set foot in high places again. "The first time I had to self-arrest was on Odell's," Hartrich says today. "I was with someone, and when we got up to the snowfield we unroped because it's pretty easy walking. As soon as I got up above the lip, there was this big gust of wind that blew me right over backwards. I was sailing down the gully backwards, and next thing I knew I just stopped. Somehow, I got myself turned around and my ice axe in the right position and self-arrested. I thought, 'I'm glad I got that right!'"

Bill Kane says of his teammate, "Mike was more experienced in the mountains than I was. I always regarded him as the one guy who went to all kinds of places in the White Mountains that none of us bothered to go to because we were too lazy to hike that far for 60 feet of clean rock."

In their acclaimed book *Yankee Rock & Ice*, Laura and Guy Waterman confirm Kane's assessment: "An even lower profile was sustained by the reclusive, introspective Mike Hartrich, a hiker as well as a climber (unlike most of his peers), who may have explored more White Mountains backcountry than anyone since Darby Field first climbed Mount Washington in 1642."

One of those who regularly joined Hartrich on these remote backcountry adventures was friend and teammate Albert Dow, who is now belaying Hartrich. "Because I'd climbed with Albert quite a bit, I was teamed up with him that day," says Hartrich. "It was fun to climb with him. He climbed quite well, and we had some shared interests. He knew a lot about antiques and I really liked history, so it was fun talking with him. We'd run around in the woods looking for cliffs. We'd do first ascents together."

"They had a great relationship," says mutual friend and MRS teammate Alec Behr. "The three of us spent a lot of time climbing together. I was involved in a couple of first ascents with them, but they both were significantly stronger climbers than I was, so a lot of times I was following along and barely making it up routes. That was such a fun time for us, in our early 20s, with a lot of freedom and very little commitment. We were all getting better and enjoying the climbing scene and the people we were with, smart people who dropped out of other pursuits to climb."

Dow also earned a lot of respect as a climber on both rock and ice. "I used to ice climb with Albert, and he was quite good at it. It was harder back then because the gear wasn't as sophisticated," says Joe Lentini. Dana Seavey, another friend and teammate who'll arrive in the ravine with the second wave, recalls the pure talent Dow possessed on anything vertical. "He was primarily a rock climber, though he enjoyed mixed rock and ice climbing as well. If you handed him two ice tools out of the Eastern Mountain Sports rental shop and said, 'Albert, go do this route,' he would float it."

Hartrich torques two Salathe ice screws into the ice in front of him and clips into them with two carabiners that are attached to nylon runners looped into his harness. He pulls any remaining slack in the rope that lies between him and Dow up to him, and yells down, "On belay!" Albert backs his two ice screws out of the ice, pulls each of his two axes out of the ice, and completes the safety loop, yelling back, "Climbing!"

Hartrich is Dow's lifeline if he falls, just as Dow is his when he's belaying. "It was kind of windy," says Hartrich about the day's conditions. "But I'd been up there hundreds of times in the wind, and you got used to it. Odell is basically two easy ice pitches and you're up in the snow."

The bond between Hartrich and Dow is as strong as the belay system that connects them to each other. "I was introverted and didn't have very good social skills," says Hartrich. "Albert could talk with anybody and would always know what to say to them, how to bring people out. He was a really articulate person. That was a very endearing thing about him. He made a lot of friends and was good at personal relationships. I'd go through stages where I'd climb and then just be bored, or I'd just sit in the house and not get out much. Albert was very good at getting me out to climb. I have a lot of acquaintances, but I don't have many close friends. Albert was a close friend."

XXXVI
SENSING DANGER

The only source of knowledge is experience.
—Albert Einstein

Mount Washington Observatory Surface Weather Observations (10:00 to 11:00 a.m.): Temperature -23°F; winds out of the west averaging 78 mph; visibility 0 miles; blowing snow/fog; windchill -70.1°F; peak wind gust: 92 mph.

Unit 2
South Gully (4,400 ft.)
Huntington Ravine
Monday, Jan. 25, 1982
10:00 a.m.

Connected by rope to teammate Tiger Burns, Joe Lentini is route-finding his way up the 650-foot snow climb that would normally include sections of low-angle ice. Today however, South Gully is loaded with copious amounts of wind-deposited snow that is waist-deep, rendering any ice underneath invisible. Two days before, during the early stages of the snowstorm, strong southerly winds blew all day, scuffing snow off the exposed terrain of the Southern Presidentials and Alpine Garden and depositing it here and on the adjoining Escape Hatch.

"I'd known Tiger my entire life," says Lentini. "He's a tough individual. We'd hiked with the team up to the base of Odell's, traversed over, and started up South Gully. We got up a pitch just underneath a little rock wall, and I started to move over and up. Above us was this giant snow slab."

Lentini is faced here with a critical decision: to continue pushing forward or respect his instincts, which are telling him there's too much risk. Although he isn't trained in avalanche detection and navigation at this point, he leans into a harrowing experience from his past to aid him in making a calculated choice.

"When I was 19 years old, I was ice climbing with a friend in Smugglers' Notch, Vermont," he says today. "We were doing a fairly long ice climb of two-to-three pitches. On the last pitch, I went over a small vertical section that was basically the end of the climb. I got into a snow slope, which was probably 35-to-40 degrees and 200 feet high, and cut over to the right where there's a rock wall. I put some pins in the wall for protection and belayed my partner up to me. When he got up, I told him to rest and that I would do the next pitch. We pulled the anchor out, and I took two steps diagonally away from the wall and said, 'I don't know about this snow.' We coiled up the rope between us so we were moving together, and he was about 10 feet below me. I took two more steps—the fracture line went left to right, diagonally up—and it let go. We both started to drop. I was underneath the snow and very aware of my rate of acceleration. I had my ice axe, went into a self-arrest position and immediately stopped myself. I looked to my left and didn't see my friend. When I finally found him, I saw that he had also been able to stop himself, but he had driven a crampon point into his leg. After we got over against the wall again, I pulled down his knicker socks and blood spurted out. We descended by rappelling, made the mile hike out of the woods, and I drove him to the hospital in Burlington."

That experience is very much in his mind as Lentini executes a few more cautious moves to test the stability of the snowpack. Burns is just behind him. "I didn't get very far," Lentini says. "Tiger and I tried different ways of going around it, and we dug into it to test it, but I just wasn't willing go forward because I knew the snow was too unstable. So we made the decision to turn around."

Lentini radios to the rest of the team and to Pinkham that they'd hit a large snow slab they considered unstable and unsafe. He wiggles the toes of his feet and clenches his teeth as his lower extremities signal alarm. His feet are clearly at risk of frostbite, and he needs to warm them as quickly as possible. He and Burns traverse cautiously across the base of Escape Hatch and begin a short descent to meet the Thiokol as it heads into the ravine with additional searchers.

XXXVII
HEAVY & SLOW

Fate follows us all.
—John Porter, climber and author of *One Day as a Tiger*

Sherburne Ski Trail
Pinkham Notch
Monday, Jan. 25, 1982
10:00 a.m.

Geoffrey May is in a better frame of mind than he was the night before. Having downed a breakfast of oatmeal with butter, dried milk, and raisins washed down with a camp mug of instant coffee, he's happy that he and companion Dave Boudreau found "the Sherbie" the night before, after a fortuitous encounter with Misha Kirk on his way back to Pinkham following the day's fruitless search for Hugh Herr and Jeff Batzer. They were able to pitch their tent about 200 feet off the trail and shelter from the raging storm.

After getting a late start in the morning, they are now making slow progress as they snowshoe their way toward the Tuckerman Trail. At one point along their route, they meet a member of the AMC crew not involved in the search but aware of what is happening. "We'd made a lateral out of the woods and over to the trail when we ran into a woman," says May. "She told us that two ice climbers ascending Huntington Ravine had disappeared, and she seemed very upset. We just didn't know what to say, so we continued on. We were backpackers, not climbers."

Although the missing climbers in Huntington are distant from where the two are headed, the woman's news hits close to home for Boudreau. Three years earlier, a close friend of his, Paul Flanagan, was killed in Odell Gully. On Feb. 14, 1979, Flanagan, age 21, and David Shoemaker, age 20, two well-known climbers and caretakers for the Randolph Mountain Club (RMS), hitched a Thiokol ride into Huntington Ravine with Lead Snow Ranger Brad Ray for a day of ice climbing. The weather forecast called for high winds and brutally cold temperatures. "Brad tried to talk them into not going, but it didn't work," recalls Bill Arnold, then an RMC volunteer and board member and later a founding member of the Androscoggin Valley Search and Rescue Team (AVSAR).

Two days later, on Feb. 16, the body of David Shoemaker was discovered by climbers on The Fan. He was frozen solid and had suffered traumatic injuries resulting from a long fall. The following day, the body of Paul Flanagan was found, also frozen. "It was a great tragedy for the mountain and the Randolph Mountain Club," says Arnold. Shoemaker was the 87th person to perish on Mount Washington, and Flanagan the 88th.

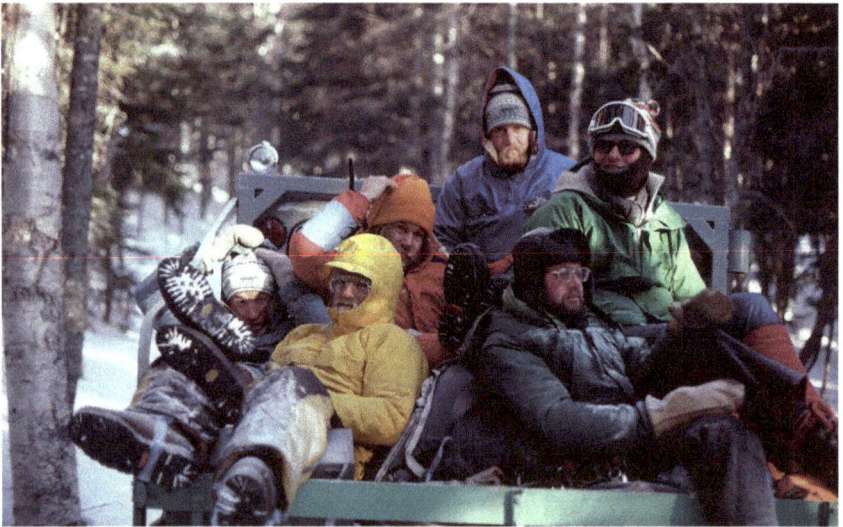

Members of Mountain Rescue Service riding in the back of the Forest Service Thiokol as it returns to Pinkham after they recovered Paul Flanagan's body high in Odell Gully.

Boudreau had befriended Flanagan in 1977 at Gray Knob Cabin during weekend trips to the Northern Presidentials, and Flanagan had taught him to rock climb. They would often enjoy outings together, in the Whites and near their homes in Massachusetts. "I was shocked and saddened," Boudreau says of his reaction to Paul's death. "I thought he was superhuman, and I could not believe he fell in an area so familiar to him. It was very sad—and still is."

These years later, after a slow but smooth descent from the Sherburne Ski Trail and Tuckerman Ravine Trail, Boudreau and May arrive at Pinkham and stand in front of the wooden trail sign behind the Trading Post: "Old Jackson Road: Auto Road 1.5 miles. Madison Hut 6.0 miles."

Now knowing exactly where they're headed, they make high steps through the two feet of fresh powder now blanketing OJR.

"I was wearing Chippewa all-leather boots lined with sheepskin, Dachstein wool socks, and liner socks," says May. "But my feet were still cold, especially my ankles. It was almost a burning sensation. That's how cold it was even below treeline."

Huntington Ravine
10:30 a.m.

Misha Kirk is back in the fight. Through his binoculars he watches as Joe Lentini and Tiger Burns walk along the floor of the ravine toward the idling U.S. Forest Service Thiokol after calling off their search of South Gully. Kirk has been designated team leader for the second wave of searchers arriving in Huntington who, along with Kirk, are piled onto the back of the Thiokol, which is being driven by Brad Ray and fellow Snow Ranger Rene LaRoche.

Following the search, Kirk wrote in his journal. "It was a struggle to get out of bed at 6:00 a.m. My body was sore and my head full of sand. I was glad I'd be able to ride up and didn't balk when I was put in charge of the Mountain Rescue Service 'B' Team. The 'A' Team was to ride up first and start ascending Odell's. The weather was better, but not by much. We rode slowly up the Fire Road. I was with Brad & Rene from the USFS. We continually searched the south side of Huntington's with binoculars, as we continued into Huntington's. By this time the teams were well into Odell's."

When Lentini and Burns arrive at the Thiokol, they toss their packs up to their teammates and climb onto the truck bed. "They told us horror stories of waist-deep drifts that prevented them from even getting to the bottom of the Escape Hatch," wrote Kirk.

Even though Kirk is happy to be leading the B Team, he is beginning to feel regret at not having a more active role in the search. "We arrived at the base of The Fan, and once again I found myself

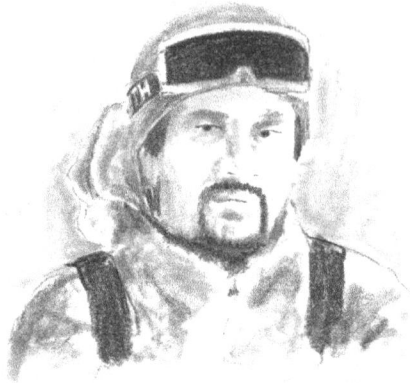

Joe Lentini

listening to the radio communications of the search teams," he wrote. "I felt left out, envious, and I wished I was up in Odell's."

Frank Hubbell emerges from the snow cave he's sharing with MRS teammate Rob Walker and hikes down The Fan to meet the Thiokol. Lentini's feet desperately need warm blood flow, so Hubbell, then training as a physician's assistant, joins him in the warm cab of the Thiokol.

"I got in the snowcat, took of my Koflach boots, and stuck my feet in Frank's armpits," recalls Lentini. "I felt almost instant relief." Hubbell will repeat this warming technique more than once that day.

As Lentini's feet begin to regain warmth, members of the MRS B Team slide off the flat wooden bed of the Thiokol to begin searching. Immediately upon stepping back onto The Fan, having searched it the day before, Dana Seavey does a double-take.

"The terrain was so different from my trip less than 24 hours before," he says. "On Sunday, the big boulders on the approach were exposed, and it was difficult weaving through them. On Monday, I actually thought we were getting off route, because the same rough trail was almost a solid snowfield right up to the base, with no exposed boulders to weave through. At that point I realized I wasn't lost because I could see the boulders were under the snow. It was now a firm wind slab. The Fan was transformed."

Seavey and two teammates are sent on their assigned route. "We were to hike up near the base of Odell in support of Albert and Michael and Steve and Doug," he says. "I can't recall if it was due to clouds or blowing snow, but I couldn't see very far up Odell's at all. I remember seeing Doug and Steve and could hear them talking and climbing. I could hear Michael and Albert but I couldn't see them. After two or three pitches, I couldn't see either team, not even the top third of Odell's. As it became obvious that they were established on the climb, I just assumed they were good or had just topped out, so we left that area."

Bill Aughton is leading a broad search when he's rejoined by Matt Peer, who's just descended from the base of Odell with Seavey. "My team searched the bases of the climbs and looked up into the gullies from the Escape Hatch, South Gully, Odell's, Pinnacle, and Central Gully," says Aughton. "I remember standing on the snow and finding a thickish crust that collapsed with my full weight. I pointed out to my team that there was something of an avalanche danger, so we kept off any steep stuff as we scoured the ravine. We also combed the base of the ravine just in case they'd bailed out or fallen off. We checked all the bushes at the bottom. Nothing. So we went back down to Pinkham."

Matt Peer, who learned to climb in the Mount Washington Valley and was brought onto the team by MRS Team Leader Joe Lentini, remembers Aughton's caution that day in the ravine. "I was gung-ho and ready to climb every gully to find Hugh Herr. But I was with Bill, and he was smarter than me and very cautious. I didn't know anything about avalanches at the time, but Bill did, and he kept us very restrained and out of the line of potential avalanches."

With Units 1 and 4 approaching the higher reaches of Odell Gully, and searchers down lower again coming up empty, Bill Kane instructs the second wave of searchers to leave the ravine. "I sent some down to Harvard Cabin so they'd be warm and ready in case we had to do anything and they needed to be back up there quickly," he says.

Seavey remembers when Kane called them off, and how difficult it was for him to leave. "My sense was we had too many people up there, and they didn't want to have to keep track of people everywhere. We'd done what we'd done. I went back to Harvard Cabin with Matt Peer and Mark Giese, Mark would often volunteer to help out during search and rescue callouts, for a while to wait … thinking we would be needed to do something else. We later got a call with instructions to return to Pinkham, and I remember being disappointed."

238

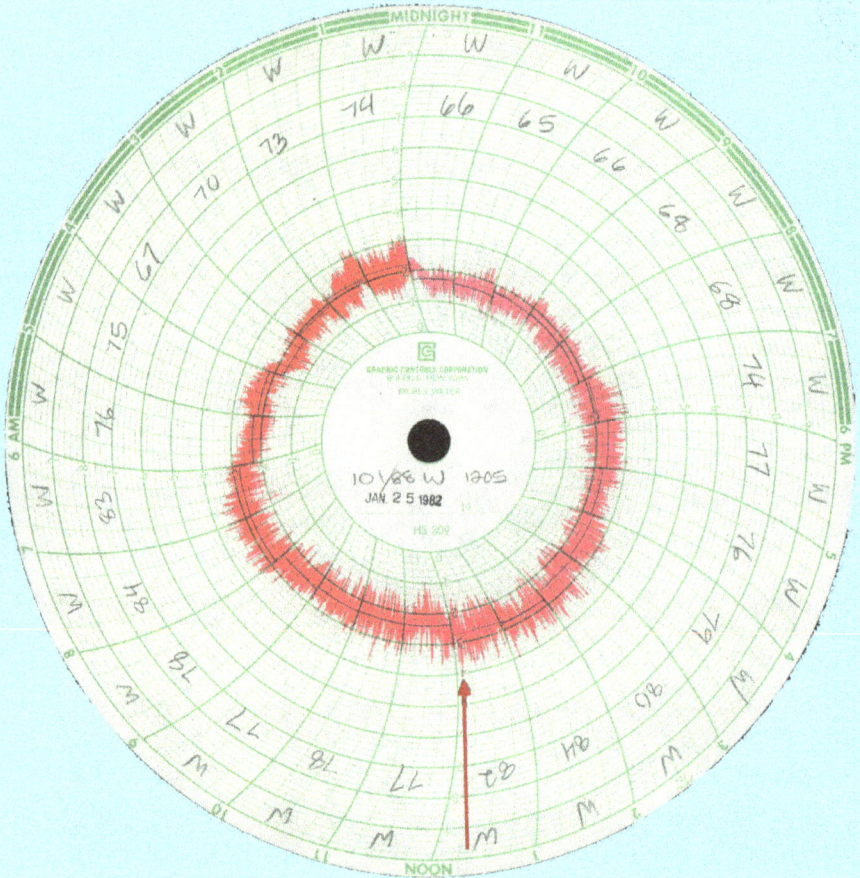

The chart from the Hays Recorder at the Mount Washington
Observatory on Jan. 25, 1982. The numbers in the outer rim represent
the time of day, the average hourly wind direction, and the average
hourly wind speed. The chart indicates a peak wind gust of 101 mph at
12:05 p.m. (see red arrow). Westerly winds throughout the day are in
the high 70s to mid 80s with gusts exceeding 90 mph. The ambient air
temperature is less than -20°F, with windchill factors reaching -70°F.

XXXVIII
INDICATORS

If you see yourself as trying to beat the mountain, eventually the mountain will win.

You don't conquer mountains; you cooperate with them.

—Stacy Allison, the first American woman to summit Mount Everest

Mount Washington Observatory Surface Weather Observations (11:00 a.m. to 12:00 p.m.): Temperature -22°F; winds out of the west averaging 77 mph; visibility 0 miles; blowing snow/fog; windchill -68.4°F; peak wind gust: 91 mph.

Odell Gully (5,200 ft.)
Mount Washington
Monday, Jan. 25, 1982
11:20 a.m.

Michael Hartrich watches as Albert Dow climbs past the top of the large ice flow and joins him on a small snow shelf from where he's belayed his teammate. With the technical portion of the climb complete, it's time to plot their next move. From here they have one of two options: to continue climbing up the snow gully to the rim of the ravine or to rappel down to the base of the gully where they started.

Hartrich remembers what was weighing on him that morning after the MRS teams were empowered to make decisions based on what they encountered. "The other team [Unit 1: Larson and Madara] climbed up the left side of the gully and rappelled back down. But they had places to put a rock anchor in and do that easily. We were on the right side of Odell, and once we got up and over the ice, we were on snow. There were ice bulges and snow, so unless we were going to make a snow or ice anchor, we were limited in what we could set up for rappelling. I was one of those people who never liked to rappel, especially on ice, and I didn't particularly like rappelling off snow anchors either."

Hartrich's hesitancy to rappel back down off Odell that morning is not uncommon in the climbing community. It is one of the riskier practices in a sport that already carries inherent risk. Setting an anchor on rock, ice, snow, or tree, having confidence in it, and then leaning back to lower oneself from it can be seen as the alpine equivalent of a one-person trust fall.

Several factors can contribute to rappel-related accidents, including fatigue, hypothermia, dehydration, improper anchor setup, and lack of focus. Technical equipment can sometimes fail, as can the terrain the anchor is placed in. In addition, weather conditions, such as low visibility, high winds, and freezing temperatures, can affect anchor placement, rappelling equipment, or the ability to see the end of the rope.

For the highly experienced Hartrich, it is a lack of confidence in the equipment they are carrying that causes him to hesitate. "When I first started ice climbing, things were pretty primitive," he says. "Back then, before the Chouinard revolution really took hold in the Whites, you didn't rappel on ice because none of the stuff was going to work."

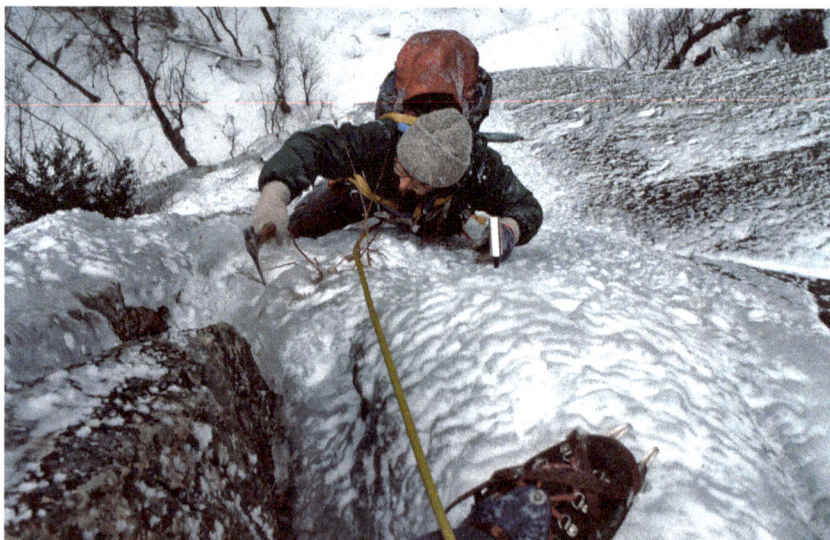

Michael Hartrich following the first ice pitch above the Cathedral Roof on Cathedral Ledge in North Conway, N.H., in 1978. Hartrich is using a combination of old and new ice tools of that time period: an alpine hammer in his right hand, and in his left a Hummingbird, which was new at the time.

If a climber has the option to walk off at the top of a route in snow, it becomes a better option than rappelling back down on ice. Hartrich and Dow have that option. Going left will bring them to South Gully or Escape Hatch. Both of these can be safe ways to descend. At present, however, they are loaded with dangerous wind slab, as Joe Lentini and Tiger Burns have reported. The other option, which is also used frequently by Huntington climbers, is the classic walk over Alpine Garden and the descent of Lion Head. For Hartrich, the decision is clear: rappelling down the ice is just too risky. "We chose to keep going," he says.

So he and Dow leave the ice flow behind them and transition to climbing the snow gully that leads to Alpine Garden. The snow is hard-packed, having been continuously hammered by hurricane-force winds. The slope is quite steep, so they remain roped together. If one of them falls and begins to slide, the other will drop down onto the snow and, with his chest and a shoulder, drive the pic end of his axe deep into the snow in hopes of anchoring himself. If the sliding teammate is unable to self-arrest, the anchored one will brace himself as the other reaches the end of the rope's slack. If the rope holds, that fall will be arrested. If it doesn't, the anchored teammate will be popped from the slope, and both will plummet.

Bent slightly at the waist and toward the slope just in front of him, Dow drives the spike end of one axe into the snow, does the same with the other one just ahead of it, and kicks the toe of each of his crampon-laden boots into the firm névé. He and Hartrich will repeat this process until the slope eases enough for unprotected movement. The closer they get to the rim of the ravine, the more they can feel the maniacal winds waiting for them just over the rim.

As he plods upward, something on the side of the gully catches Hartrich's eye. The silver object appears in contrast to the dark rock that it lies against. Hartrich traverses toward the wall to get a closer look. "I found a carabiner at one of the belay stances and footprints here and there," he says. "The carabiner was clipped to a piton wedged into the rock."

From this belay point, Hartrich and Dow see that the footprints rise up the slope to the rim. "There were tracks, and they were going everywhere. Up there, tracks can last for weeks. So we figured we'd start following them."

Since Misha Kirk found the pack that Hugh Herr and Jeff Batzer stashed two days earlier, this is the strongest evidence that the missing pair might be found in the vicinity of the search. Hartrich and Dow radio their intentions to teammates and to Pinkham. Though not definitive proof that Herr and Batzer are still in the area, Odell Gully remains the point where they were last seen. The footprints Dow and Hartrich have spotted are indications that their search must continue, so they follow the kick-steps in the snow and arrive at the rim of the ravine, where they unrope.

The footprints they've been following out of the gully continue onto Alpine Garden toward Lion Head. "It's well known that anybody who climbs Odell's goes left at the top and comes down South Gully or the Escape Hatch or goes over to Lion Head and down," says Hartrich. "So we decided to follow the tracks because nobody had any idea where Hugh and Jeff were, and to me it was pretty obvious that they were going to head over to Lion Head as a way to come down."

That kind of assumption has been the problem with the search since it started: no one can fathom that Herr and Batzer left Huntington and ended up in Great Gulf, since that is beyond anyone's experience.

Buffeted by winds approaching 80 mph, and now fully exposed to the searing windchill, Hartrich and Dow continue to follow the tracks out onto Alpine Garden until they disappear in the ground blizzard that the two are about to walk into in pursuit of the missing climbers.

XXXIX
LOSING HOPE

I wish this could've been any other way.
But I just don't know, I don't know what else I can do.
—Nine Inch Nails, "Every Day Is Exactly the Same"

Great Gulf: Temperature: -10°F; windy; visibility daylight.

Emergency Bivouac Site (2,247 ft.)
Great Gulf Trail Junction
Monday, Jan. 25, 1982
12:00 p.m.

Jeff Batzer is trashed. As he gingerly makes his way down the embankment to the large boulder where he and Hugh Herr are bivouacking, the cramping in his legs is almost unbearable. Over the course of Batzer's three-hour solo attempt to reach Pinkham, which is 4.5 miles away, he's traveled just under a mile, most of which was in disoriented circles.

"The winds were cutting hard through the woods," Batzer recalls of his ordeal. "Without my frozen parka, it was penetrating the layers on my upper body. I was feeling pretty miserable when gusts were rolling through. My left foot in the mitten was starting to get really cold, and I think it was completely frostbitten by noon."

Just as he and Herr had encountered while they followed the West Branch of the Peabody River out of the deeper reaches of the gulf, Batzer found impenetrable clusters of thick vegetation during his self-rescue attempt. "Along the river there were balsam firs a foot and a half apart and just tangled together. It was like a barrier and impossible to get through, so I'd go around them."

He was also struggling through waist-high and deeper snow. "I was following the painted blazes on the trees and fighting my way through, but it was so dense. Snow was covering the trees and the blazes. Where was the next blaze? At several points, I knew I was off trail. The snow was blowing really hard. It was cutting right through my clothing and feeling like death at that point. I just could not find the trail. I was going in circles, and terrified of getting lost and separated from Hugh."

Batzer ultimately decides to turn around and follow his errant tracks to his starting point at Great Gulf Trail junction. "Making it to Pinkham would have been the last thing we were going to be able to do for ourselves, and I knew what it meant to fail at that," he says. Unbeknownst to Batzer, he'd gotten to within a mile of the two-mile mark on the Mount Washington Auto Road.

When Batzer arrives at the bivouac boulder, he has the impression Herr hasn't moved since he departed hours ago. An already critical situation has gotten even worse for his friend.

"When I got back at about noon on Monday from trying to get out, Hugh was sitting on the boughs partially in the cave," he says. "He was hugging himself trying to stay warm, and his toes were sticking out of the ends of his socks, and they were discolored. His feet were on their way to being frozen like rocks. He wasn't covered with the frozen parka I'd left behind."

Batzer tells Herr, who cannot walk by this point, that he's so sorry he failed. "We both knew what that meant," he says of the painful moment. "Hugh told me, 'That's OK, Jeff.' There were no tears, only silence."

They are seriously dehydrated, and Batzer has an idea of how to get water to ease the feeling of having dry sponges in their mouths. "I made a fishing pole-type implement using slings and runners and put them on my ice axe. I walked down to the water and threw the slings into the river so they'd get soft. I then dragged the runners back through the snow to Hugh so we could drink the water out of the snow sticking to the runners. It was really hard work, and even though we drank desperately, we couldn't quench our thirst. I did that a couple of times and then just stopped."

They rest together for a time on top of the spruce and fir boughs, continuing to hug one another to stay as warm as possible. Suddenly, Batzer sits up, and Herr wills himself to stand as well.

"I felt this rally of strength," Batzer recalls. "OK! I've got one more trail to do: Glen House. Let's try to do this,' I said. I made it about five feet out of the hole, but I just couldn't get myself up that little hill onto the trail. I was too weak. I turned and looked at Hugh. He was standing just outside the hole and then collapsed back into the sitting position. And that was it for the expedition to Glen House."

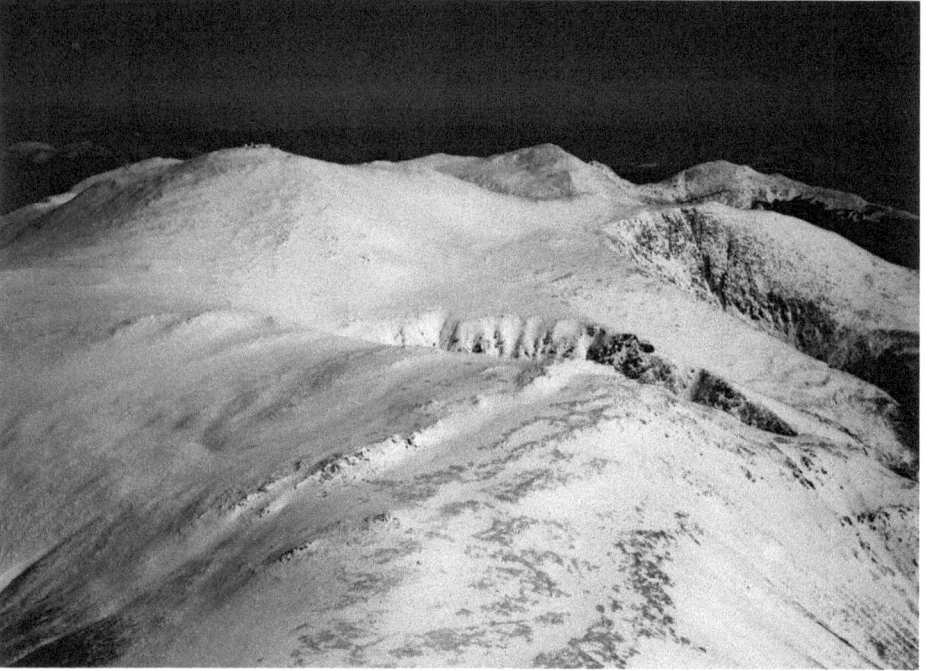

Alpine Garden from the air lies between Tuckerman Ravine (scar in the foreground) and Huntington Ravine (scar above and to the right).

XL
WORRY AND WAIT

Mountains know the secrets we need to hear.
—Tyler Knott Gregson, author/photographer

Mount Washington Observatory Surface Weather Observations (12:00 to 1:00 p.m.): Temperature -21°F; winds out of the west averaging 82 mph; visibility 0 miles; blowing snow/fog; windchill -67.8°F; peak wind gust: 101 mph.

Alpine Garden (5,000 ft.)
Mount Washington
Monday, Jan. 25, 1982
12:20 p.m.

Michael Hartrich executes a hard stop. Since leaving the belay stance high up in Odell Gully, where he and Albert Dow discovered footprints and a carabiner an hour before, they've struggled to keep the thinning indentions in the snow in view. Dow follows his teammate's lead and also pauses. He is careful to stay close enough to Hartrich to keep him in sight in the ground blizzard but far enough away to avoid being driven into him by rogue gusts. Winds exceeding 90 mph are blasting down the eastern snowfields above them. Fifteen minutes earlier, a 101-mph blast, the day's highest, rolled through.

The gusts and devastating windchill are forcing Hartrich and Dow to squint, raise their heads to scan the terrain around them, and quickly tuck their faces back into the lee of their right shoulders for relief. After a handful of attempts, they stop this painful game of peek-a-boo. The frozen footprints that have led them here are gone. Hartrich radios that they've lost sight of the prints and are continuing toward Lion Head.

Tuckerman caretaker Joe Gill, who led a team up the Lion Head Winter Route the day before, believes the prints Hartrich and Dow are seeing in Alpine Garden are the ones he and fellow members of Unit 24 left behind. "Nobody else was up there then, and we now know that Herr and Batzer went the other way," says Gill. While no one can ever know if Gill's assumption is accurate, we do know that Unit 24 did not descend into Odell where the tracks Hartrich and Dow are following originated. Because tracks on the rim of the ravine can last several days, even in extreme weather, there is no way to pinpoint their timing.

As Hartrich and Dow leave Huntington and move south toward Lion Head, the eastern slopes off to their right increase in height. There in the shadow of the summit of Mount Washington, winds are relenting from hurricane-force gusts of 90 mph or more down into the 70-mph range. But Hartrich knows this temporary "reprieve" will end as they pass by the apex of the summit cone and approach Lion Head.

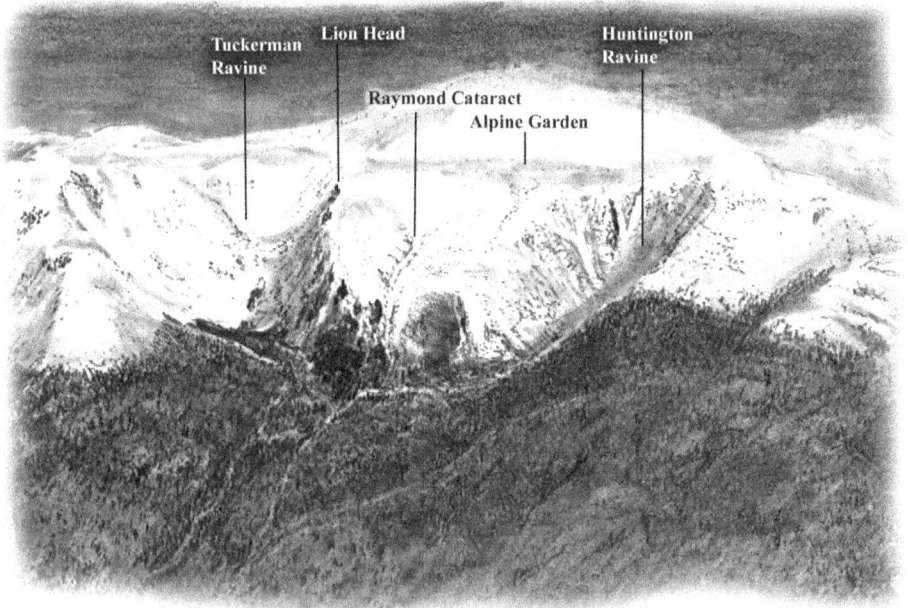

The two continue moving in hopes of reconnecting with the prints. Hartrich has their climbing rope coiled over one shoulder and around his upper torso, known as a climber's coil, and both wear backpacks. When westerly gusts collide with them, the packs act as sails and spin the men directly into the headwinds. Thick, frozen fog and blowing snow are making navigation over Alpine Garden a challenge. Deep pockets of snow conceal undulations in the terrain, causing them to drop into knee-deep holes. Sastrugi, wind-driven snow dunes created by constant winds and ample amounts of unconsolidated snow, force them to thread their way through scores of drifts. The alpine zone begins some 300 feet below them and extends to 500 feet above them, encompassing more than 200 acres. Today Hartrich and Dow can see no more than one-eighth of a mile in front of them.

For Hartrich, the harshness he and Dow are experiencing on Alpine Garden early that afternoon is in sharp contrast to the meditative beauty he has previously enjoyed there. "I used to guide the Pinnacle Rock Route in Huntington in the summer and head across the Alpine Garden," he says today. "I particularly liked doing that in the spring when all the flowers were in bloom."

Before winter causes most mammals, human or otherwise, to avoid Alpine Garden and remain below treeline, the expanse is rife with fauna. Rodents such as the red-back mouse, the masked shrew, and the eastern short-tailed shrew make homes among the massive scree fields that blanket the mountain. Porcupine, snowshoe hare, squirrels, and chipmunks also make their homes here.

Plant life is also abundant. You can find three-forked rush, labrador tea, mountain cranberry, and black crowberry among other flora in the garden, some of which are rare and endangered. Patches of krummholz—stunted, windblown specimens of black spruce and balsam fir—abound along boulder-lined trails and the cairns that guide travelers through the alpine zone. In this cold, wind-shaped terrain, trees no more than a foot tall spread out horizontally rather than vertically, hugging the ground.

Hartrich and Dow have covered approximately half of the .68-mile distance between Huntington and Lion Head. They are about 15 minutes away from its Winter Route down the mountain. Because visibility is so low, they are unable to see the massive rock structure named for the apex predator it resembles. Shortly after leaving Huntington, they choose a line that will allow them to traverse the upper slopes of Raymond Cataract. Known as contouring, this strategy will keep them at a consistent elevation and on track to link up with Lion Head, while also permitting them to visually search a place known for collecting those who find peril in Alpine Garden. Raymond is also known to collect heavy amounts of wind-loaded snow when winds are westerly, as they have been since Saturday night.

The slope Hartrich and Dow are contouring is not very steep, less then 30 degrees. However, a terrain restriction known as a choke lies below them. The upper portion of Raymond is wide at the top and narrows toward the bottom. Picture a funnel cut in half. One hundred feet above this choke point is where the terrain steepens significantly. When the slopes of Raymond are loaded with snow, as they are now, large wind slabs can break at the point where the slope steepens. When a slab lets go, it will funnel down into a tree-constricted area. This area is known as a terrain trap because as the slide slows and stops, debris will continue accumulating as it funnels downward. A person caught in such a terrain trap is at risk for deep burial and traumatic injury because of the trees. Hartrich and Dow stay high enough on the slope to avoid getting too close to the known slide path below them.

While still hoping to find signs of Herr and Batzer, they are doing everything they can to avoid getting snared by the dangers surrounding them. Because Raymond Cataract is loaded with wind-deposited snow and has a well-known reputation for letting go when it is, they determine that it would be too risky to drop any farther down. "Albert and I didn't see any evidence that Hugh and Jeff had been there and didn't want to go down into Raymond's because you do not want to go down there in winter," says Hartrich. "It didn't make any sense that they would have stayed in Alpine Garden, so we decided to bag it and go down Lion Head."

Huntington Ravine
12:35 p.m.

Doug Madara and Steve Larson (Unit 1) join Bill Kane, Paul Ross, and Todd Swain (Unit 5), who are waiting for them at the base of Odell Gully. Joe Lentini and Tiger Burns (Unit 3), having attempted South Gully before encountering wind slab, are waiting for all of them on the floor of the ravine with Snow Rangers Brad Ray and Rene LaRoche. As Madara arrives at the base of the gully, Kane notices the toll that the weather had taken on the climbing teams. "Doug's balaclava was frozen to his neck, and I helped him peel it off," Kane recalls. "I had blisters under my eyes from frostbite."

At 12:30 p.m., Misha Kirk (Unit 17) departs Huntington for Lion Head. He knows from their radio reports that Hartrich and Dow plan to descend there and feels strongly that someone should be there to meet them. Excerpts from his journal offer an insider's glimpse of what is happening that time:

> Albert and Mike were going over the top and over to Lion Head. Steve and Doug had gone up and down Odell's in 3 hours. Impressive, considering the cold temps, blowing snow, and poor visibility. I was now outside the Thiokol, letting other people defrost and doing the two-step jog to keep warm. At times. I could see halfway up Odell's, which was five times as far as yesterday. As I saw Doug and Steve nearly down, I got this feeling I should walk over to Lion Head and make sure Mike & Albert got down safely. I didn't understand this gut feeling or bother to. I'd been active too long in mountaineering and emergency medicine not to act on intuition. I told some people and [Pinkham] of my plans and left down the trail.

Five minutes after Kirk's departure, at 12:35 p.m., Hartrich radios that he and Dow are beginning their descent of Lion Head. Ten minutes later, the Thiokol driven by Ray and LaRoche, carrying Kane, Larson, Madara, Ross, Swain, Lentini, and Burns, leaves the floor of the ravine and stops briefly at Harvard Cabin.

"We drove to the cabin and told everyone who was waiting there to start down to Pinkham, and that we'd take the Thiokol over to Tuckerman's to pick up Michael and Albert," says Kane. "And then it was worry and wait, wait and worry."

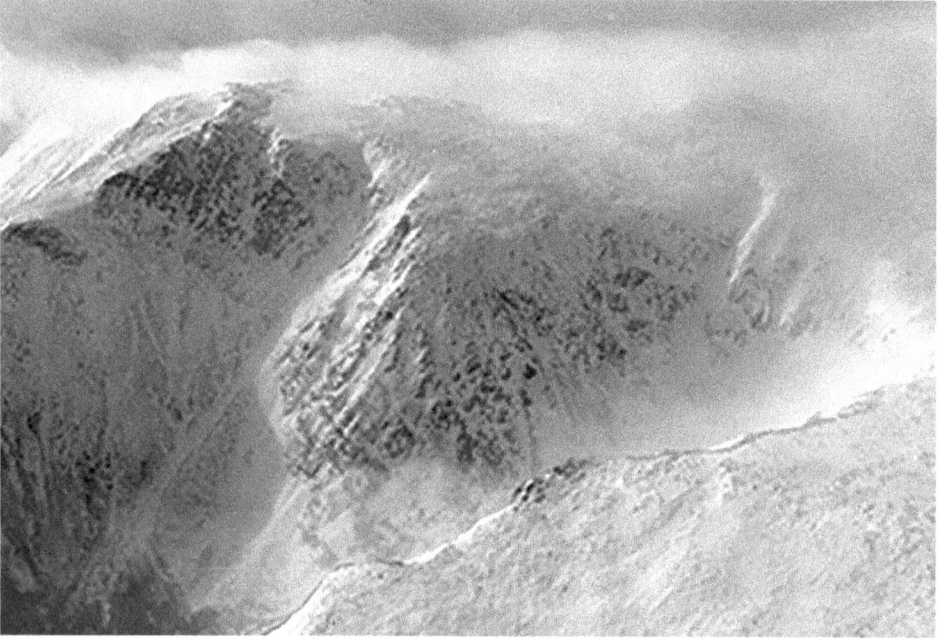

Lion Head (foreground) with Tuckerman Ravine and Boott Spur in high winds. Photo was taken on Jan. 26, 1982.

XLI
THE LION IN WINTER

[T]hey all felt that the adventure was far more dangerous than they had
thought, while all the time, even if they passed all the perils of the road,
the dragon was waiting at the end.
—J.R.R. Tolkien, *The Hobbit*

Mount Washington Observatory Surface Weather Observations (12:00 to 1:00
p.m.): Temperature -21°F; winds out of the west averaging 82 mph; visibility 0
miles; blowing snow/fog; windchill -67.8°F; peak wind gust: 101 mph.

Lion Head (4,240 ft.)
Mount Washington
Monday, Jan. 25, 1982
12:45 p.m.

As Michael Hartrich and Albert Dow move south past the crest of the summit and arrive at a point roughly parallel with the parking lot of Mount Washington State Park, they experience the full force of the winds. When westerly winds barrel through this section of the mountain, which lies between Alpine Garden Trail and the precipice of Lion Head, they submit anyone hiking up or down to a severe test of physical strength and emotional control. This is gloves-off behavior for Mount Washington.

Hartrich and Dow's eyelashes are caked with thick frost. Their anoraks and pants are plated with ice and snow. "My beard was frozen inside my anorak hood," recalls Hartrich. "That would happen every time I'd go ice climbing or lead a trip up to Washington. It probably would have been smarter to shave it off!"

Through frozen fog and blowing snow they can see the dark forest below them. The long line of ice-encrusted conifer and spruce stands between them and the relative security provided by the forested trees. Below treeline, at least, they'll be out of the wind.

Once they decided it was too risky to descend into Raymond Cataract, they've followed the bowl to Raymond's southern flank, bringing them onto the Summer Route at 4,400 feet and close to the snowfields perched above a cliff band on the northern face of Lion Head. This portion of the route is known as the Summer Traverse because it is prone to avalanche when wind-loaded with snow in winter. Hartrich and Dow are 700 feet northeast of the Winter Route, their intended target for the descent.

Hartrich is intimately familiar with Lion Head, but because of limited visibility, he is unable to get his bearings. "I had led winter hiking trips on Lion Head quite often," he says. "I'd been up there countless times. But you can still get lost because every year it's different."

At 12:45 p.m., Misha Kirk, who is at approximately 3,700 feet, notices something abnormal about the terrain above that alarms him. Having hiked across the Fire Road, he is approaching the intersection of Tuckerman Ravine Trail and Lion Head Trail. From this vantage point, Kirk is able to see the snowfields of the summer traverse approximately 500 feet above him. Kirk will later write in his journal, "Unlike yesterday, I was able to hike fast. I approached the sharp left turn, just down from the start of Lion Head Trail. I stopped and looked up. There where the summer Lion Head [Trail] traverses south at treeline hung a huge snowfield on top of a slide, like a double-decker ice cream cone ready to topple over. I quickly expressed my fear to [Pinkham] for Mike and Albert."

As Kirk looks at the slope as far as the cloud ceiling will let him, he knows exactly what he's seeing. As a caretaker at Hermit Lake Shelters, he's grown accustomed to the constant changes in the contours of the snow surface high above. The mid-to-upper slopes of Lion Head's Summer Route are loaded with wind slab that is massive and dangerous.

After hearing from Kirk, Pinkham radios Hartrich and Dow, alerting them to the avalanche hazard high up on the Summer Route and suggests they stay on the Winter Route. The Winter Route is to their right, and they continue trying to locate it in the swirling snow and frozen fog. According to the official report, the two are "proceeding with caution, carefully avoiding potential avalanche slopes," including the one that Kirk has warned them about.

Even with the adjustment Hartrich and Dow have made in response to his concern, Kirk is unnerved by the situation. "Mike and Albert could see what I was talking about and relayed that they would be careful," he wrote in his journal. "I felt a pit growing in my stomach. I asked [Pinkham] to call Joe [Gill] from Tucks to come and keep me company. Five minutes later, I was at the bottom of Lion Head waiting for Joe. I tried to wait, but I was getting cold and tense. So I began to climb, which due to waist-deep snow wasn't too fast. Soon Joe met up with me. He was on skis."

Meanwhile, Hartrich and Dow have dropped below treeline and are descending in a southeasterly direction and at an angle, hoping to link up with the elusive Winter Route. "We were below the cliffs for a time looking for a place to go down, plodding through snow," says Hartrich. "In retrospect, I wish we'd gone down elsewhere, but I didn't want to head straight down and wallow a long distance through deep snow."

Hartrich is aware of the snowpack conditions but feels some relief now that he and Dow are below treeline. "I knew there was a lot of snow there," he says. "But I wasn't thinking about it because we were down in the trees. It wasn't a big priority in my mind because the big thing for us was just trying to find a way down. We were tired and we wanted to get back. It was pretty deep powder snow, but when you're in the trees, you're not worried about it."

The two continue moving at an angle in the direction of the Winter Route, which they are hoping to take down to safety, but blazes on the trees are covered by snow. "I had no idea where we were," Hartrich acknowledges. "I couldn't see anything. We were down in the trees and there were clouds. The one thing that came into my mind was that the day before, a team went up the Winter Route. So we wanted to drop down and slab over until we get to their tracks. I was still thinking we were going to find the packed-out snowshoe rut where they went up. But I didn't realize it was completely obliterated by then. I lost sense of where we were, so we kept going and going, still looking for Hugh and Jeff."

Because they are out of the winds and trudging through deep powder, Hartrich and Dow are overheating. "Once we got down lower, we stopped for a while to get something to eat and drink," says Hartrich. "We were pretty comfortable at that point. But I finally said,

'We've got to go down.' I couldn't see anything, and you couldn't see anything above you."

Hartrich and Dow move along the slope and continue decreasing their elevation. They unknowingly cross over the Summer Route again at the switchbacks. They then cross over the 1969 avalanche path, which Hartrich is familiar with. But because vegetation has regrown within the massive avalanche scar, he doesn't recognize it. Shortly thereafter, they reach the Winter Route at the 4,000-foot mark, but unfortunately the limited visibility prevents them from realizing it. "We had to get out," says Hartrich. "I felt like we were getting pretty close to the trail, so we could head down."

After missing their intersection with the Winter Route, they will descend in the direction of Tuckerman Ravine and continue to try to find a safe way down the mountain.

When Joe Gill, having left the caretaker's cabin in Tuckerman after Kirk's request for support, arrives at the Lion Head Trail entrance to catch up with Kirk, he cannot see Hartrich and Dow descending. "They were off trail at that point," he says. "They had moved to the right and were beelining toward [Hermit Lake] in Tuckerman. I thought they were either headed to the snow ranger's cabin or the AMC cabin. Those would have been the closest to them."

Hartrich and Dow are approximately 100 yards south of the Lion Head Trail. As they move toward Tuckerman Ravine, they are still trudging through deep snow at an elevation of approximately 4,000 feet just below a cliff band. With Hermit Lake and the AMC shelters just over 100 feet in elevation below them and to the left, they are now only minutes away from the warmth and comfort of the burning woodstove in the caretaker's cabin—if they could only see it. "I couldn't see Hermit Lake because of the visibility, so I still couldn't tell where we were," says Hartrich. "But the approach into Tuckerman Ravine is like a triangle and narrows, so I knew we'd eventually come to something there."

At this point, even though they've missed the Winter Route, they have a plausible way down if they can orient themselves. As they cross a relatively narrow snow slope, Dow is above and slightly ahead of Hartrich to the right. Seventy feet above, a small cliff band runs parallel to them. Below them, a glade of white birches signals new growth and renewal.

"Albert was just above me," says Hartrich. "We still couldn't see anything above us. There was this one small, open snow slope to go across to get back into the trees. There was a foot of powder. We walked across the small area underneath the little cliff, which didn't look like very much. It was basically just a little runnel coming down, a snow slope with trees in it. I was just walking down into the trees when all of a sudden, I heard Albert yell."

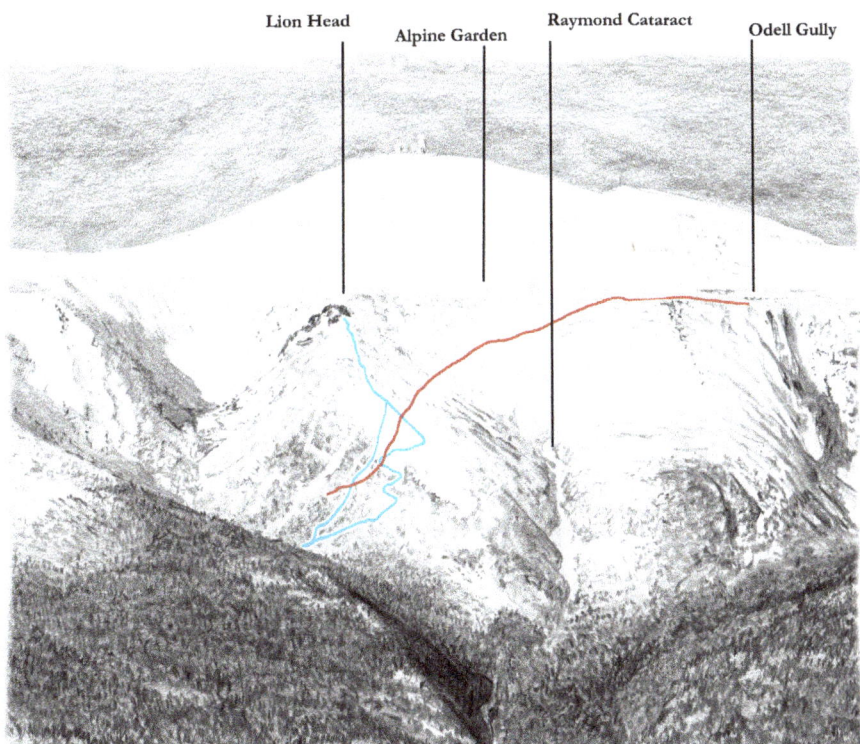

The red line shows the approximate route taken by Albert Dow and Michael Hartrich as they topped out on Odell Gully, traversed Alpine Garden, and contoured Raymond Cataract before descending Lion Head.

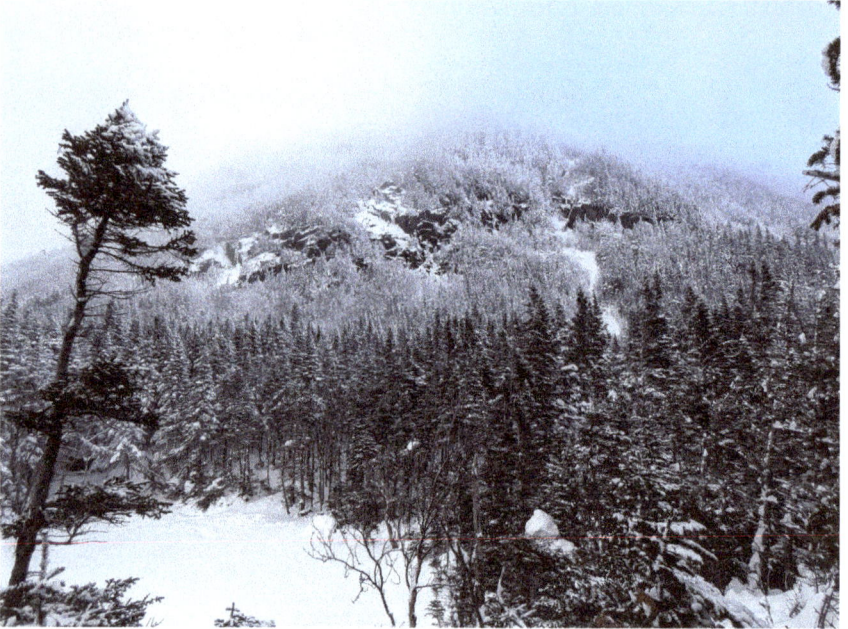

This photo, taken during the winter of 2022, shows the remnants of the avalanche scar just below the cliff line on Lion Head where Albert Dow and Michael Hartrich were buried.

XLII
THE DRAGON

So comes snow after fire, and even dragons have their ending.
—Bilbo Baggins, in J.R.R. Tolkien's *The Hobbit*

Lion Head (4,000 ft.)
Mount Washington
Monday, Jan. 25, 1982
1:45 p.m.

Albert Dow is the first to know something is going wrong. His sympathetic nervous system, sensing that an external force has taken control of his balance, sends an immediate stress response. In an instant, adrenaline and cortisol release into his bloodstream, putting his brain and body on high alert. He is prepared to fight or flee. But he isn't granted time to choose his course of action. He can't confront the threat nor run from it; all he can do is let out a yell.

At the mercy of the collapsing and accelerating snowpack, Dow loses his footing. Defenseless, he is knocked headfirst onto the slope by a wall of cascading snow and is quickly enveloped.

Michael Hartrich, who is traversing the slope just below and to the left of Dow, has no time to process his friend's cry. "I didn't have time to think or to turn and look. I was knocked forward onto my chest," says Hartrich. "I managed somehow to turn onto my back. I was trying to swim in it."

Dale Atkins, an internationally recognized expert on avalanches who for decades has worked as an avalanche forecaster, researcher, and instructor, pictures the scene as it unfolded: "As the fracture started, it was as if Michael and Albert were standing on a rug when someone pulled it out from beneath them. In this case the rug was the two-to-three-foot slab of snow sitting atop the weak layer with an ice crust underneath. When the rug was pulled out, you'd think they would have fallen backward, but they were on a 30-degree slope or steeper, so gravity pulled them downhill. As the rug was pulled, they moved with it until it knocked them over. They were literally going with the flow of the avalanche."

This avalanche was weeks in the making. The soft wind slab that is plummeting down the shallow gully started to form overnight during the snowstorm on Jan. 23, the day Hugh Herr and Jeff Batzer went missing in Huntington. As winds shifted from southerly to westerly, large amounts of windblown snow from Alpine Garden and points beyond had been loading here. As snow continued to accumulate, it packed the crystals together, creating a soft, cohesive slab.

Below this slab is a two-inch weak layer of soft snow that formed early on as winds shifted westerly and temporarily decreased in speed before ramping back up. This weak layer is hidden below Hartrich and Dow's boot strikes and sits on top of an icy crust poised to let the weak layer slide over it and down. Just before the slab lets go, Hartrich and Dow are crossing it simultaneously. Two people traveling together over unstable snow increases the impact, so it is impossible to know whether it is Hartrich or Dow who triggers the slide.

When their boots strike the slab, microfractures throughout the layer of weak snow coalesce into larger fractures that spread throughout the unstable snowpack. As these fractures break through the surface, they become visible. But that happens in a fraction of a second, and because the snow is soft, the collapse of the slab is silent. Hartrich and Dow have no idea what hits them.

The slab fractures approximately 40 feet above them, just below the cliff line. The fracture line or "crown" is 70 feet across, and the slab that lets go is 100 feet long. So Hartrich and Dow are in the middle of a 70-by-100-foot snow slab weighing 397,000 pounds, the weight of a fully-grown Antarctic blue whale.

"The avalanche happened relatively low down in the terrain," says Atkins. "Especially if you were a climber, you wouldn't think of where they were as scary avalanche terrain at all. It's terrain they'd had to suffer through to get where they wanted to go. But that can sometimes be some of the most dangerous terrain, not the real steep gullies and high faces, but those transitional slopes like the one they were traversing."

Joe Gill, then the Tuckerman caretaker, responded to the scene that day and returned to the site a day or two later to assist with the investigation. "I could push my fist through the soft slab with no problem," he says, referring to his second visit. "But when I reached the two-inch weak layer underneath it, it was so soft that I could slide my arm underneath the soft slab. The weak layer was like air. It just didn't take much for the slope to let go on them over that solid layer of ice."

The soft slab that envelops Hartrich and Dow is moving so quickly and with such force that they cannot process what is happening to them. "Once the snow started moving, the acceleration was almost instantaneous," says Atkins. "They would have reached maximum speed in the first 20 to 30 meters, traveling somewhere between 45 and 56 miles per hour. They were getting pushed along the flow and were at its whim. Getting swept into a tree would have been the equivalent of a pedestrian being hit by a car going that speed. Trees will act like fences and capture snow and sometimes people. You don't break bones in an avalanche; what breaks bones is colliding with a tree or rock. Being in an avalanche is like being in a river—you're going along with the flow."

As they plummet downward, Hartrich and Dow are funneled into the glade of birches that line the lower portion of the shallow gully. It is a deep terrain trap that increases the possibility of traumatic injury and/or a deeper burial once the flow stops. "I really don't remember anything, but I must have hit a tree or something because I had a gash above my left eye that I had to receive stitches for," Hartrich says.

The avalanche will travel 350 feet, only 10 feet short of a football field. It will slow before it stops completely. "Eventually I came down into kind of a flat area and stopped," says Hartrich. "All of a sudden, the snow just started coming down over me and covered me. I thought, 'Oh, I'm screwed now. This is it.'"

"Michael and Albert are in a traffic jam," says Atkins. "They are moving along with traffic and they suddenly stop, but what is behind them plows into them. Surface snow and moving debris travels faster than what's in front of it, so it's going to continue to flow and overrun what's already stopped. That's what Michael experiences."

Atkins offers advice for those who might find themselves in a similar situation:

> We tell people that when you feel the avalanche start to slow down, you should put your hand in front of your face or reach your arms up. Once an avalanche slows, it reacts less like a flowing river and more like a solid block. When it transitions from fluid to block, you are completely trapped in it. It's not rock hard; it's just interlocked and moving as a single unit. Avalanche victims will say, "I felt it starting to slow down but then I couldn't move my hands. I couldn't get them in front of my face.' So it's important to try to raise your arms before you get trapped.

Ryan Driscoll, a certified mountain guide, member of MRS since 2015, and Level 2-certified by the American Institute for Avalanche Research, corroborates Atkins advice: "I think trying to swim at least initially is effective. Anything you can do to try and stay on top is good. When you realize you are going under as the debris is slowing down, you throw an arm across your face to create an air pocket and hope for the best."

As overwhelming as the situation is, Hartrich does not give up and manages to do exactly what Atkins and Driscoll recommend. "I kind of woke up and started to punch away at the snow with my left arm as it was still going over me, and I was able to open up a hole. I couldn't move the arm very much, because the snow was all set up. I was unable to move any other part of my body at that point. But I had this little hole in the snow and one arm free. I don't know how deep down I was. I was just lying there buried, looking at the hole, and I figured, 'Well, I hope nothing else comes down.' It was a stressful situation, and basically my mind just turned off because it didn't want to deal with what was going on. I have no idea how much time I was there, but it was a while."

Dr. Nicole Sawyer, a New Hampshire-based psychologist who specializes in critical incident stress and resiliency within the first-responder community, says Hartrich is in "survival mode." "When you're in that state, your body shuts every unnecessary function down. Only the bare necessities remain. Your emotional experience of your entrapment is not a necessary thing. So your brain very kindly shuts that down for you to prevent the panic."

With his left arm barely movable, he uses his forearm and fist to hack away at the heavy snow that entombs him. With enormous effort, he creates a small gap between his chest and the snow, just enough space for him to reach the chest pocket of his frozen anorak. He pinches the flap of the pocket in his Dachstein mitten and pulls. As he peels the flap open, the sound of releasing Velcro signals his success. He pulls the brick-like portable radio he's carrying out of the pocket, slides it across his chest, brings the speaker to his balaclava-covered mouth, and depresses the transmitter button.

"I radioed that Albert and I were caught in an avalanche on Lion Head. And then it seemed like forever."

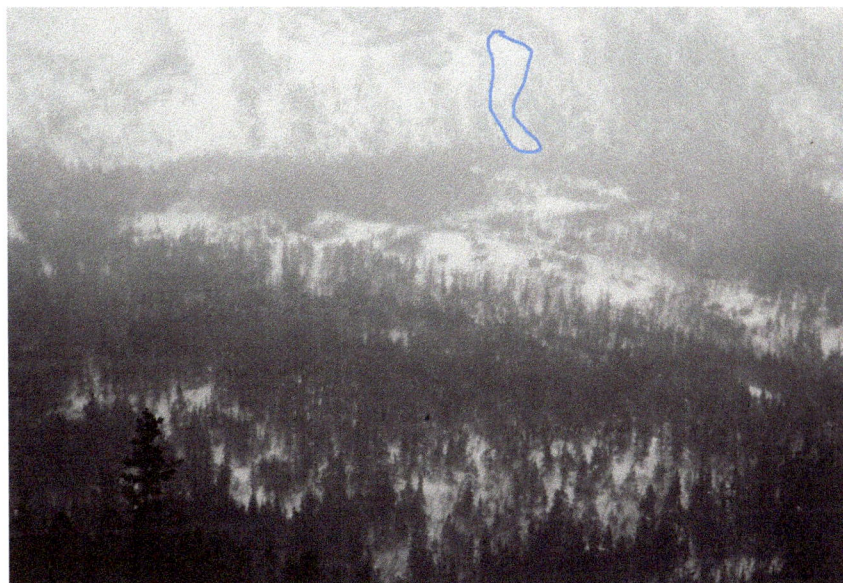

Two days after the avalanche on Lion Head, backpackers Geoffrey May and David Boudreau climb the Boott Spur Link Trail in Tuckerman Ravine. May stops to take a photo of Tuckerman Ravine and unknowingly captures the avalanche site.

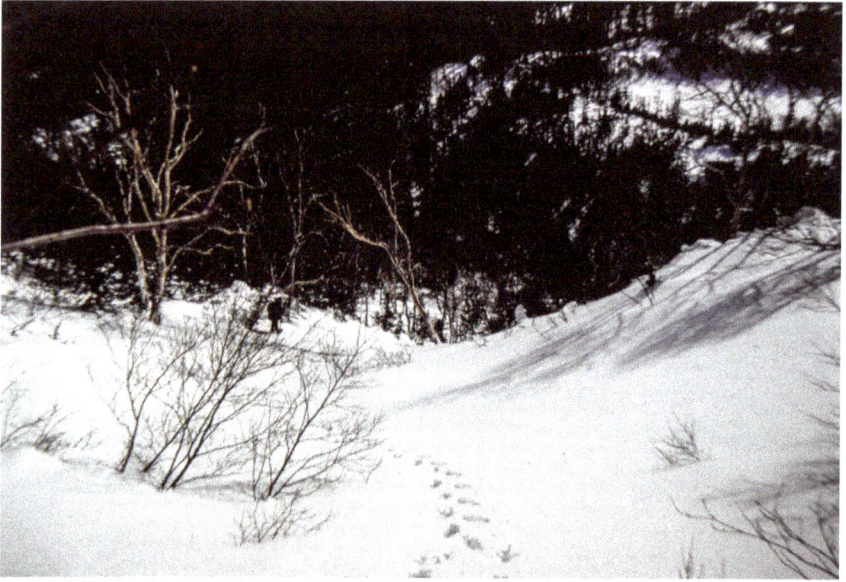

Two photos of the avalanche path on Lion Head taken by Tuckerman caretaker Joe Gill in the days following the tragedy. The top photo was taken near the crown line looking down the shallow gully. On the left side of the gully, in the middle of the frame, is an individual who is standing at the approximate location where Michael Hartrich and Albert Dow crossed. The bottom photo shows the location of the crown line just below the cliff band.

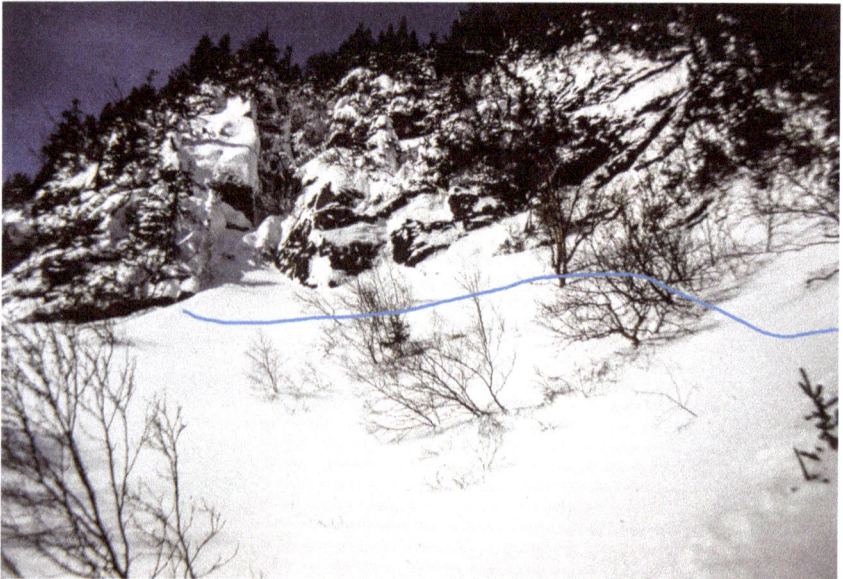

XLIII
UNIT 4 IS DOWN

Two hundred miles to clear.
Chasin' a sound I hear.
When the call brings them all to tears.
And the hopes they all turn to fears.
—Kings of Leon, "The Bandit"

Lion Head Trail (3,800 ft.)
Monday, Jan. 25, 1982
2:00 p.m.

Joe Gill is on the fast track. When Misha Kirk radioed him from the base of Lion Head asking that Gill meet him at the trail junction, he sensed Kirk's worry and felt his quickest way to the trailhead was on skis. But on reaching the junction, Gill realizes that Kirk has already started up in the hope of meeting Hartrich and Dow on their way down. He quickly catches up to Kirk and sees that he is struggling.

Because he has rushed over to Lion Head from Huntington Ravine, Kirk isn't wearing skis or snowshoes. Gill looks on as a determined Kirk drives through waist-deep snow. "As we climbed, Joe and I took different paths," Kirk wrote in his journal. "Suddenly I heard some yelling. I called to Joe to see if it was him. He said no but that he had heard it too. I notified base that I was suspicious, and that something wasn't right!" Shortly thereafter, Kirk and Gill receive the news: Hartrich and Dow have been avalanched.

"I told Misha what I'd found for snow conditions up there the day before, and we decided to go off in different directions," says Gill. "We followed our individual hunches as to where the slide had happened. Misha went right and headed up the Summer Route, and I went left because I felt the greater avalanche potential was under the ledges on our left, and because someone had radioed that Mike and Albert were beelining it to the cabin, which was in that direction."

Standing motionless on the Summer Route, Kirk listens as the haunting sounds of distress surge and fade away. He cannot get an accurate read on where the cries are coming from. "We heard yelling, but it sounded like they were coming from the porch at Tuck's," wrote Kirk. "We thought someone was seeing something from there that we couldn't see."

Fire Road (3,538 ft.)
Huntington Ravine
2:00 p.m.

As he rides on the exposed truck bed of the Forest Service Thiokol, Team Leader Bill Kane holds a heavy portable radio close to his ear, fearing that the throaty engine of the Thiokol might drown out an important radio transmission from Hartrich and Dow. A few minutes earlier, Kane, Rob Walker, Paul Ross, Todd Swain, Joe Lentini, Tiger Burns, Steve Larson, and Doug Madara had loaded onto the back of the Thiokol at Harvard Cabin for the 15-minute ride over to Lion Head to meet their two descending teammates. Brad Ray and Rene LaRoche, who are in the front cab of Thiokol, bring the total number of passengers to 10.

"We were always aware we were on the edge," Kane says today. "At that point, we felt we had dodged a bullet as we were riding in the Thiokol and waiting for the guys to come down. We'd done our job. We'd cleared the fact that Hugh and Jeff were not in Odell. They were somewhere else, but not in the gully. But I was still terrified. We knew where Michael and Albert were, and I remember speaking to Michael by radio when they were at the top of Lion Head. I was thinking to myself, 'They should be down by now. Why aren't they down by now?'"

Madera recalls hearing intermittent transmissions from Hartrich and Dow as the group was moving across the connector trail in the Thiokol. "It got to the point where I thought something was wrong," he says.

Shortly after the Thiokol leaves Harvard Cabin, caretaker Matt Pierce writes in the log:

"The cabin is empty now. Just me now. MRS has left having done all that could be expected in these conditions. Climbing in these conditions, below zero and blowing 60 bastards, is difficult for the best. The faces of several & the toes of a few [are] garbed in shades of frostbite. Evidence of the severity & the risks taken."

Joe Lentini remembers a jovial mood in the truck bed as he and his teammates jostled along the Fire Road toward Lion Head. Although they were all cold and tired, they shared a sense of warmth and comradery for a difficult job done well. "We were getting out of there, and we were so relieved because it was unsafe up there," says Lentini. "We were laughing and joking until that crackle on the radio, and it was like the switch just flipped. I can remember we were right where you make the traverse over to Tucks when Michael started screaming on the radio, 'Avalanche, avalanche!' And that was it."

Hartrich's desperate screams slam into the chest of each man, eliciting a systemic stress response throughout the Thiokol. Cortisol and adrenaline pump through their bloodstreams, causing heart rates to spike and respiration to accelerate. Hands shake and shoulders shudder as their bodies prepare for a response. Unlike Hartrich and Dow, who had no time to feel or process the adrenaline dump they experienced on the slope as it collapsed below and around them, the Thiokol's occupants feel all of it. "It was horrible," says Kane.

As exhausted and stunned as they are, these first responders will move toward the crisis without hesitation. The distance between them and their two teammates in trouble cannot be closed fast enough. No longer searching, they are now in rescue mode.

"Brad Ray accelerated the Thiokol, and we shot over," says Lentini. "Our minds were going 100 miles per hour. It's one of those things where you're in one mood and really happy, and then all of a sudden it's like 'Holy shit!' The world just turned."

Even with the throttle pegged, the Thiokol can only achieve a running pace at best. Everyone riding in back has the urge to jump off and run toward Hartrich and Dow. But they know that in deep snow they won't get very far before flaming out.

Frank Hubbell, who had been sitting in a snow cave in Huntington Ravine on standby during the morning climbs, is descending from Harvard Cabin to Pinkham when he learns of the trouble on Lion Head and heads that way. "I was on foot when I learned of the avalanche," he recalls. "I immediately kicked into prayer. 'Everything's going to be OK,' I told myself."

Harvard Cabin (3,520 ft.)
2:00 p.m.

Matt Pierce is startled out of his attempt to decompress at Harvard Cabin after the departure of the Thiokol when he hears Hartrich's chilling radio transmission, which shatters the cabin's short-lived calm.

Pierce grabs his pen and makes an entry in the cabin's log: "The last unit #4 caught in avalanche!! Rescuers must be rescued. Mike is on the radio & says he is half buried. Will this weekend ever end? I'm just waiting by the radio. ... The other group of MRS is on the way in the snow-cat. Joe Gill & Misha are nearly at the scene."

Unable to restrain himself, Pierce throws on his jacket and gloves and slams the heavy wooden door shut behind him. As he points in the direction of the Spur Trail, he has the wherewithal to grab a critical tool. "I left the cabin with a snow shovel and started running uphill to where they were rendezvousing at the base of Lion Head," he says. "I remember it was sunnier, but it was really cold. I think I got frost nip on my lungs that day."

Jeff Moskowitz, an AMC crew member who'd searched trails in the vicinity of Harvard Cabin on skis before hunkering down there during the search in Huntington, is mindlessly gliding down the Huntington Ravine Trail when his portable radio yanks him into alertness. "I had started down from Harvard Cabin to Pinkham," he says. "I had finished what I had been asked to do. All of a sudden, the radio just blew up, and everybody was frantic. It was really alarming and scary to listen to. Somebody was screaming, and you had no idea who it was. There was a huge amount of urgency once someone figured out who it was, where they were, and what had happened to them. I remember thinking that I could be helpful, but I got the strong feeling that because of the assumed location and the fact that there was an avalanche, Pinkham didn't want people up there who weren't on Mountain Rescue Service."

Pinkham
2:00 p.m.

As a former member of the British Special Air Service, Bill Aughton has been schooled in the belief that you do not leave a dangerous situation until every last member of the team returns from a mission. "We were at Pinkham when word came down that Michael and Albert had been avalanched," says Aughton, who was sitting with fellow Brit, longtime friend, and MRS teammate David Stone when the word arrived. "I can remember running around Pinkham trying to find snowmobiles because the Thiokol was already up there, and I wanted to get some of us up there fast. I couldn't, so we grabbed our packs and ran over to the construction shed. We managed to get three big snow shovels, strapped them onto our packs, and legged it up to Tucks at breakneck speed. I was with David and Dana [Seavey], who was a good friend of Albert's."

Seavey recalls that team members at Pinkham were told to just stand by, since there were others on the way. "When the avalanche call first came in, no one at Pinkham thought it was that bad," recalls Seavey. "I said to myself, 'Fuck that! And I headed to the avalanche site."

For his part, fellow MRS member Matt Peer recalls that in his urgency to act, he headed off in a different direction from that of teammates. It is a poignant example of how individuals react to stressful events. "I started running back up there on the Huntington Ravine Trail as fast as I could, until I learned the avalanche was actually more toward Lion Head," he says. On realizing his error, he headed in the direction of the call.

Mike Waddell, an AMC crew member who had searched Old Jackson Road with Jeff Tirey and Jack Corbin the night before, also refused to wait around when trouble struck. "I was in the radio room at Pinkham," he says. "There was a crowd of us when the call came in. That was tough. There was a lot of screaming into the radio. You could hear the wind howling over the radio and if the intention was to electrify anyone who heard it, it succeeded. Those of us who were in the room just blasted out of there with little or no preparation. We grabbed whatever gear was lying about and ran up the Tuck Trail."

Lion Head (4,000 ft.)
2:20 p.m.

Joe Gill traverses the slope on skis in the direction he believes the yells are coming from. Threading through thick tree cover, he watches as the canopy ahead eases and the terrain brightens. Soon, a shallow gully within a glade opens up before him. "I heard Mike hollering as I was approaching," he recalls. "I traversed across to the voice and came on what was an obvious avalanche path. There were birch glades all along the ledges there, and birches were sticking out of the slide path everywhere. Above the glade, I could see there was an open slope where Mike and Albert had probably started into it. The snow was churned, but it wasn't blocky at all because it had passed through a bunch of trees. It was basically just a rough patch of snow. I can remember thinking I had never seen that area slide before."

Gill plants his ski poles into the slope and conducts a quick scan of the debris field. Almost immediately, his eyes are drawn toward frenetic movement. "I basically came out of the woods right on top of Mike," he says, though in the moment he could not tell if he was seeing Hartrich or Dow. "I found him in the deposition area of the avalanche. I saw his gloved hand sticking out of the middle of it, and he was holding his radio, which seemed like a miracle. He was on his back and his head was downhill. He was completely buried except for his hand."

When he realizes he's found Hartrich, Gill notifies Pinkham but adds that Dow is missing. "I could see Mike's face, and he had one arm free," recalls Gill. "He was glad to see me but also kind of panicked. He was talking to me when I got there."

Using his mittened hand, Gill shovels snow away from Hartrich's face until it's fully exposed. Then he places what he hopes is a reassuring hand on Hartrich's shoulder as he explains that he must leave him for a time in order to find Dow. "Mike, I've got you, there's more help on the way, but I've got to find Albert," Gill recalls saying. "Misha showed up shortly after that and went to work digging Mike out as I set off to look for Albert."

Kirk will write in his journal, "I arrived and saw Mike's Dachstein waving up in the snow. What a great sight as I whooped in joy. I ran down and started to check and dig Mike out. As people started to

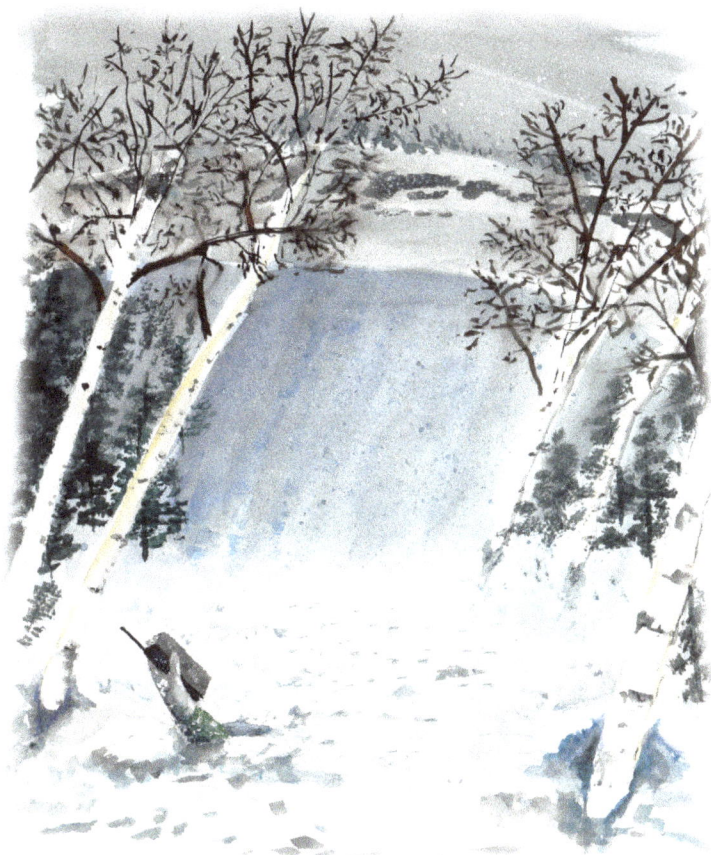

arrive, I told them to start looking for Albert. Mike was OK but cemented in with heavy, wet snow. I looked around and just couldn't believe this slope had avalanched with so many trees around. Mike told me that Albert had shouted out a warning, and he thought Albert was somewhere above him. Digging out Mike with just my hands was hard, so eventually I had to use a shovel."

A bit earlier, as Kirk was making his way to the avalanche site, he was joined by the responding members of MRS who had ridden over from Harvard Cabin in the Thiokol. While the rescuers traversed in single file across the slope, the snowpack offered a not-so-subtle warning that the slopes near the avalanche site were still primed. "By this time other members of MRS were beginning to arrive," wrote Kirk. "I was in the lead, traversing with Joe Lentini and others behind me. Suddenly, we heard a great loud 'Arrumph' on a steep slope covered with lots of trees. I looked at Joe and he looked at me. We were scared, but we didn't slow down. Our friends were in trouble."

While Kirk works to extract Hartrich from the deposition, and others arrive at the site, Gill leverages his avalanche training in hopes of locating Dow. "I did a visual search back and forth of the avalanche path," he recalls. "I was looking to see if there was anything fetched up in the trees. I started the ground search by doing a big loop, and then I fine-tuned it until other people showed up to take over. We had people there pretty fast. It was cold, and although it wasn't particularly windy, it was still a bad day."

XLIV
THE GLADE

Loaded with ice a sunny winter morning
After a rain. They click upon themselves
As the breeze rises, and turn many colored
As the stir cracks and crazes their enamel.
Soon the sun's warmth makes them shed crystal shells.
Shattering and avalanching on the snow crust—
Such heaps of broken glass sweep away
You'd think the inner dome of heaven had fallen.
—Robert Frost, "Birches"

Avalanche Site (4,000 ft.)
Lion Head
Monday, Jan. 25, 1982
2:35 p.m.

It is a place where the phrase "off the beaten path" could have been coined. At most a 10-minute walk from Hermit Lake and the shelters lining it, this birch glade is beautiful but holds no great attraction for hiker, climber, or bushwhacker. Claude Monet painted more than 100 winter scenes in his lifetime, and this spot could have easily been one of them.

By mountain risk standards back then, tree-laden terrain like this one was considered benign, unthreatening, and sleepy. Encountering a glade of birch trees does not cause the hairs on the back of the neck to rise or a chill to run down the spine. The only known avalanche hazard in this area at the time was on the headwall in Tuckerman Ravine. On Lion Head itself, it was believed any such hazard had been mitigated by the designation of a specific Winter Route up and down the mountain. Even one of the largest avalanches in Mount Washington history, which occurred on Lion Head in 1969, was far to the right of this one. With over a decade of regrowth within the scar left by that avalanche, its slide path was indiscernible. This moderately steep slope in the glade of 30-to-35 degrees had always held on to the snowpack. It was a small plot of relatively gentle terrain that stretched briefly from Tuckerman Ravine to Lion Head or vice versa.

"I was incredulous that a tree-filled slope could avalanche," says Todd Swain. "It never occurred to me that was a possibility." Paul Ross, who along with Swain and Bill Kane stood high on a perch in Odell that morning as climbers searched it, recalls being equally flabbergasted. "When we got to the avalanche site, I just couldn't believe it had happened there among those trees."

Rene LaRoche and Brad Ray approach the site with probes and shovels they retrieved at the Hermit Lake rescue cache after dropping off the MRS team. LaRoche, who'd been a snow ranger in Cutler River Drainage since 1965, still marvels today at how rare an event he and others were witnessing that afternoon in such an unlikely spot.

Although it is true that no avalanche had been witnessed in the birch glade by any of the experienced climbers on the rescue team, avalanche expert Dale Atkins says today that trees don't always provide refuge from such an event. "Trees are a perception of safety," he says. "But when you have weak layers of snow, the trees might not provide enough support to hold on to it. And when an avalanche does happen, the trees become like baseball bats or battering rams."

Here in the lee at 4,000 feet, the weather is less extreme than searchers have faced over the last two days, but it is still harsh. Westerly winds pouring down off the summit of Mount Washington, known as down-sloping, approach 40 mph. When combined with the ambient temperature of -15°F, the windchill is still a caustic -49.7°F. Snow is sloughing off Lion Head above the searchers, giving the impression it's still snowing. "It was a typical windy day," says Joe Lentini. "We were feeling it blowing around us, but we were completely oblivious to it."

It is the first time the members of MRS have been asked to probe for an avalanche victim. Up to this point, the limited number of callouts have been for victims on top of the avalanche debris field, not buried under it. "Nobody knew what to do with the probes they gave us," recalls Steve Larson. "So Brad and Rene told us what to do, and we quickly started probing."

The goal of this early stage of the search is to probe as much of the debris field as quickly as possible in hopes of getting a positive hit. Asphyxiation of a buried victim can occur within 10 minutes, so every second counts.

"We started probing in the avalanche debris set," Kirk wrote in his journal. "We first probed in the obvious spots that would tie up a body: trees, mounds of snow, etc. Every once in a while, someone's probe would catch. He'd call out for a shovel and start to dig. With the first one, we were just about set to jump over to help dig. But as more people called for the shovel, and more false alarms ensued, the calmer and more frustrated we became. As the minutes ticked by, I started to feel the worst had happened. I started saying aloud, 'C'mon Albert, where are you?' Someone mentioned, 'Well, he might have popped out below and gone for help.' 'No,' I said, 'he'd never leave Mike.' We all agreed."

The false alarms Kirk is describing are known as false positives. The debris field often includes chunks of ice, trees, rocks, and branches. Anything in the path of the slide when it lets go is subject to being scraped off the terrain. "The thing you're looking for with a positive strike is that a body has a little bit of rebound to it, a little bit of squish," says avalanche expert Ryan Driscoll. "If you think you have something you then do a comparison probe off to the side."

Bill Kane recalls the challenge of doing probes among the birches, especially in such a time-sensitive search. "A body caught in an avalanche will come around a tree to the other side," he says. "The first thing we did was to go up between every rock and tree and probed below it to see if we could find Albert in there. Of course we didn't during the hasty search. The wind was still going strong at the site. So we always had this background noise, but we were all completely focused on what we were doing."

Ryan Driscoll further explains the challenges rescuers were facing that day: "In a gladed environment, the debris is going to strain through the trees. Some of it is going to build up on the uphill side of the trees. If there's any sort of bench feature in the terrain or scoop in the slope, it's going to be deeper there. In treed terrain you can get sucked under a log and you might have an air pocket."

At 3:00 p.m., nearly an hour after his near burial, Hartrich is extracted from the debris. Approximately 600 pounds of snow has been removed to free him. "Once Mike was free, I gave him a quick going over," wrote Kirk. "I was pretty sure all he had were contusions and bruises, but I asked him to lie there quietly while I conferred with Frank Hubbell, who then took Mike to Tucks for a better exam."

When they dig him out, Hartrich is in a state of shock and very concerned about Albert. "I told them he had been just above me to the right. I was hoping they'd find him up there." In the stress of the moment, someone suggests that Hartrich join the search. But having been compressed by the snow for almost an hour and then released, he is in danger of keeling over at any moment, and Hubbell is eager to get him to safety and warmth.

"Michael had been encased in ice," Hubbell says today. "We decided that Joe [Gill] and I would walk him over to the caretaker's cabin to get him out of his wet clothing. We wanted to check him out to make sure he was OK. We were very happy that Michael could walk under his own power. As we were rewarming him, I remember him saying, 'I'm positive I'm OK. Let's hope Albert is OK.' He was very focused on Albert."

With Hartrich rewarming and stable, Gill heads back to the avalanche site to assist with the search. "It was dead calm at the site," he recalls. "Everybody was calm and professional. There was no screaming or yelling."

With the hasty search yielding no results, Ray and LaRoche direct searchers to the base of the slide to conduct a more targeted search of the debris. Despite the tremendous urgency, their approach must be methodical if they hope to succeed. Ray stands at the base of the deposition and directs rescuers to line up. They will begin on the right side, and he will walk forward with the line to keep them together. LaRoche stands above everyone to give verbal directions so that the line moves and probes simultaneously.

"We started at the bottom of the debris," says Kane. "We lined up to the left and to the right from the point where Michael was found. We'd step up, probe four to six holes, and step up again. It wasn't really a wide debris field, maybe 100 feet across."

"By this time I was going over CPR in my head as I probed," wrote Kirk. "I felt calm but scared. I knew I'd do my job. I was just afraid for Albert."

It has been 50 minutes since the first rescuers arrived at the site and began to search. LaRoche continues to call cadence. With the exception of a few false positives, the group remains totally silent. LaRoche drives his probe into the snow to use as a marker for the probe line and detects something beneath the snowpack. "I wasn't quite sure if I'd hit a little spruce tree," says LaRoche of that moment. "You're supposed to know what it feels like to find a person. In training, we'd bury a mannequin in the snow and try to locate it. It feels a little different from snow or a tree or a rock. When I felt something there, I had somebody dig."

"Rene called out for the shovel," wrote Kirk. "I half paid attention as I watched out for my position on the line. Then Rene shouted. He had found something blue."

"That's where Albert was, by that little spruce tree," says LaRoche. "The tree stopped him, but the snow kept going a little bit, and he was right on the edge of it, right on the edge of the slide."

For Joe Lentini, it was a life-altering moment that remains seared in his memory. "Our adrenaline was going full tilt as we probed," he says. "We took a step up to probe. Then off to my left I heard, 'I've got him!'"

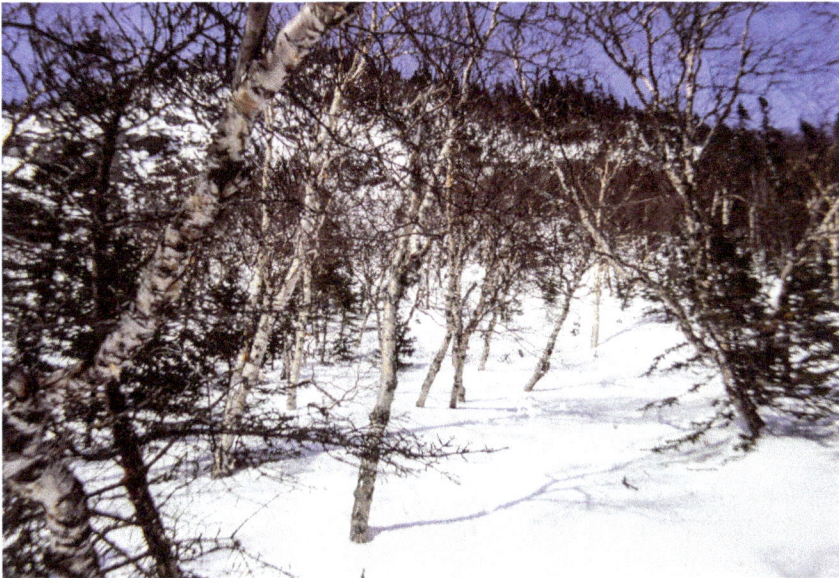

This photo, taken by Tuckerman caretaker Joe Gill looking upslope at the slide path, shows the glade of birch trees where Albert Dow and Michael Hartrich were found.

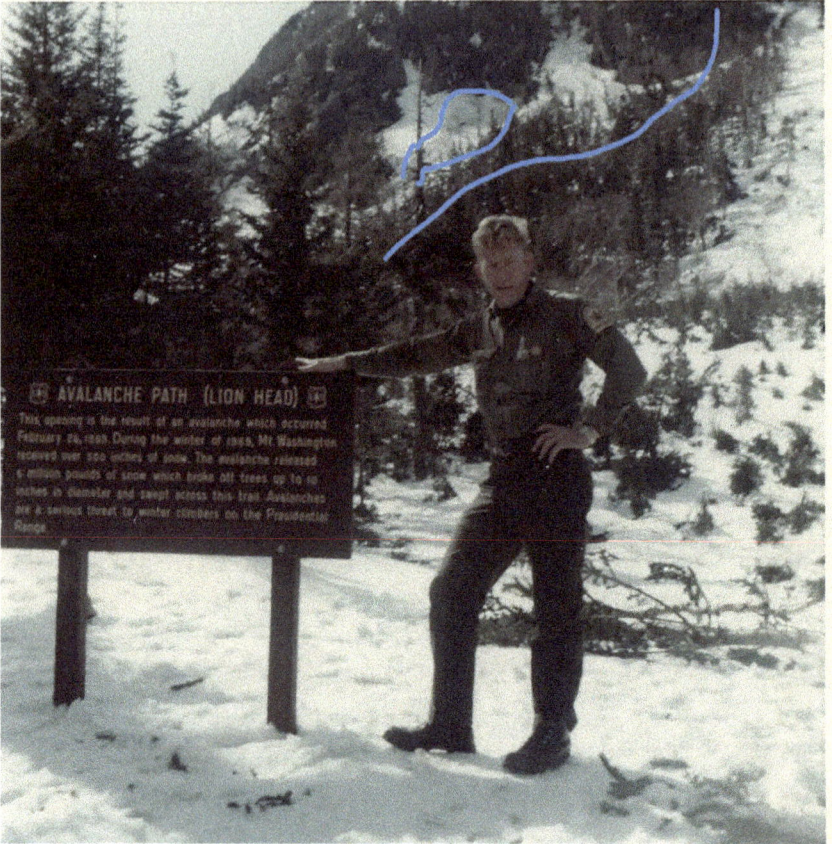

Snow Ranger Rene LaRoche, in an early 1970s photo taken from another angle than the photo on page 164, at the site of the 1969 slide path on Lion Head. By 1982, when Michael Hartrich and Albert Dow hike across the 1969 slide path, it had experienced heavy regrowth of trees and other vegetation, making it indiscernible. Shortly after crossing here, they unknowingly cross the Winter Route (blue line). The circle (top middle) is the location of the avalanche that overtook them.

XLV
FULL MEASURES

When you're part of a team, you stand up for your teammates. Your
loyalty is to them. You protect them through good and bad,
because they'd do the same for you.

—Yogi Berra

Avalanche Site (4,000 ft.)
Lion Head
Monday, Jan. 25, 1982
3:15 p.m.

The once rigid probe line implodes as members of Mountain Rescue Service rush toward Snow Ranger Rene LaRoche. His avalanche rescue training has yielded the result all had hoped for 50 minutes earlier when rescuers first arrived at the avalanche site. LaRoche's positive probe strike has located Albert Dow approximately three feet beneath the snow.

"We had been probing for five or 10 minutes," says LaRoche. I moved one of the searcher's backpacks that was lying on top of the debris because it was in the way of the probe line. I then probed and found Albert directly under the place where the pack had been. He was very close to the spot where Mike had been partially buried."

Joe Lentini recalls the searchers dropping their probes and forming a shovel line next to LaRoche. "One person would shovel as hard as they could for 30 to 40 seconds, and then just fall off to the side, exhausted. While someone dug, others were behind him pushing the snow away. And then the next person shoveled. You shoveled until you couldn't any longer. We were all pretty fit back then, but it was just like you were at 100 percent of your ability."

Michael Hartrich had been able to create a hole at the surface of the debris through which he could breathe and notify rescuers. But Dow, who is found about three feet away from his teammate, is buried much deeper. With their mittened hands, some rescuers kneel and dig violently while others keep shoveling. Some remove their mittens and claw their way downward bare-handed. They are fueled by adrenaline and desperation, which render them oblivious to the emotional and physical punishment being exacted upon them.

"A typical burial requires removing 2,000 to 2,600 pounds of snow, which is one ton of snow," says avalanche expert Dale Atkins. "To completely free a buried person, a single rescuer who is fit and uses a typical backcountry avalanche shovel can clear that much snow in about 15 minutes. It would take about five minutes to reach the person's head and chest, and another 10 minutes or so to uncover the rest of the person. Lacking a shovel, one person using their hands would take about an hour." Because there are so many rescuers here at the avalanche site, they will reach Dow in minutes.

Fellow avalanche expert Ryan Driscoll says that avalanche rescue techniques he and others teach today were not known to those on Lion Head in 1982. "When you get a positive strike, you should leave the probe in and move one step downhill to dig," he says of the strategy that has developed over time. "This is the shortest way to the victim. Digging straight down can cause the walls of the hole to collapse into the hole. When you do get to the victim, you should go for their airway as fast as you can. Ideally, you want to get them out in under 10 minutes and start treating them."

Matt Pierce, who'd bolted out of Harvard Cabin and across the Fire Road to help, says, "It didn't take us very long to get to Albert. Everybody just started digging, and at times there were too many people digging in one spot. We only had so much room."

During his digging cycle, Doug Madara works himself to exhaustion and then moves off to the side for the next person in line. "I was thinking that if Albert was alive, we were going to need a litter, so I ran down to the hut and grabbed a litter and took it back there. By the time I got back, they were down to the body."

Steve Larson, who along with Madara had searched Odell Gully earlier in the day along with Hartrich and Dow, is the first to reach his stricken teammate. "I was digging with my hands, and I found Albert's foot, just the sole of his boot," says Larson, as he solemnly recalls the moment. "It was the first sign of Albert we found. I can remember that he was lying on his stomach and then we just had to

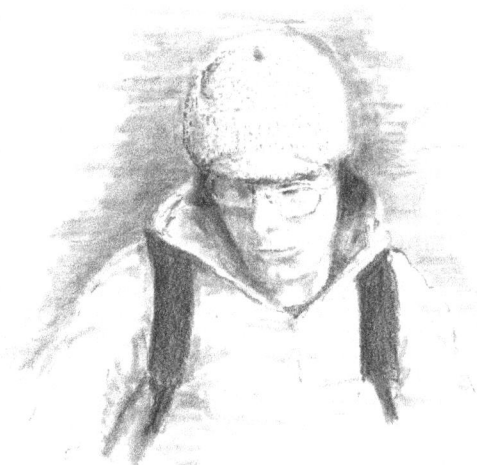

Doug Madara

follow along. We started digging for his head, which was much deeper than his boot."

Joe Lentini, a close friend and teammate of Dow, recalls the moment Larson revealed the boot. "And then there Albert was," he says. "We dug down and cleared around him. It was clear to me that Albert wasn't breathing. We were trying to clear the debris away and get him up onto the snow safely." In minutes, rescuers removed approximately 1,850 pounds of snow to extract him.

As Dow's teammates remove debris on and around him, Misha Kirk prepares everyone for the next phase of the rescue attempt. "I shouted out, 'Who's going to do CPR with me?'" he wrote in his journal. Larson remembers Kirk's ability to make decisions amid the total chaos. "Misha was battle hardened," he says.

Even before they get Dow out, Kirk begins working to save him. "I was able to get my ear to his mouth; no breathing," he wrote. "I got no carotid pulse. I got two fingers in his mouth, no snow. In fact his mouth was warm to my bare fingers. He had a huge gash on his lower jaw, but absolutely no blood in the snow. Finally, he had no ice mask around his face. I knew then he had died instantly, and we didn't have a chance. But we had to try. He was our friend."

When rescuers find evidence of an ice mask, it indicates that a buried victim was breathing underneath the snow. "The snow around your face is permeable for a bit," explains Ryan Driscoll. "As you breathe, the snow freezes and becomes impermeable, forming an ice mask." The fact that there is no ice mask present at Dow's face signals that he did not asphyxiate.

"As soon as Albert was completely dug out, Bill [Kane] and I began CPR," wrote Kirk. "Initially I couldn't get a patent airway, so I tried back blows and other measures. Finally, I was able to go mouth to nose. I was still in bare hands, and after 10 minutes they were in bitter pain. I had to ask for relief, and Rob Walker jumped in."

"We got Albert up on the snow and we tried to get a breath in, and it wouldn't go in," says Lentini. "We repositioned him, but a breath still wouldn't go in, so we radioed Pinkham for an airway to be relayed to us." Plans were put in motion to have the Gorham Police Department relay an endotracheal tube (ET tube) from the Gorham Medical Center. An ET tube is placed between the vocal cords through the trachea to ensure that oxygen delivered by a rescuer reaches the victim's lungs.

Kane was also alternating with Kirk and Walker as they applied CPR. "Albert had indications of significant trauma that I ignored because I told myself we were going to save him," says Kane. "I had been doing CPR with Rob for at least 30 minutes. It was when Frank [Hubbell] arrived that he did a physical assessment and found a devastating gap in Albert's cervical spine."

His hands freezing from a combination of digging without mittens and performing CPR, Kirk recognizes the stark and painful reality of the situation. "I held my hands in Joe Gill's armpits, inside his jacket, and closed my eyes to the tears," Kirk wrote. "I had seen death many times, and I knew as soon as I saw Albert that we couldn't do anything. We had found an obvious C-3 neck fracture and as the minutes ticked by, the mood of fearing the worst rose. We avoided saying anything and looked into each other's eyes for hope."

Hubbell, who arrived with first-aid supplies after being summoned back to the site from the caretaker hut, recalls the emotional weight of the moment he realized nothing else could be done for Dow. "When I got there Albert was lifeless. Someone was doing chest compressions on him, and Bill Kane was managing his airway. This went on for a few minutes and I said to Bill, 'Let me take over the airway.' When I slid my hand behind Albert's neck I felt the separation of the cervical vertebra. I could put two fingers in the space. Albert's cervical spine was completely severed between C1 and C2."

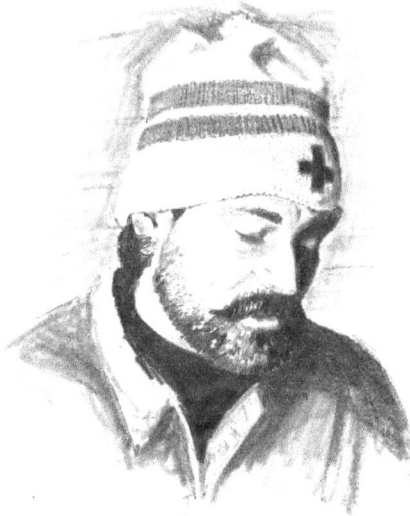

Frank Hubbell

Before long, Hubbell realizes the dreadful extent of the injuries Dow has sustained. "His neck was broken in four places, he had multiple fractures, a flailed chest, and internal bleeding," says Hubbell. "I finally told them, 'He has no chance at survival; he was killed on impact.' There was absolutely no question that Albert was killed instantly. So I stopped everybody at that point."

Though incredibly difficult to hear, the news Hubbell relays offers a shred of comfort. "We all had tragic consolation that Albert didn't die under the snow waiting for us to reach him," says Kane sadly.

Ken Rancourt, who works at the Mount Washington Observatory and who had transported MRS members up the Auto Road the day before, is on standby at Pinkham with a snowmobile awaiting the arrival of the endotrachial tube. He remembers the moment he was notified that it wouldn't be needed after all. "I was frustrated," he says. "One of the phrases you hear frequently is 'Don't hurry,' meaning that no effort is warranted in the circumstances. I knew 'No hurry' meant that someone didn't survive."

Matt Pierce remembers the grief that swept over everyone at the site, especially those who were closest to Dow. "When I saw him, I realized I'd met him that morning at breakfast at Pinkham," says Pierce. It was hard because there were a lot of people there that knew him really well and were good friends of his. They were taking it really hard. Everybody was in shock. "

Lentini is one of those who is gut-punched by the loss of his good friend and teammate. "When we knew it was all over for Albert, we just stopped, and people started crying. It was just devastating. It's something I will never forget. I was crushed. My friend was dead, and there was nothing I could do. We put him on the Stokes litter and prepared to carry him down."

"The snow was really deep," says Kane. "So we made a trail straight out to the Thiokol for the carryout."

Hubbell's experience in wilderness medicine and safety has caused him to begin worrying about the rescuers who are being exposed to the extreme cold while trying to save Dow. "It was eerily silent," he says. "Everyone was just holding their breath. I knew there were going to be secondary cold-injury problems if we didn't stop working. To this day, I carry the weight of having had to call it. But we had to start treating the people who had taken their gloves off. I can remember that Doug Madara's hands were stiff and almost frozen. We had to get hands covered and into armpits. We had to get people out of there."

XLVI
IN TATTERS

Albert Dow remains the only member of an organized backcountry search and rescue team in New Hampshire to be killed in the line of duty. He was the fifth avalanche fatality and the 94th person to die on Mount Washington.

Tuckerman Ravine Trail (3,800 ft.)
Mount Washington
Monday, Jan. 25, 1982
Shortly after 4:00 p.m.

Grief-stricken and exhausted, MRS rescuers make final preparations to escort Albert Dow off the mountain. As they encircle the rescue litter that holds their fallen teammate, they try to contain the disbelief and confusion that threatens to overtake them before they complete their task. Down-slope winds howl and buffet the group as they stand in silent vigil, jolting them into action. It's time to go.

For the first time in 55 hours, snow is no longer blowing above treeline on Mount Washington. Everything that's fallen here since Saturday morning has been scuffed from exposed terrain and transported onto the eastern aspects of the mountain or remains as a mosaic of drifts chiseled by relentless westerly winds.

The adrenaline that fueled the rescuers as they desperately tried to liberate one teammate and resuscitate the other has long worn off. Emotional trauma exacerbates the extreme fatigue and aching muscles each man is enduring.

"When it was time to transport Albert, it was kind of an odd situation," recalls Joe Gill of the initial moments of the carryout. "All of his teammates who'd dug him out were in complete shock. I was the only one pulling the litter. They fell in line, in two columns, behind the toboggan. Not a word was spoken as we hiked out; it was eerie."

When they reach the Thiokol, they lift the litter and slide it across the wooden bed. At this point, they are faced with the unprecedented challenge of how to handle the death of one of their own. During missions that have forced them to contend with a stranger's death in the mountains, they have used emotional distance to see them through. That's not possible now.

"I didn't want to ride down to Pinkham in the Thiokol," says Bill Kane. "But because I was there at the time when Albert was found, Frank [Hubbell] said I should in order to maintain custody of Albert's body."

Steve Larson tells the others that he intends to walk down. "I remember not knowing what to do," he says. "I just wanted to be alone, and I thought a peaceful walk by myself might be the best thing. Joe [Lentini] came over to me and said, 'Listen, we came up here together, and we're going to go down together.' So I got into the back of that Thiokol. Joe took a leadership role that day, and he was right."

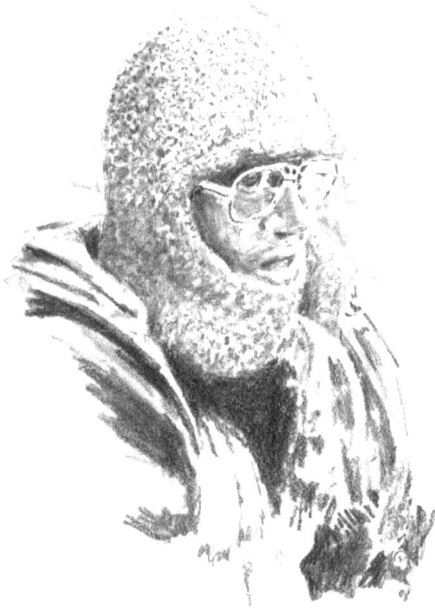

Steve Larson

Psychologist Dr. Nicole Sawyer, who has studied the aftereffects of trauma in the search and rescue community, says, "For a lot of first responders, especially in a situation like this one, they're trying to find some sort of justification or meaning because so much of their volunteer service is based on their own sense of meaning, purpose, and duty to their fellow outdoorsmen."

Sawyer adds that back in 1982 there was not a lot of attention paid to the mental health of rescuers. "No one is going to say, 'Hey, how are you feeling?' So people are going to try to apply what they know to the situation. They're going to try to find some greater meaning around the loss or tragedy. This is when statements like 'He died doing what he loved' come in. Those statements are not helpful. They are the patch people try to put over their wounds because they don't know how to make sense of the loss. They're trying to find some way to reconcile the loss in a way that makes sense to them."

On this afternoon, the immediate response to Dow's death is profound sadness and quiet pain. "It was somber," says Bill Aughton, who had run up with others from Pinkham. "Sadly, we got there just as they were bringing Albert out of the woods. I can remember that Dana [Seavey] was crying and very upset. Frank Hubbell had tears in his eyes as he tapped the body bag and—very, very softly—said to me, 'This is Albert.' It just shook everybody."

Even as he adopts a leadership role, Joe Lentini is struggling with his inability to put Albert into the category of other victims he has encountered during search and rescue missions. "This was totally different," he says. "I'm standing right there, and it's personal. Albert was a friend, and it had all unfolded in front of me. I'd been part of it. It sucked."

Dana Seavey, a close friend of Dow who had carpooled with him to Pinkham that morning, recalls being overcome with disbelief. "There was never a thought that one of us was going to die," he says. "We were young and superhuman. I never felt like the number one risk was avalanche. I was shocked when I heard there was one. I was on the Tucks Trail when the Thiokol was on the way down. I stood off to the side. I knew Albert was in there, so I walked down on my own."

The Thiokol is making the 30-minute, 2.4-mile descent to Pinkham. "On the ride down there was a lot of emotion," recalls Matt

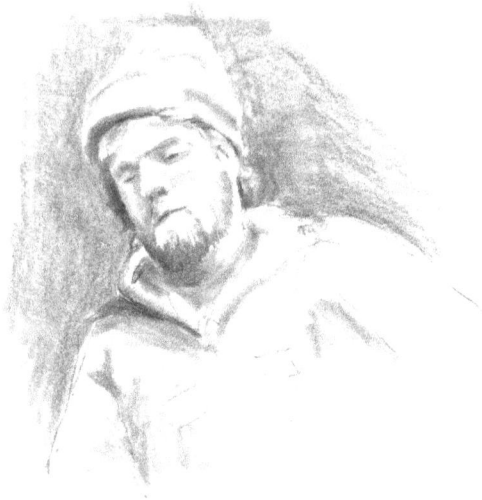

Dana Seavey

Pierce. "People were crying, which at 30 degrees below zero doesn't work well. There were people looking at the faces of others and saying, 'Cover up; you're getting frostbite.' It was a cold and miserable ride down."

In addition to tears and sadness, anger is the next emotion to manifest itself among some. "I remember some people being pretty angry," says Doug Madara. "That's just how they were expressing their emotion. I do remember somebody saying they were going to walk down. They wanted to be separate from the group, and someone said, 'We're a team, we should stay together.' It was one of our friends. But it wasn't just one of our friends; in some people's minds, Albert had been out there risking his life to find somebody, and it didn't go well."

"You have to find a reason," says Dr. Sawyer. "If you can't find a reason, you feel lost. We blame and finger-point because finding fault gives us some sense that there was control over the situation, and that control failed. That seems better than feeling like it was fate. So blame and fault are often the initial responses to these types of incidents. What we understand better today is that we need to accept those feelings and move on to what's really underneath them. With anger, it's more about a person reconciling the mistakes that were made so they can say, 'We're never going to let that happen,' when really, it's always going to happen again. It's always hanging there in the balance."

Second-guessing oneself is another common response and almost always impossible to avoid. Michael Hartrich says today, "In retrospect I wish I'd made different decisions. Being the more experienced, it was up to me to make decisions. Whenever you're involved in a situation where there's a fatality, you feel responsible for it. You carry that until the day you die. You wish you could bring it back and make better decisions. But, you know, I don't think we would have. Part of the thing about avoiding avalanches is that you make basic assumptions about them based on the situation you're in and you follow through on those assumptions. The thing is, I never would have been there if it hadn't been for a rescue."

When the Thiokol arrives at Pinkham, New Hampshire Fish and Game informs Frank Hubbell that the press has arrived. "Word had gotten out that a rescuer had been killed," says Hubbell. "So instead of going to the Trading Post, we decided to send Bill Kane over to talk with them. Thankfully, Fish and Game brought us off in another direction."

Dow's teammates remove him from the back of the Thiokol and carry him to a Gorham ambulance for transport to Mount Washington Memorial Hospital in North Conway. He will be pronounced dead on arrival shortly after 5:00 p.m.

For many at Pinkham, however, the mission is not complete. It is time to notify Dow's family, friends, and loved ones.

XLVII
SHOCK WAVES

*And perhaps the most beautiful paradox of all is how a human soul
is heartbreakingly fragile and unbreakably strong at the same time.*
—Anonymous

Pinkham
Monday, Jan. 25, 1982
5:00 p.m.

Dave Warren watches as Pinkham descends into near-chaos. The
AMC manager and member of the search planning team has spent
the past two days coordinating the search for Hugh Herr and Jeff
Batzer from the radio room at the administration building. As
stunned and grief-stricken rescuers file into the Trading Post,
members of the media converge on anyone they think will offer
details of the tragedy that has just occurred.

"The team came back to the operations center, and the mood
changed at that point," recalls Warren. "I stopped thinking about
Hugh and Jeff and where they were. Obviously, they were still lost,
but everybody was focused on Albert's death and the need to notify
his family. We still had to look for those two missing climbers. But we
hadn't had any breaks. It was a horrible mood."

Returning rescuers weave through members of the press in an
attempt to get inside and try to re-establish their bearings. "They
parked the Thiokol over by the Forest Service building so it wouldn't
be in the bright light of the media," says Matt Pierce. "Walking back
toward the lodge at Pinkham there were reporters and cameras, and
they were trying to interview us. Instead of heading back up to
Harvard Cabin, I ended up spending the night at Pinkham. I was
soaking wet, freezing, and not feeling well because of my run over to
Lion Head. I was emotionally and physically spent."*

News of the tragedy is hitting every corner of the camp, shaking up anyone in its path. "I was working in the Pinkham Notch shop at the time and recall going over to the Trading Post," says then-AMC crew member Paul Cunha. "The MRS team had just come down after Albert was killed, and the sadness and grief were palpable. In the dining room, there might have been a dozen people, maybe more, with their heads in their arms down on the table. With the number of people in the space, there was a heavy quietness. They had lost a friend. "

With emotions so high and grief so raw, questions are being raised about whether or not to continue the search for Herr and Batzer. "A lot of us were thinking that maybe we weren't going to find those guys at all," says crew member Mike Waddell, who had just returned from the base of Lion Head "That was the reality that was starting to dawn on everyone. But it was still confusing. They had just disappeared into thin air. It does happen up there, but usually you have some indication."

In between shifts at the front desk, Dave Moskowitz had spent the past two days searching the lower portion of the eastern side of Mount Washington on skis. "I remember the Pinkham entrance and dining room the evening Albert died," he says. "It was a tense mix of emotions, very somber, and there were some emotional outbursts. There were packs and gear strewn everywhere, and it seemed as though all that had been expected had come undone."

Some members of MRS leave for home, others sit alone in the far corners of the dining room, and some find comfort standing together. Team Leader Bill Kane, who's just finished a quick briefing with members of the press, goes over and over in his mind the details of a tragedy no one saw coming and starts to beat himself up with thoughts of how he might have prevented it.

Through his own grieving, Steve Larson notices Kane's state of mind and asks to speak to him alone. "Bill was having a hard time," he says. "I felt the need to let him know that I didn't think he was in the least bit responsible for the outcome. I also wanted to tell him that if he wanted to go out again tomorrow to keep looking for Hugh and Jeff, that I was ready and willing to go." To this day, Kane remains grateful to Larson for his supportive words.

Those in charge of notifying others of Dow's death are finding the task monumental, especially in an era when communications are still slow and tedious. There are no cellphones or texting or social media to get word out instantaneously to massive numbers of people. The 24-hour news cycle doesn't yet exist. No cable news networks, no apps, no internet. News is consumed by reading the newspaper or watching the evening news on television. In addition to their first priority of reaching members of the Dow family, notifiers must contact the Carroll County Attorney's Office and other officials, write and send out press releases, and manage the media. It is a challenging task at any time, but given the exhaustion and grief of this moment, it feels overwhelming.

Despite the low-tech communications available at the time, news began spreading by word of mouth. Even before MRS set foot back in Pinkham's parking lot, people in this close-knit mountain community were getting in touch with each other to share the few details they had heard. "The word back in North Conway was that two of our climbers were in trouble, but they were unnamed. So loved ones were wondering who was missing," recalls Dana Seavey. Because this often happens when word of accidents circulate without the details, one of the first priorities of the searchers when they come down from the mountain on this sad day is to contact their families and assure them, "I'm OK. It wasn't me."

Seavey decides to go directly to his car when he arrives at Pinkham to get as far away from the chaos as he can. As he opens the car door, he notices the gear Dow had left in the back seat that morning. "Your climbing partner's gear is like an extension of your own," he says. "You're always sharing ropes, racks, or maybe using only one pack on hard climbs. So getting back to my car after the accident and looking in the back seat really hit home. Driving back alone in the dark through Pinkham Notch with only his stuff in the back was painful. I will never forget it."

One of Dow's close friends and fellow MRS teammate Alec Behr has been working across the street from Pinkham at Wildcat Mountain all day. Hearing that something has happened, he walks across to the Trading Post and hears the sobering news. "Michael [Hartrich] walked in with a bunch of people while I was there," he recalls. "He was in shock. It's a hard thing to digest whenever somebody you know dies. It affects you strongly no matter what your initial response is. For me, it has never gone away."

Bill Aughton and David Stone leave Pinkham together and drive to Stone's home. It has been hours since David's wife Lin and Aughton's partner Peggy got word of trouble with the search. They had decided to wait through those uncertain hours together. "When David and Bill returned, David just stumbled through the door, speechless," says Lin Stone. "They were just devastated, gray and white with cold. It all became a blur. David knew Albert very well. It was a tight community and Albert's death was a huge loss. He was such a kind and engaging young man."

Brenda Monahan, a friend and coworker of Dow's at Eastern Mountain Sports, was working there on that Monday. She remembers that her late husband Jim was planning to meet Dow at Pinkham at the end of the day's search. "We knew the search was going on because the climbers were going," she says. "Jim was so optimistic that they were going to find the missing climbers because they had always come through. But when he got there, they were bringing Albert down. Someone came over and told him what happened, and he just about collapsed. He didn't know what to do, so he came to the store. Jim had it in his head that he wanted to tell Albert's girlfriend Joan. So we started toward Brownfield, Maine, where she lived."

On getting back to Pinkham, Joe Lentini has the same impulse as Jim Monahan: to inform Joan Wrigley in person. "I realized it was going to be a shit show," he says. "I knew reporters were around, and I decided I had to get to Joannie before she heard it on the radio. So I drove to Brownfield Road in Maine. All of a sudden, I saw her car stopped in the road. Then I saw the Monahans' car. As I got to Joannie, she was standing there in the road just screaming and crying. I stood there crying myself. There was nothing I could do."

With word traveling through the community, concern is growing that the Dow family needs to be notified. "Because I knew Albert better than most of the team members, they were suggesting that maybe I should get in touch with them," says Alec Behr. "Then somebody with a clearer head said, 'No, no. The state police will do that,' which was a good thing because—good Lord!—that's not something I would have wanted to do."

Tuftonboro Corner
Tuftonboro, N.H.
5:50 p.m.

Albert Dow Jr. sits down at the dining room table and thanks his hosts for the invitation to join them for dinner while his wife Marjorie is away in Bradenton, Fla., caring for her mother. Neither Albert Jr. nor Marjorie knows that their son has been involved in two days of searching for Hugh Herr and Jeff Batzer on nearby Mount Washington.

"It was evening, and the neighbor Dad was having dinner with looked out the window and said, 'There's a police car in your yard,'" says daughter Susan. "So Dad got his coat on and went across the street to see the officer. It was a state trooper who had been sent to tell him Albert had been killed on the mountain. The trooper was also there to pick him up and bring him to North Conway. My dad made the trooper wait while he went to tell the neighbors what had happened, and then went into the house to call us."

When she receives the phone call from her husband, Marjorie—devastated and confused—immediately books a flight home to New Hampshire that night. Unfortunately, her return does not go as planned. "The plane blew an engine on takeoff and had to abort," says daughter Caryl Dow, recalling her mother's agonizing efforts to get home to her family. It was all just a twisted mess. Mom had to call my grandmother to come get her at the airport, and after not sleeping all night, she had to start over the next day. By the time she got to Boston on Tuesday, she was a worn-out dishrag. I wasn't any better. We all just wanted to get home to Daddy."

Caryl, who lives in Manchester, N.H., isn't home when her father tries to make contact. "I went grocery shopping on my way to my boyfriend's house," she says. "My father called my apartment and told my roommate what had happened and asked how to get in touch with me. My roommate gave him my boyfriend's number, so my dad had called and told my boyfriend before I arrived. I can remember that my boyfriend just didn't know how to tell me. I remember screaming at him, 'You have to tell me what's going on!'" And then he finally told me that Albert was killed. I couldn't call my father because he had left. It was just wrenching. I remember rolling around on the bed in agony. My dad did end up calling me back, maybe from the hospital. My mother was going to come into Logan Airport, so he asked me to stay in Manchester to meet my Uncle Bill, who was going to pick her up there."

When her father calls, Susan is at home in Scott Township, Pa., where she lives with husband Charlie and daughter Amy. "I was pregnant at the time and fixing dinner," she says. "Dad told me that my brother had been killed on Mount Washington in a rescue attempt, and that he didn't have any details. He was going up to the hospital to identify Albert, and he was going to meet Joannie there. He said he had just told my mother in Florida, and she was making arrangements to fly home. He asked me what I wanted to do. My husband returned home and found me on the floor, holding Amy and crying. Charlie took the phone, talked to my father briefly, and started calling airlines. He ended up booking a flight for us into Logan Airport the following morning."

The Memorial Hospital
Mount Washington Valley Medical Center
North Conway, N.H.
6:00 p.m.

After driving to Brownfield, Maine, to notify Joan Wrigley, of Albert's death, Joe Lentini is running on fumes. He and mutual friends grieved with her for a time, and then he drove off to attend a meeting with some of his teammates at the Eastern Mountain Sports Climbing School in North Conway, located on the second floor above the retail store in the lobby of the Eastern Slope Inn.

"The team meeting was that same night," says Lentini. "We felt there was nothing else we could do for the search for Hugh and Jeff. We'd covered all the terrain we could cover. We told planners at Pinkham that if they needed us, they could call. But there was nothing obvious for us to do at that point."

Lentini then drives to Mount Washington Memorial Hospital in North Conway to support Wrigley and the Dow family. "I was heading into the hospital, and I ran into a dear friend of mine walking out," Lentini recalls. "She had given birth prematurely a couple of days earlier, and she was being released as I walked in. There was this

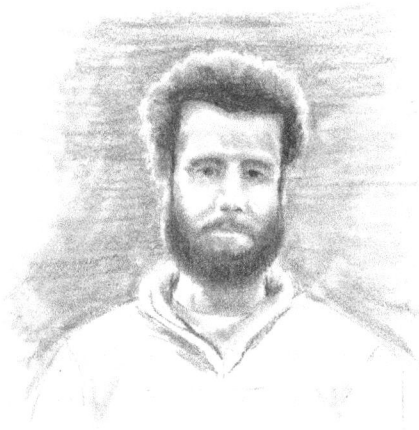

Alec Behr

weird juxtaposition of me going one way to see Albert, and her going another with her newborn. I can remember drinking a lot of bourbon that night."

Michael Hartrich is in the Emergency Department at the hospital receiving stitches for the laceration on his face that he suffered in the avalanche. He recalls the efforts of staff to help him process his loss and the kindness of an anonymous benefactor. "They asked me if I wanted to go see Albert, and I didn't," says Hartrich. "They told me it was supposed to be good for me, but I couldn't deal with it. As I was getting ready to leave, they said, 'Somebody has paid for your medical bill.' That was a very big thing, because at the time it would not have been easy for me to cover any big medical bills."

Sitting quietly in the lobby, Alec Behr awaits Joan Wrigley's arrival. Behr remembers the moment Albert Dow's father arrived to confront every parent's nightmare. "I was sitting on a bench in an entryway when Albert's dad came in," Behr says. "He and I knew each other pretty well. He'd driven Albert and me to ski races several times when we were younger. As he walked by, I greeted him, but he barely acknowledged me. He was there to identify Albert, and even today, I can't imagine what he was going through."

---

* In the early morning hours of March 9, 1982, during a moonlit ascent of Central Gully in Huntington Ravine, Matt Pierce and Harvard Cabin guest Luc Groulx of Quebec were caught in an avalanche and swept 700 feet down the gully and over The Fan. They came to rest at the base of the ravine. Both were buried up to their waists. Groulx was uninjured, but Pierce suffered broken ribs and developed bronchitis, taking him out of caretaker duties for three weeks during the 1982 winter season. Pierce told reporter Charles Townsend, "It felt like I had fallen down a flight of stairs holding a safe."

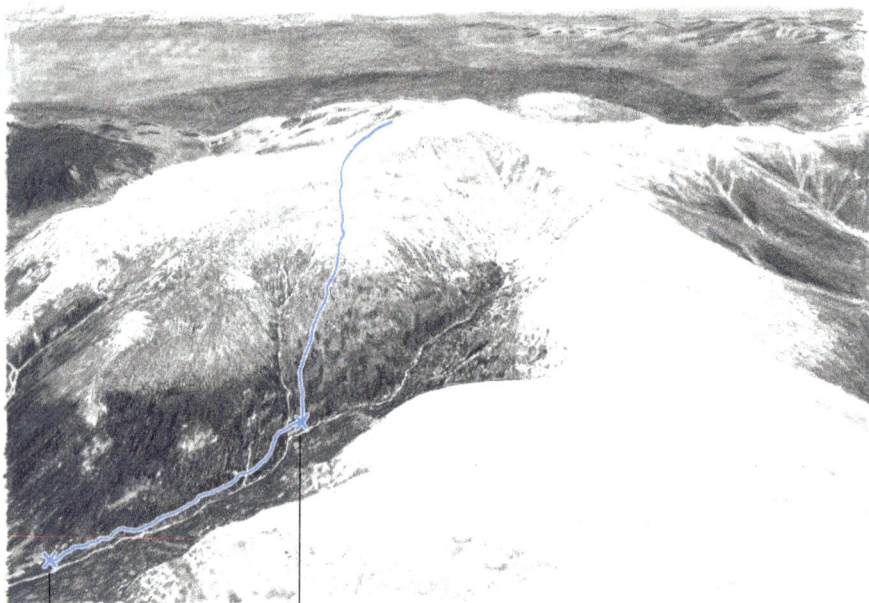

Hugh Herr and Jeff Batzer's bivouac on the night of the 23rd

Bivouac on the night of the 24th and 25th

XLVIII
JUXTAPOSITION

So this is the difference between telling a story and being in one: the fear.
—Patrick Rothfuss, *The Name of the Wind*

Great Gulf: Temperature: -10°F; windy; visibility darkness.

Emergency Bivouac Site (2,247 ft.)
Great Gulf Trail Junction
Monday, Jan. 25, 1982
6:00 p.m.

Hugh Herr and Jeff Batzer abandon the nightly hugging strategy they've employed since they arrived in Great Gulf on Saturday afternoon. Though Herr had been harboring thoughts of death ever since they landed in Great Gulf, Batzer's failed attempts to reach Pinkham and then Glen House has led both of them to accept what appeared to be the inevitable.

"When Jeff failed to get out, that's when we both resigned ourselves to our impending death," says Herr. "We stopped making any efforts to live. We'd lost track of time. We thought maybe a day had passed. In my wildest imagination, I didn't think there was a rescue effort going on. We didn't think anyone was looking for us. In my mind, we were alone."

Batzer has held on to hope for a bit longer than his friend, but he is also sinking into despair. "I became more and more concerned by Monday afternoon when I came back from trying to get out," he says of his waning optimism. "I was becoming fearful. I knew we might not make it out because it seemed like we were so far in. At that point, it was a constant battle trying to keep our hands warm. Our fingers were literally freezing. We were losing feeling in them; they were

300

tingly, burning, and then after a while all feeling went away."

As they lie separated on the bed of spruce and fir boughs, Batzer's frostbitten feet are nearly frozen solid as well. His earlier attempt to reach Pinkham wearing only one boot has resulted in catastrophic cold injury. "My feet felt like cinder blocks connected to the sensitive part of my legs that I could still feel," he recalls. "I was carrying these weights through the woods, but they had no feeling."

They are too weak and broken to create a thicker layer of spruce and fir boughs to add warmth, and on some level they know that any additional warmth will only prolong their suffering. "It was uncomfortable that night," says Batzer. "There was physical pain as my hands and feet transitioned to freezing. I had no internal pain, but I remember being desperately thirsty. My urine was dark brown and black from dehydration."

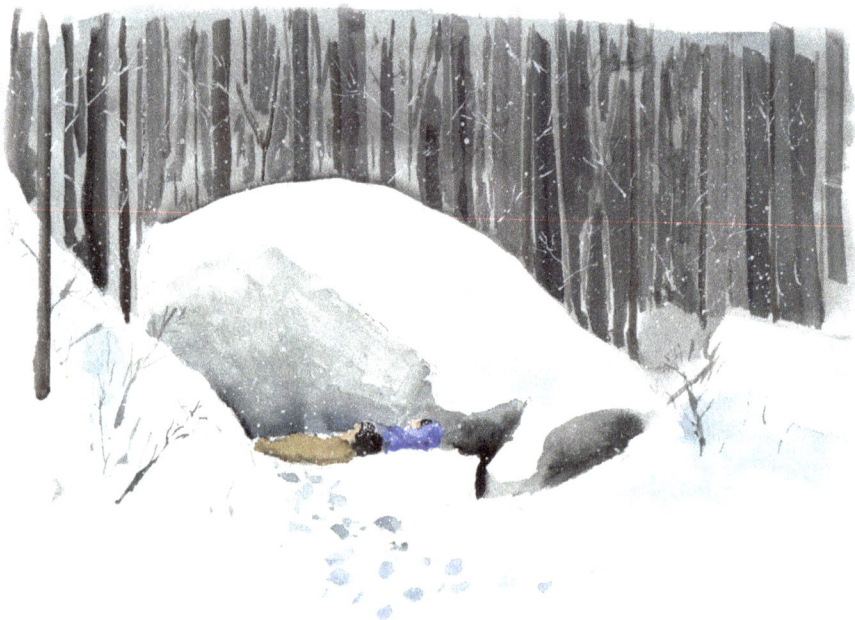

Cold-injury expert Dr. Gordon Giesbrecht says that the responses Herr and Batzer are having at this point are common. "With any kind of potentially fatal stress, if fighting is too painful, too difficult, people die because they give up. Part of survival is the mental will to live."

Batzer says today, "I had been praying from the first night on, 'Lord willing, if it would be your will, please get us out.' But that Monday night, I didn't think that was God's plan for us. I thought we were going to die. Throughout the night I would have trouble breathing at times. At one point I stretched out straight and was gasping for air. I thought, 'I'm dying.'"

Madison Gulf Trail
Mount Washington
6:00 p.m.

David Boudreau is basking in the warmth of his insulated sleeping bag. It's been a long slog toward Great Gulf Wilderness. "We had finally got our shit together and were on Old Jackson Road," says Boudreau, referring to their slow start that morning. "We hiked for five or six hours before eventually stopping. Daylight was so short that time of year, so we stopped an hour before the sun went down. The weather had gotten better, but it was still really cold."

Over the course of the day, he and Geoffrey May, who is encased in the sleeping bag beside him, maintained a slow and steady pace. "I remember being upset at the lack of progress we were making," says May. Because of the below-zero temperatures, they stopped only briefly to refuel on granola bars and squeeze tubes filled with peanut butter and jelly.

At one point, they reached the intersection of the Old Jackson Road and the Mount Washington Auto Road at the two-mile mark. This is where searchers Jeff Tirey, Jack Corbin, and Mike Waddell turned around late in the afternoon on Sunday and returned to Pinkham. Then the two crossed the Auto Road, stepped onto Madison Gulf Trail, and hiked north following white blazes dotting the trees. They stopped for the day at a point just north of Lowe's Bald Spot.

After setting up their tent, they fired up their cookstove and enjoyed a freeze-dried dinner and potato buds with butter. They are less than two miles from Hugh Herr and Jeff Batzer's bivouac site. This is the closest anyone has come to the missing pair. The following day, they'll try to get a much earlier start so they can finally reach their intended target of Madison Col near the boarded-up Madison Hut. If

Mother Nature allows, they'll traverse the Northen Presidentials. It is an itinerary for which they are well prepared. But they have no idea that fate will intervene and turn their intended plan on its head.

XLIX
ARRIVALS

Grief is not a disorder, a disease, or sign of weakness. It is an
emotional, physical, and spiritual necessity, the price you pay for love.
The only cure for grief is to grieve.
—Rabbi Earl Grollman, pioneer in the field of
crisis intervention

Pinkham
Tuesday, Jan. 26, 1982
2:00 a.m.

Misha Kirk is suffering from sleep deprivation. As a former Army Special Forces medic, operating in a cold-weather environment without sleep is all too familiar to him. He's been awake for at least 24 hours and knows how to "embrace the suck" but he also knows he must rest soon. As the search for Hugh Herr and Jeff Batzer enters its fourth day, however, his mission isn't yet over.

At this early hour, not only does Kirk feel the effects of severe fatigue, he is also grieving the loss of Albert Dow. The first time Kirk met Dow was in Tuckerman Ravine, not far from the site of the avalanche that took his life. That first contact sparked a friendship, and the two would participate in rescues together.

Kirk and AMC crew member Jack Corbin are waiting for the arrival of Richard and Joan Batzer, Jeff's parents, who are driving the 500 miles to Pinkham from their home in Holtwood, Pa. At around 2:00 a.m., they arrive with Jeff's older brother, Richie, and Kirk and Corbin walk them over to the administration building.

"Jeff's mom looked as if she had cried the whole ride up to PNC," wrote Kirk in his journal. "His dad was being supportive and realistic. Jeff's brother was optimistic but looked lost. It was hard to present a positive picture, especially when all the gear Jeff and Hugh had was now accounted for. Which meant they had no bivy gear. I went to bed feeling sad and not looking towards tomorrow."

John and Martha Herr, Hugh's parents, had decided to wait at their home in Pennsylvania to see how Monday's search would play out before heading north to New Hampshire. They will arrive later on Tuesday. In her book *Second Ascent: The Story of Hugh Herr*, Alison Osius writes of their journey, which was punctuated by an unsettling discovery:

> Hugh's parents were on the highway. They would drive for an hour or two, then phone [their son] Tony at home in case he heard any news. When they crossed into New Hampshire on Tuesday morning, they stopped at a roadside diner. They parked right in front of a phone booth but in their distressed state never saw it. ... A waitress approached, and John asked about a phone. "Phone's outside," she said. Just then a seated man lifted his newspaper to read. John saw its headline: "Rescuer Killed in Washington Avalanche While Searching for Two Missing Climbers." He turned and walked out. Martha had been right behind him. She had seen the headline, too. It had jumped out at her, looking like a huge banner. "That can't possibly be this rescue," she thought. As they walked back across the parking lot, she asked, "You don't think that could be the boys, do you?" "I'm afraid so."

After settling Jeff Batzer's parents in for the night at Pinkham, Kirk crawls exhausted into bed. He anticipates another long day of searching and is now not optimistic that they will find Herr and Batzer alive. He shuts off the lamp next to his nightstand and almost immediately falls into a deep sleep. As he drifts off, he has no idea how critical his role in the final throes of the search will become later that day.

Boston Logan Airport
9:00 a.m.

Bill Holmes has his hands planted firmly at 9 o'clock and 3 o'clock on the steering wheel of his car as he drives toward the airport terminal. In front of him, emergency vehicles, TV satellite trucks, buses, and cars clog the roadway, making it difficult for him to weave through. Fifteen million travelers pass through here annually, a figure that will double four decades later.

Bill and wife Beverly, who live in nearby Reading, Mass., are impatient with all the traffic, desperately wanting to get to the terminal where Bill's sister, Marjorie Dow, is arriving from Florida.

Logan is still reeling from the effects of an airliner accident that occurred during a snowstorm on Saturday night when a World Airways DC-10 slid off the end of the runway and into Boston Harbor. It is the same storm system Hugh Herr and Jeff Batzer disappeared in on Mount Washington that morning. As the Holmeses park their car, the Massport Safety Office is overseeing the removal of the severed cockpit section of Flight 30 from the harbor.

When they finally arrive at the terminal, and Marjorie Dow walks through the door to meet them, they are shocked by her appearance. "My aunt told me that even after 42 years, she will never forget the look of grief on my mother's face," says Caryl Dow. As she walked toward them her head was down, she was bent over at the waist and could barely move. My Aunt Bev said, 'It was as if I was watching a broken woman walk off the plane. Your mother collapsed into her brother's arms and said, 'I just can't believe this. My boy is gone.'"

The Holmeses drive Marjorie Dow to Manchester, N.H., where Caryl is waiting. She and her mother will drive to the Dow home in Tuftonboro and await the arrival of Susan Dow-Johnson, husband Charlie, and their 5-year-old daughter Amy. They, too, are flying into Logan and will rent a car.

"It was snowing out, and my mother and I had to drive to Tuftonboro in my frozen Volkswagen Bug," says Caryl today. "The defrost didn't work, and my mother kept saying, 'We're getting rid of this car and getting you something safer!'" Though that might have seemed like a light comment, Marjorie's insistence on safety was not lost on her daughter.

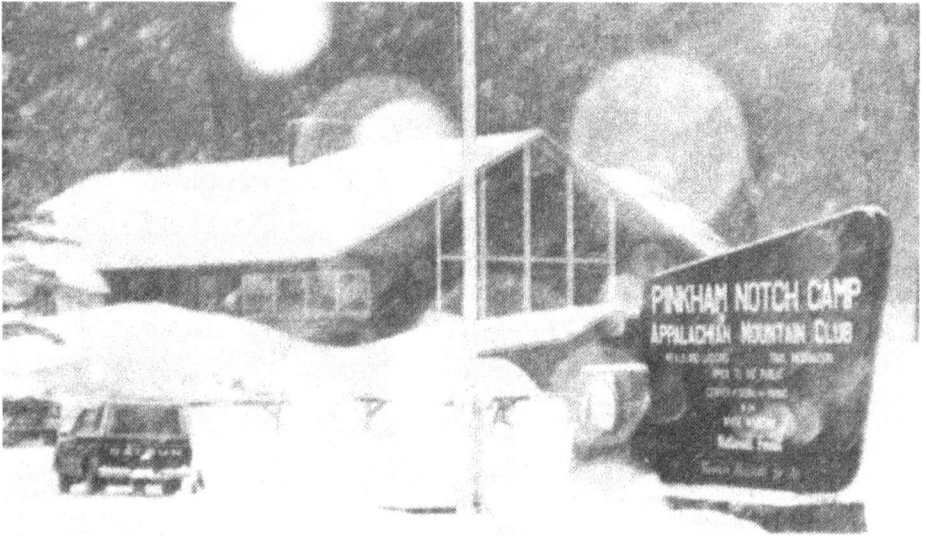

After looking at this photo recently, Jeff Batzer believes this may be an image of his Datsun pickup truck that he parked there on Friday, Jan. 22, 1982, before he and Hugh Herr made their beeline to Harvard Cabin.

L
LAST RESORT

Don't let what you cannot do interfere with what you can do.
—John Wooden, basketball star and coach

Mount Washington Observatory Surface Weather Observations (7:00 to 8:00 a.m.): Temperature -20°F; winds out of the west averaging 65 mph; visibility 0 miles; fog; windchill -63.1°F; peak wind gust: 71 mph.

Great Gulf: Temperature: -9°F; windy; visibility daylight.

Pinkham
Tuesday, Jan. 26, 1982
7:45 a.m.

AMC Manager Dave Warren pauses briefly to look up at the sky. It's been days since the sun has shown itself in Pinkham Notch, but patches of blue indicate that skies are clearing. Feeling the effects of the still-bitter cold, Warren continues toward the administration building where he's coordinating the continuing search for Hugh Herr and Jeff Batzer. On this third day of what has been a frustrating and tragic search, the loss of Albert Dow is on everyone's mind, even as they keep trying to make sense of where Herr and Batzer might be.

"I'd worked for a long time at Pinkham," says Warren. "We experienced a number of fatalities—people who were standing where they shouldn't and slipped and fell, people dying from exposure and heart attacks. But this was the first time a rescuer had died. It was a completely different dynamic. The anguish of losing Albert made it even harder for us to deal with the frustration of not knowing where Hugh and Jeff were. The obvious places where they could have been, they weren't."

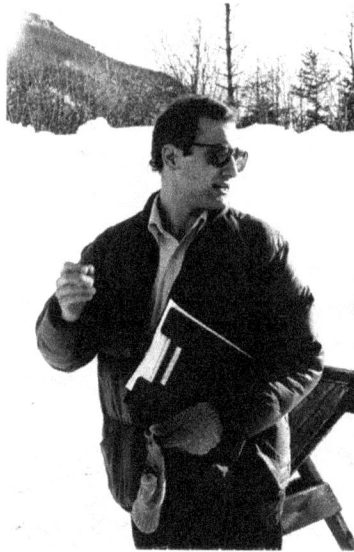

Appalachian Mountain Club Manager Dave Warren in the parking lot at Pinkham holding his search and rescue notebook on Jan. 26.

The broad area of low pressure that traversed in from Quebec and brought with it an arctic air mass is now meandering over Mount Washington. But a ridge of high pressure is building, which will cause the low to slide offshore into the Gulf of Maine. Skies will gradually clear after dawn, but winds will remain at hurricane force until around noon, then decrease as they shift from westerly to northwesterly. At this early hour, Mount Washington is entertaining sustained winds in the 60-mph range and gusts in the 70s.

David Moskowitz is working the front desk for the AMC that day and remembers the blue skies and high winds. "From our vantage point at Pinkham, what would otherwise have been a crisp view of the high peaks was out of focus the day after Albert died," he says. "There was a huge amount of sadness. I think some people were feeling anger toward the missing climbers, believing that their decisions led to Albert's death."

The media and members of the public are asking Warren if he holds Herr and Batzer responsible for Dow's death, but Warren has too much experience in these and other mountains to oversimplify the situation. "Local newspapers were writing stories and interviews were happening," says Warren. "Because a rescuer had died, something no one could remember ever happening before, the search attracted media attention from everywhere. People would ask me if I thought Hugh and Jeff had caused Albert's death. As sad as I was, I felt it was just a tragedy. Did Hugh and Jeff make some errors in judgment? Yes. But were those errors in judgment the direct contributor to Albert's death? No. Things happen, and it doesn't make sense to try to tie them together or to try to create a causal chain. People get in trouble on mountains all the time, everywhere in the world. If anything, it was a true showing of the climber's code: You go out and you willingly and knowingly take risks. You try to be aware of those; you try to manage them; you try to use your best judgment. If you get in trouble, your friends will try to help you, just as you would try to help them. That's the code climbers live by."

Barbara Tetreault, a correspondent for *The Union Leader* at the time, recalls that the dynamic of the missing climbers story changed dramatically after the tragedy on Lion Head. "I was still a little green on the job," she says. "I did a short piece on the two missing climbers, but it really started to get massive attention when Albert was killed in the search. That just catapulted the regional event into a national story. There was a lot of attention on the rescue and on the question of whether those two young guys should have been out there at all in those conditions."

But amid all the media attention and widespread grief, Warren knows he must focus on the day's plans. With the technical routes searched by Mountain Rescue Service the day before, the scope of today's search will expand to areas that haven't been reached. Planners know that a ground search of a much wider area will take too long, and the snowpack is still hazardous. Tetreault quotes Warren as saying, "Snow conditions are very unstable. We are waiting for a break in the weather so we can get a helicopter in."

Warren says today, "MRS was on standby in case we needed them, but we felt if we were going to find Hugh and Jeff, it would be in a place we hadn't been looking on foot, so we sought aerial assistance."

Moskowitz recalls that the mountain was essentially shut down in the aftermath of Albert Dow's death. "They basically closed the whole range after the avalanche," he says. "We were told not to go out. I was working at the front desk and was glad to have a purpose."

At this time, the only people still searching on the ground are Snow Rangers Brad Ray and Rene LaRoche, who are doing so on snow machines. The Forest Service Thiokol, which was used heavily on Sunday and Monday, is inoperable due to radiator problems. With Ray and LaRoche in the field, Snow Ranger Walter Winturri will assume Forest Service command of the day's search.

At 8:00 a.m., Sgt. Carl Carlson of New Hampshire Fish and Game contacts Maj. Mason Butterfield at Fish and Game headquarters in Concord to make a formal request for aerial search assistance. Shortly thereafter, Maj. Butterfield contacts Maj. John Blair at the New Hampshire Army National Guard (NHANG) to request a helicopter search of Mount Washington and notifies Gov. Hugh Gallen's office that NHANG has been asked to assist.

At 9:15 a.m., a Bell UH-1 Victor, known also as a "Huey," takes off from the NHANG Aviation Support Facility in Concord and points north toward Mount Washington. The aircraft is piloted by Capt. John Weeden and copiloted by Chief Warrant Officer 4 Ronald Boyer, with Staff Sgts. James Halub and Walter Lessard serving as crew chiefs.

Staff Sgt. Joseph Bourque and Sgt. David Patch leave NHANG base in a ground support fueler carrying 1,200 pounds of jet fuel. They will take I-93 north to Pinkham Notch and refuel the Huey later that day. Sgt. Ronald Bellerose is with them and will maintain flight and radio operations during the mission.

As the Huey descends toward the temporary helipad in the parking lot at Pinkham, onlookers know this is a last-ditch effort to find Hugh Herr and Jeff Batzer. Both time and hope are running out. If the two missing climbers or signs of them are not discovered today, the active search will likely be suspended. It will then take the form of an ongoing directive: "While you're out there, keep your eyes open for them."

LI
EDGE OF DARKNESS

The fight for survival was not so much a quest for life as an ever-constant vigil against death.
—Rob Taylor, *The Breach: Kilimanjaro and the Conquest of Self*

Great Gulf: Temperature: -9°F; windy; visibility daylight.

Emergency Bivouac Site (2,247 ft.)
Great Gulf Trail Junction
Tuesday, Jan. 26, 1982
8:00 a.m.

Jeff Batzer tosses aside the birch bark he's trying to eat and spits out most of it. With his frozen fingers, he scrapes out what remains in between his cheeks and gums. His mouth is so dry from dehydration that he cannot generate any saliva to aid in the breakdown of the paper-like substance.

"I was always trying to hang on," says Batzer. "As the morning went by, we were just sitting up against each other but not holding one another like we had been. I said, 'Lord, if there's any way you can rescue us, please do,' but I didn't think that would happen. I also whispered, 'But Lord, if you're going to take me, please do.' I still wanted to be rescued, but there was that tension."

Hugh Herr sits in complete silence. He cannot walk, nor has he attempted to stand since mid-day yesterday. Though they are touching, each might as well be alone.

Both men are in the deep throes of frostbite and incapable of slowing its spread. Some of their appendages are frozen solid. "On the last day there were no tears, but there was a deep sense of grieving," recalls Batzer. "I knew I was probably not going to make it. I knew I had to get ready for that, but I still had hope."

Batzer knows that Herr's severely weakened state puts him in even greater jeopardy. At one point, he engages Herr in hopes of getting some reassurance from his dying friend. "When sunlight came, I said, 'Hugh, I'm a believer in Jesus, and I'm trusting Him that I'm going to go to heaven. Are you a believer?' and he said, 'Yeah, I am.' I said, 'OK, good.' I just wanted that covered."

They will not talk again until an unexpected turn of events changes the tenor of their day—and their lives.

Old Jackson Road
Pinkham Notch
8:55 a.m.

The AMC's Cam Bradshaw is breaking trail. Pinkham has tried to inform everyone at camp that they cannot go out because of the aerial search and unstable snow conditions. Fortunately for Bradshaw—and others—she did not get the memo.

Bradshaw has night watch at Pinkham in 13 hours and is getting in a good long hike before work. Every hour and 15 minutes from 10:00 p.m. to 6:00 a.m., she will check each of the buildings and parking lots at the camp

Bradshaw lives at Pinkham, which allows her to get outdoors and into the backcountry quickly. Before taking on the night watch role, she worked as a member of the AMC trail and kitchen crews, was caretaker at various summer shelters, and assisted with search and rescue-related activities when the AMC was called upon. In addition to night watch, she fills in for the caretaker at Hermit Lake Shelters, when needed.

"Cam was super shy and treasured her alone time," says fellow crew member David Moskowitz. "We were in one of the most incredible places in the world, and we all went out all the time. But nobody went out as much as Cam did, and she always went out by herself. That Tuesday was a terrible day at camp, which was probably why Cam bolted to get the hell away from it."

On this morning, Bradshaw is well prepared for a long day out in the cold. "I was wearing my snowshoes, and I packed a walking ice axe, extra clothes, food, and water," she recalls.

Bradshaw snowshoes along Old Jackson Road heading north. Her only agenda that day is to be in the backcountry. "I was not involved with the search," she says. "I don't remember how or when I heard about Albert, but it was devastating. I was not looking for Hugh and Jeff because nobody expected they could still be alive. My itinerary was Old Jackson Road to Madison Gulf Trail, then Great Gulf Trail to the [recently abandoned] Osgood Trail. From there I'd hike back up to the Auto Road to OJR and home to Pinkham for supper."

Though strictly out for a bracing and therapeutic day on the trails, Bradshaw is unknowingly on her way to becoming intensely involved with the search for Herr and Batzer. In fact, her intervention will not only be helpful, it will prove critical.

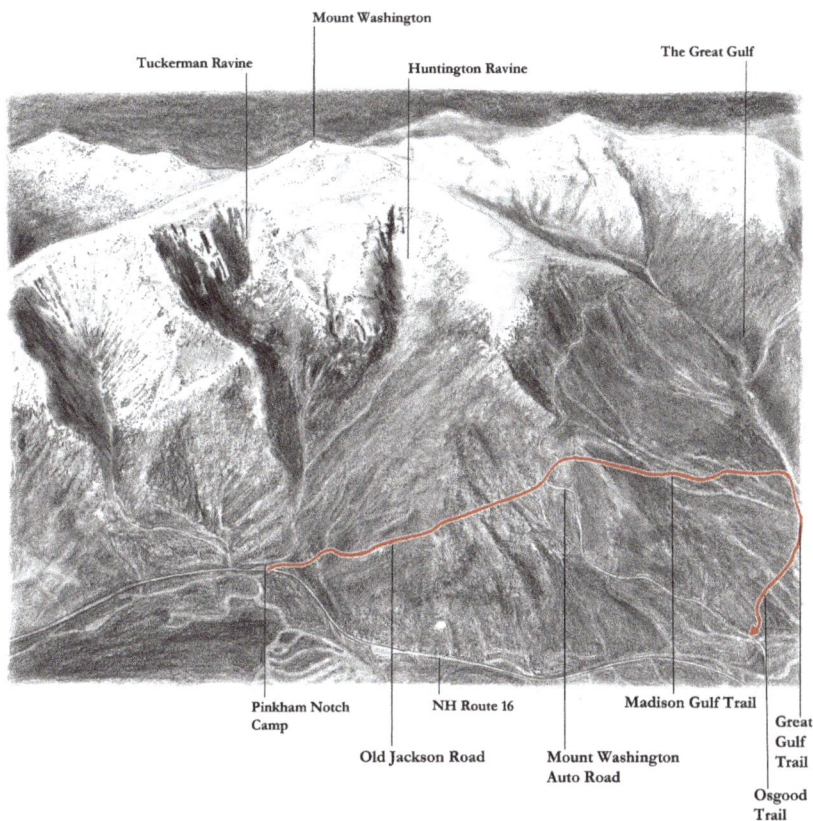

Cam Bradshaw's planned hiking route on Jan. 26.

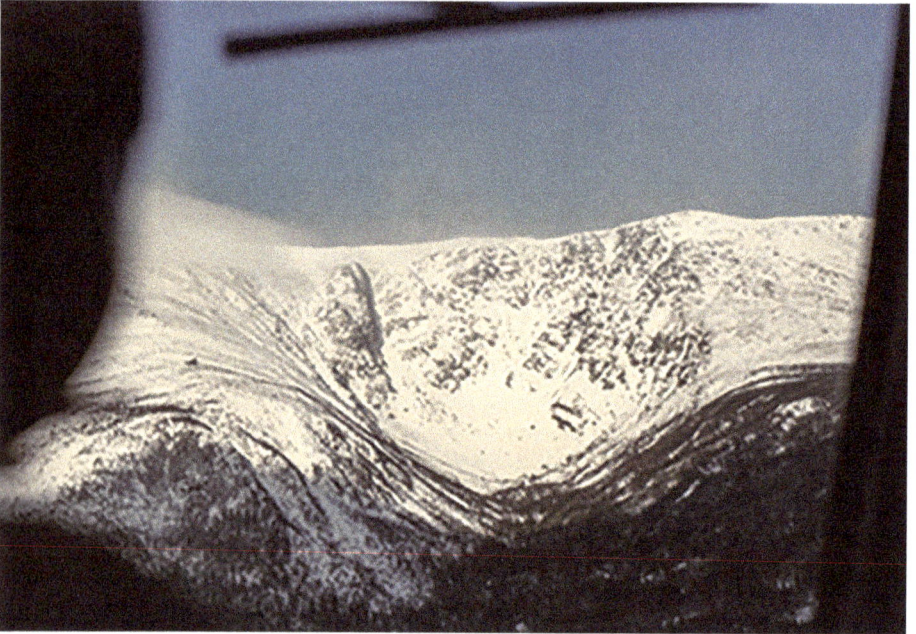

This photo, taken by Misha Kirk, shows Capt. John Weeden as he flies the Huey helicopter toward Huntington Ravine on Jan. 26. Shortly after this photo was taken, the aircraft experienced severe mountain turbulence.

LII
GUARD UP

Skillful pilots gain their reputation from storms and tempests.
— Epictetus, speaking of boat pilots

Mount Washington Observatory Surface Weather Observations (9:00 a.m. to 12:00 p.m. Tuesday, Jan. 26): Lowest temperature -20°F; winds have shifted out of the northwest averaging 65 mph; visibility 0 miles; fog; lowest windchill -63.1°F; peak wind gust: 74 mph.

Great Gulf: Temperature: -9°F; windy; visibility daylight.

Pinkham/Airspace over Mount Washington
Tuesday, Jan. 26, 1982
9:45 a.m. to 12:00 p.m.

Misha Kirk wolfs down his breakfast and readies himself for the next phase of the search for Hugh Herr and Jeff Batzer. While Brad Ray and Rene LaRoche search between Tuckerman and Huntington Ravines on snow machines, Kirk will join the crew of the inbound Huey helicopter and search from overhead. On his way to the parking lot to meet the arriving aircraft, he runs into Bill Kane of Mountain Rescue Service, who is wearing the emotional and physical weight of the past two days.

"I met Bill Kane that morning," wrote Kirk in excerpts from his journal. "He had come up to talk to the press. It was hard for Bill, and I tried to give him support. When I told him I was going up in a helicopter to search the ravines, he told me he thought it would be scary in there with the high winds, and that he would pray for me."

Kane has no desire to talk to the press at this time about what happened to Albert Dow but knows they will just find someone else to interview. "I was trying to be calm and forthright," he says.

Kirk shields his face as the burly, 57-foot, rotary-wing aircraft with its 48-foot wingspan approaches the snow-covered parking lot. Although this portion of the lot was plowed prior to the helicopter's arrival, the twin rotors powered by its single Lycoming T53-L-13 1,400-horsepower turboshaft engine generates a violent ground blizzard at the improvised landing pad. For Kirk, who is trained in casualty evacuation, it's business as usual.

Kirk guides the helicopter to a landing but has trouble maintaining visual contact through the swirling snow. "It was an intense whiteout, and all I kept hearing was the huge roar of the spinning blades," he wrote. "As I continued to back up to avoid being hit, the chopper kept advancing. ... Finally, the chopper was down as I heard them cut the rpms."

The New Hampshire Army National Guard first assisted New Hampshire Fish and Game with a ground search in 1951. Seven years later, it conducted its first aerial search and has assisted Fish and Game with aerial search and rescue missions ever since.

"We were on call every weekend year-round," says Capt. John Weeden, the pilot for this mission. "We had a good working relationship with the Fish and Game Department, so we were the primary helicopter rescue operators and were called in quite frequently. Ron Boyer, my copilot on this one, came in and we all pre-flighted. The crew chiefs were cross-trained to operate the rescue hoist and attach Stokes litters."

The Bell UH-1V (V for "Victor") is ready-made for aerial searches and rescues in the White Mountains. The model was configured for medevac (medical evacuation) use by the Army, and the first units were supplied to the New Hampshire Army National Guard. The upgrades installed for medevac use included a radar altimeter, distance measuring equipment, an instrument landing system, and a rescue hoist known as a "jungle penetrator." The Victor also had a landing light and searchlight that worked independently of each other. The searchlight operated on an axis and was controlled inside the cockpit. "At night we would use both," says Weeden. "Back then, we didn't have infrared capability or the technology found in the Black Hawk helicopters used today."

"We didn't have anything for cold weather in those days," says copilot Ronald Boyer. "We only wore regular flight suits, gloves, and regular uninsulated combat boots. We didn't have the heavy-duty flight suits like they do today."

The Huey, as it is affectionately known by Army pilots, has an empty weight of 5,210 pounds and a cargo capacity of 3,880 pounds. Gross capacity is 9,039 pounds, so when the 209-gallon fuel tank is full of JP-4 jet fuel weighing 1,358 pounds, cargo weight is an important consideration. Its maximum and cruise speeds are 127 mph, and it can climb 1,600 feet per minute to a maximum of 12,600 feet. Its maximum fuel range is 318 miles, but there are several factors, like weather, that impact fuel burn rate. Its maximum endurance on a full tank of fuel is 2.4 hours.

"With the endurance of that helicopter, we always planned on two hours of flight time before we needed to look for a place to land and refuel," Weeden says. "It's pretty much a constant rate of fuel burn. In the case of a headwind, your ground speed is reduced, but your fuel consumption shouldn't be affected. It varies depending on the nature of the weather or the demands you're putting on the engine. Hovering requires more torque, more engine power."

As he lands, Weeden takes the torque out of the rotors but does not shut down the aircraft. He exits, leaving the other three members of the crew—Boyer and Crew Chiefs James Halub and Walter Lessard—with the aircraft. He meets with Kirk and Lt. Bill Hastings of New Hampshire Fish and Game in the parking lot, where they quickly plot a search pattern.

"We planned to fly a grid search based on the itinerary Hugh and Jeff filed," says Weeden. "They weren't sure where these two gentlemen were because of the nature of the storm. We talked about the direction of the wind and where they could have gone. That's where we started with our search."

In in his official report, Weeden wrote: "It was decided that the best area to search was Huntington Ravine, specifically the Odell ice flow located therein. It was surmised that there was a good probability that the two young climbers would have been located there or in the Lion's Head area. Without shutting down the aircraft, the crew commenced an aerial search, assisted by Lt. William Hastings of New Hampshire Fish and Game and Misha Kirk, an AMC paramedic who was finitely familiar with the search area."

Kirk and Hastings follow Weeden to the idling aircraft. The

sliding door to the cargo/crew area opens, and they climb in to join Halub and Lessard. With the ceiling approximately four feet high, they won't be able to stand upright. That suits them just fine, because mountain turbulence is expected to be severe, so all four will remain buckled to the bench-like seat during the search.

"It was decided we'd go up to take a quick look with what fuel they had left," Kirk wrote. "We left the ground, and Bill Hastings handed me a pair of binoculars and patched me into [communications]. We were just above the trees heading directly for Huntington when we hit the wind. It spun us around, we shook as if we're going to break apart, and we were driven toward the north rim of the ravine flying diagonally on our side. I hadn't been gripped like that for a long time. The pilot calmly said, 'Well, we won't try that again,' as he climbed higher. Due to the high winds, we couldn't get lower than 700 feet or over 2,100 feet over the top of Huntington."

In his two-part piece in *Yankee Magazine* (Jan./Feb. 1983), "The Rescue That's Still Being Debated," Evan McLeod Wylie wrote of the harrowing moment for the Huey's crew: "Northerly winds crossing the summit of Mount Washington were accelerating as they barreled down the eastern slope, creating a zone of extreme turbulence. Abruptly the two seasoned pilots felt their aircraft becoming

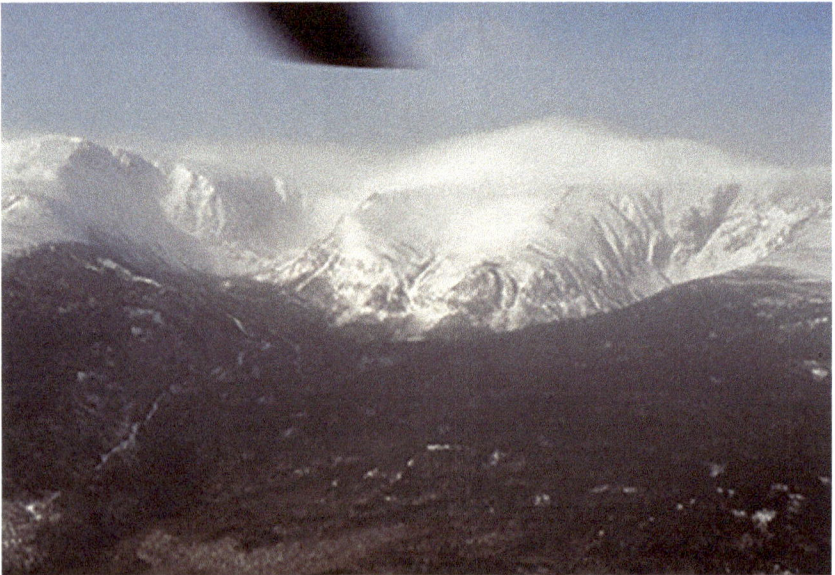

Taken by Misha Kirk on Jan. 26, this photo shows the Cutler River Drainage and the summit of Mount Washington in high winds. Note the Huey's rotary blade (top middle).

unmanageable. The airspeed instruments fluctuated wildly. The helicopter bucked and shook, and wind-shear forces threatened to send the aircraft out of control and plummeting toward the rocks."

Kirk noted in his journal that he was "calmly scared" during that turbulent ride but "exhilarated by the view" and trying his best to focus his vision through the jerking binoculars. "Feeling like a cork bobbing in an ocean on a rough day," he wrote. "It was just so neat to see this mountain I had climbed so many times from the air. There is an indefinable beauty in a dangerous mountain scene."

As difficult as flight conditions are for Weeden, he brings extensive experience to the cockpit. He enlisted in the Army in 1968. After completing basic training, he attended flight school and was commissioned as a "warrant officer with wings." Weeden flew helicopter gunships for a year in Vietnam and served as an instructor pilot as well. He was discharged from active duty in January 1971 and that year joined the New Hampshire Army National Guard as a full-time instructor and operational pilot. He graduated from Plymouth State College in 1973, and in 1974 was commissioned as a first lieutenant. In November 1979, he was promoted to flight operations officer and executive officer of the 397th Medical Detachment. At the time of this mission, Weeden had logged 4,200 hours of flight time.

Weeden's copilot, Ronald Boyer, started his military career as a mechanic. He attended flight school in 1957 at Fort Rucker, Ala., and had flown a few search and rescue missions in the White Mountains before this one. "What was really surreal about this mission is that Albert Dow's sister, Caryl, went to the University of New Hampshire with my son," says Boyer. "She had visited my house the summer before Albert's death."

The presence of the helicopter has greatly expanded the search area. Weeden is beginning to fly beyond the ravines and into Great Gulf Wilderness, where Herr and Batzer are trapped. "Visibility was great that day," says Dave Warren. "The helicopter searched a lot of the ridges, went up and down the Auto Road, and started to peer into Great Gulf as much as it could. But Great Gulf is enormous, and most of it is wooded, mostly with firs."

Having found no signs of Herr and Batzer during the morning search, Weeden turns the aircraft back toward Pinkham to refuel. Wind conditions are making the approach problematic, however. "We began our descent," wrote Kirk. "It took 20 minutes. We had to slowly descend in a wide arc toward Carter Notch. At 600 feet the pilot warned us to hang on as we hit turbulence and shuddered all the way down."

At 11:15 a.m., after an hour of searching, the Huey lands and shuts down. The crew will hit the dining room at Pinkham for lunch, and the aircraft will be refueled and serviced when the ground support crew arrives at 12:30 p.m.

It is not lost on anyone involved that dusk will descend here in just a few hours. If a breakthrough in the search for Herr and Batzer is to come, it will have to be soon. Aerial assets are not in consideration for the following day.

"During lunch I avoided [Hugh and Jeff's] parents," wrote Kirk. "With each passing hour, I was getting more and more sure we should give up. I didn't want to convey this to their parents, as I wouldn't lie to them."

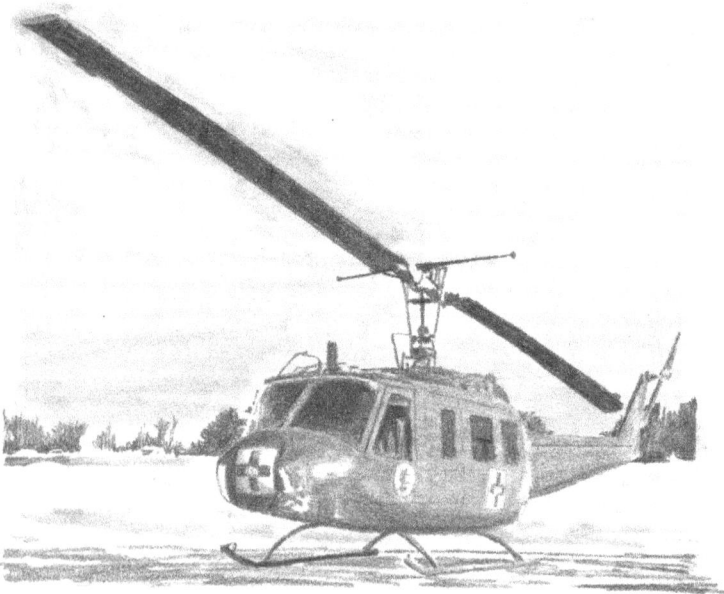

LIII
ALIGNING

Sometimes when things are falling apart, they may actually be
falling into place.
—Unknown

Mount Washington Observatory Surface Weather Observations (12:00 to 2:00
p.m.): Temperature averaging -19°F; winds out of the northwest averaging 61
mph; visibility 0 miles; fog; windchill averaging -60.8°F; peak wind gust: 73
mph.
Great Gulf: Temperature: -9°F; windy; visibility daylight.

Madison Gulf Trail
Tuesday, Jan. 26, 1982
12:00 to 2:00 p.m.

Dave Boudreau and companion Geoffrey May have gotten plenty of sleep and have broken into their stash of bacon, which now sizzles in their cooking pan. But the "thump, thump, thump" they are hearing from above is confusing them. "We had seen a helicopter go by and were wondering why," recalls Boudreau today. "It's amazing how sometimes you don't think as clearly as you'd like when you're in a dangerous environment. We were probably seeing the same helicopter making multiple passes, but from where we were sitting that morning, it didn't occur to us that it was just one helicopter trying to search a grid. We thought we were seeing multiple helicopters from the National Guard all trying to do some type of exercise."

The two friends are having another slow morning before heading out for the day. "We were more into the process than anything else," says May. "So we took our time over our breakfast."

Nearby, Cam Bradshaw is making good time in her efforts to visit Great Gulf before returning to Pinkham for the start of her

10:00 p.m. shift on night watch. Shortly after she passes by the trail for Lowe's Bald Spot, she finds a wide trough on the trail ahead of her. "I was surprised to find fresh tracks there," says Bradshaw. "Then I came across a couple of backpackers eating breakfast and breaking down their camp."

Boudreau recalls Bradshaw's unlikely appearance and remembers feeling a little sheepish at the late start they were having. "She said, 'Hey, how are you guys?' and gave us a nice greeting and chugged on past. She didn't mention that anyone was missing. We were breaking camp at noon, and darkness would be coming at about 4:30. What were we thinking?"

Mount Washington Airspace
12:50 p.m.

Having finished their lunch and with the aircraft refueled, the Huey's crew of six takes off from Pinkham for their second round of searching. They'll fly over the northern flanks of Mount Washington, including Great Gulf Wilderness. At this hour, they find weather conditions to be much more tolerable than what they encountered that morning, as indicated in Lt. William Hastings' report. "Diminishing winds allowed us a closer approach over the Nelson Crag area (as close as 600 feet), with visibility steadily improving."

Madison Gulf Trail
1:15 p.m.

Cam Bradshaw is still enjoying her solitary walk when she comes across a disruption in the flat snowpack ahead of her. "It wasn't long after leaving the campers that I came across postholes in the snow," she recalls. "At first I thought it was a moose, but it soon became clear that it was a person."

Bradshaw follows the tracks intently and realizes that whoever made them must have been disoriented. "The person clearly had trouble following the trail, so I had to check out each diversion," she says.

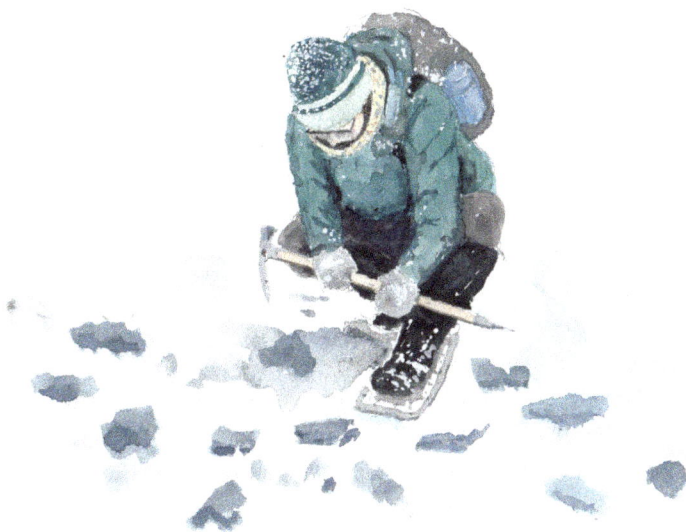

Cam Bradshaw takes a closer look at the footprints in the snow.

As she heads off trail, she encounters thick tree scrub. It is obvious to her that the person had a difficult time threading clusters of firs and large blowdowns. "At that point, I pretty much knew it was the lost climbers. After all that time, I really thought they were surely dead by then."

The fitful trough she is following rejoins Madison Gulf Trail heading toward Great Gulf. "I followed the tracks to the junction of Great Gulf and Madison Gulf Trails," she recalls. "I noticed they dropped off the trail to the river, but I didn't follow them because that just looked like where the person had gone to the stream for water."

At this moment, Bradshaw is within feet of Hugh Herr and Jeff Batzer, who remain hunkered down over the embankment and out of sight. "I crossed the bridge spanning the West Branch of the Peabody River and followed the tracks up Madison Gulf Trail. There were no bodies at the end of those postholes, so I doubled back toward the junction."

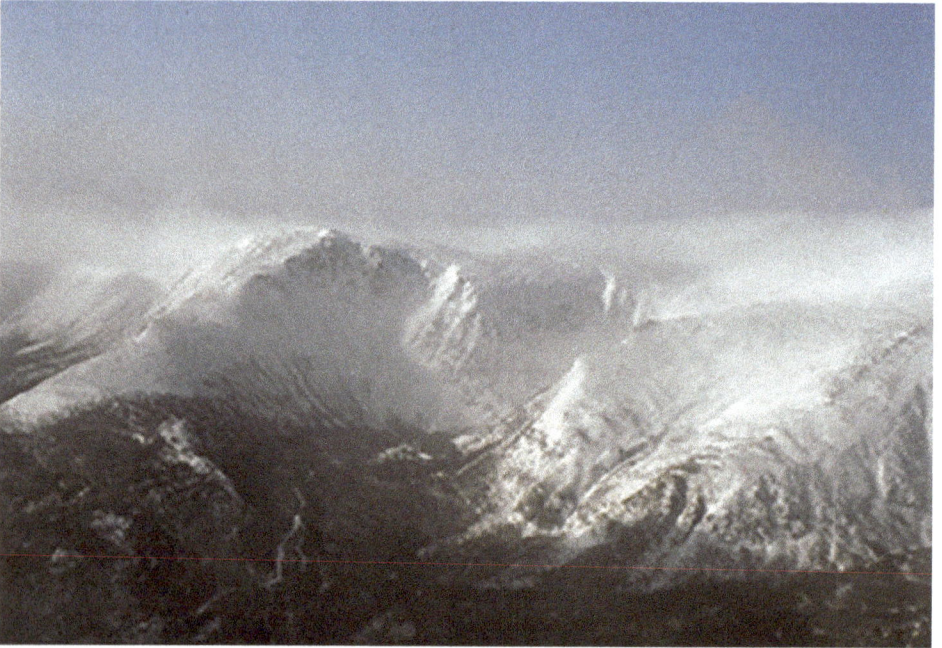

This photo of the Boott Spur, Tuckerman Ravine, and Raymond Cataract was taken by Misha Kirk from the Huey on Jan. 26.

LIV
CONVERGENCE

Place and a mind may interpenetrate till the nature of both is altered.
—Nan Shepherd, Scottish mountaineer and poet

Great Gulf: Temperature: -5°F; visibility daylight.

Emergency Bivouac Site
Tuesday, Jan. 26, 1982
2:00 p.m.

Jeff Batzer rolls onto his right side, plants his right hand on the spruce bed beneath him and pushes himself up to a standing position. His left foot, still covered only by a wool sock and his Gore-Tex mitten, is frozen and resists any attempt to bear weight. Batzer looks up through the thick tree canopy. The muffled "thump, thump, thump" he and Hugh Herr have listened to for most of the day seems a little louder. They have no way of knowing that the Huey from the 397th Medical Detachment has flown a grid-search pattern over the Cutler River Drainage and is now working its way northward toward them.

"Earlier that morning we'd heard the sound of the Huey off in the distance," says Batzer today. "Hugh and I thought, 'Could that be somebody looking for us?' because 24 hours earlier we had started processing the possibility that maybe we were being looked for by then. But as the morning went on, we ruled it out."

Batzer latches onto his rigid ice-encrusted parka and limps his way over to a spot near their bivouac that seems to have less tree cover. He turns the tan hooded coat inside out so the dark red inside fabric is visible. The thumps are so close now that Batzer can feel the power of the Huey's twin rotors in his chest.

"We didn't know the helicopter was for us, but I was waving my jacket and trying to position it in a small clearing, so they'd see it," says Batzer of his desperate efforts to be found as a declining Herr looked on from his prone position. "It passed over us a few times, and I was trying to wave the parka when it went by. There were no indications they saw us."

Even with the ability to fly at 600 feet because of improving weather conditions, the likelihood that the Huey's crew can see anything beneath the thick tree cover is remote. Unlike the crews of today's Black Hawk helicopters, which are equipped with infrared technology capable of detecting heat signatures on the ground, this crew can only rely on binoculars to detect the presence of a human.

Batzer lays the jacket over a bush near the river and returns to the spruce bed to rest. "I'd say it was around 2:00 p.m. when Hugh became delirious," says Batzer. "He was in kind of a drunken state. I just sat next to him with my eyes closed. I still felt I was clear of mind, but I wasn't able to move much at all." At this hour, they are in such pain that communication is reduced to a continuous volley of low, dreadful moans.

Herr remembers that he harbored no hope that afternoon that the presence of the Huey in Great Gulf would lead to their rescue. "We didn't think it was for us," he says. "We believed if we weren't self-sufficient in getting out of there ourselves, we were dead, and that's where we were at that point."

Trail Junction
Great Gulf Wilderness
2:30 p.m.

Cam Bradshaw pauses at the snow-clogged footbridge spanning the West Branch of the Peabody River. The trail junction leading back toward her home base of Pinkham lies on the opposite side of the river. Even wearing her wooden snowshoes, Bradshaw has been forced to trudge through snow depths of four feet or more as she's followed the frenetic tracks leading nowhere. At times, she pauses to call out to anyone who might be out there in the forest beyond her sightline. Nothing. Just the sound of a mild wind moving over and through the forested terrain. Bradshaw has seen that whoever she's been tracking seemed to be trying to follow each of the trails that intersect here.

Bradshaw has altered her own plan in an attempt to find the source of the tracks but has had no luck and realizes it is time to head back to Pinkham. She removes her backpack and takes out a snack. She knows she needs to replenish the many calories she's burned since passing by Geoffrey May and David Boudreau an hour and 15 minutes earlier.

For a moment, Bradshaw stands at the bridge, taking in the stillness. As the Peabody flows beneath the ice in its easterly journey toward its main branch, she revels in nature's white noise. Her response is in sharp contrast to what others might consider to be the "white hell" of this side of the mountain. And her pleasure is certainly at odds with what Herr and Batzer are experiencing only yards from her. She traverses the bridge, her feet at the height of the handrail because the snow is piled so high. When she reaches the intersection that will lead her out of Great Gulf, she makes one last attempt to call out to the missing climbers.

"I heard snapping branches and this voice calling out one or two times," says Batzer of that moment. "I called back and could see her standing there above us. I thought to myself, 'This can't be real,' and I said to Hugh, 'We're going to see our moms and dads after all.'"

Herr also recalls the moment they make their initial contact with Bradshaw: "We went from this emotional state of just preparing for death to, 'Oh my gosh, we might live.' So the elation was very profound. But we were hallucinating a lot, too. As we had made our way down Great Gulf on Sunday, we thought we saw so many bridges that were in fact just fallen trees across the river. So when we saw Cam Bradshaw, we both looked at her in silence because we were sure it was an illusion."

Bradshaw, who sees the frozen coat Batzer placed over a bush before seeing the men themselves, also has difficulty processing what she has discovered. "I found the two of them tucked under a boulder at the intersection," she says, adding ruefully: "If I had been a better tracker that day, I wouldn't have wasted so much time."

Shocked that Herr and Batzer are still alive, Bradshaw says their ultimate survival owes a good deal to luck. "It was a good job by Jeff and Hugh to get as far down out of the Gulf as they did. Otherwise our tracks would not have crossed."

Leaving Great Gulf Trail, Bradshaw quickly makes her way through a heavy entanglement of 10-foot trees and down the steep embankment in order to reach the two men "Are you the guys from Odell Gully?" she asks them.

Batzer tells her they are and asks her to alert rescuers. He adds that he thinks they can follow her out if she leads the way.

Bradshaw drops her backpack and rifles through it for for food and clothing. "I had already eaten most of my food and had drunk my nice warm tea," she says. "So I gave them some raisins and some ice-cold river water. They were so thirsty!"

Although Batzer believes they can walk out on their own, Bradshaw is realistic about the grim situation they're in, especially Herr. Their exposed feet are the color of milk and grotesquely swollen. Their faces are ashen and badly chapped from wind and exposure. Bradshaw tells Batzer she will arrange for a rescue party to come to them. She finds that she cannot communicate with Herr. Though he is coherent at times, he is responding more to Batzer than to her. Even though she can see the damage their long exposure has done to them, she is hopeful that if they can be evacuated that night, they will live.

"Cam was with us for between five and seven minutes before she went off to get help," Batzer says "She left us some light garments and water. I remember a Hershey bar, which was awesome! And drinking water was amazing."

Batzer recalls Bradshaw telling them that it would take her about five hours to get to Pinkham and enlist help. "She told us to hang in there, that they were going to come back for us. What a great lady!"

Herr says he wasn't discouraged by the amount of time it would take for help to arrive. "I thought to myself, 'We're going to live! Oh my God, I can't believe we're going to live!'"

Bradshaw hoists up her backpack, now a little lighter without the down vest, wool shirt, mittens, gloves, and food she's leaving behind for the stricken pair. "She went sprinting off," Batzer recalls.

"There's a lot to be said for Cam putting two and two together," says Michael Hartrich of Bradshaw's tenacity. "That's a one in one thousand thing. Hugh and Jeff should have been dead. The chance of them being there and her finding them. No one even thought about sending a search party there to look for them."

As they prepare for their long wait, Herr and Batzer lie next to one another on the spruce bed trying to grasp the completely unexpected turn of events. Batzer turns to his friend, who is fading in and out of delirium. "Hugh, we've got to stay with this," he says. "Someone is coming to get us." But he knows that time and hope are slipping away. "I was worried we wouldn't make it that long," he admits.

Madison Gulf Trail
2:45 p.m.

David Boudreau feels like the past couple of days have been a forced march toward the planned waypoints they have yet to reach. Trailing close behind, Geoffrey May finds the going to be tolerable, since Cam Bradshaw had done part of the work of breaking trail and Boudreau is doing the rest. May is thankful he's not having to break trail while carrying his 70-pound pack.

About 100 yards down the trail, Boudreau sees someone moving quickly toward them. "We're walking along, and we see Cam coming back," he remembers. "She was red-faced and running in her snowshoes. As she got closer to us, she yelled out, 'I found them, I found them!'"

"Found who?" Boudreau asks. Both he and May are unaware that anyone is missing.

"I found the climbers!" she replies and goes on to explain the situation.

In response, May retrieves the trail map from the deep front pocket of his jacket. "This is where the wilderness first-aid course I took while in graduate school came in," says May today. "I pulled out my map and said to Cam, 'Show me exactly where you found them.'"

Bradshaw indicates the point on the map where the three are standing on the Madison Gulf Trail and traces her finger along the black line into Great Gulf where it intersects with other trails.

"She showed us where they were," says Boudreau. "She said they were alive and in very, very rough shape. She told us they had been out for three nights without overnight gear and asked us to go to them and do what we could while she went for help."

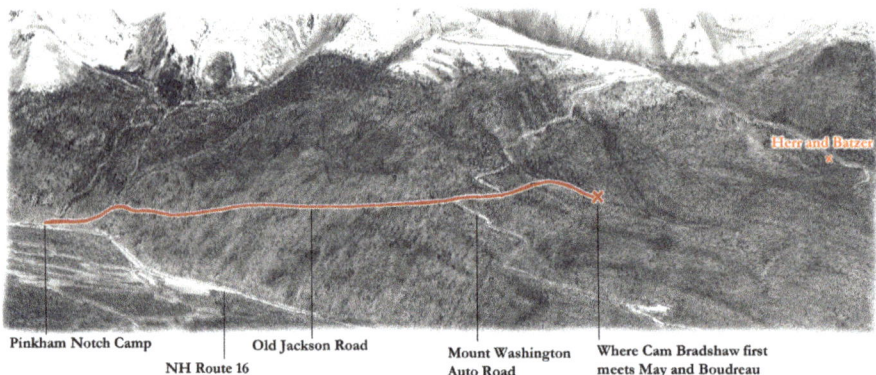

Pinkham Notch Camp | Old Jackson Road | Mount Washington Auto Road | Where Cam Bradshaw first meets May and Boudreau

NH Route 16

Bradshaw leaves them and continues toward the Mount Washington Auto Road about a mile away. Boudreau and May move in the opposite direction toward Great Gulf and the intersection where Herr and Batzer are bivouacked.

"We double-time it to get over there as fast as we could," recalls Boudreau. "We were concerned about what we were going to find, but we were singularly focused. We knew these guys were going through every climber's worst fear, getting stuck in the mountains and anticipating a slow, painful death. We felt a strange sort of excitement as we moved in their direction. I guess I felt, 'Hey, I've got an opportunity to do some good here.'"

Even with their adrenaline pumping and their sense of urgency, Boudreau and May remain conscious of the heavy loads they are carrying and the importance of managing their energy. "We made sure we didn't go too fast so we couldn't jeopardize ourselves," May told reporter Donna Lombardi of *The News Tribune*. "We didn't want to be tired and out of breath when we got there. We wanted to be useful."

At just before 3:00 p.m., Cam Bradshaw can see ahead the junction where Madison Gulf Trail meets the Auto Road. She's done well to cover this much ground after all she's already gone through. There's a lot more to be done to bring this rescue to a close, but she feels some comfort in knowing Herr and Batzer will soon have the company and aid of two competent outdoorsmen. "It was a relief to know Jeff and Hugh would have someone there with them while they waited."

LV
BREAKTHROUGH

I remember Brad [Ray] saying if we found these boys alive
after being out for multiple nights, he'd never give up on a search again.
—Misha Kirk, journal excerpt

Great Gulf: Temperature: -4°F; visibility daylight.

Pinkham
Tuesday, Jan. 26, 1982
3:00 p.m.

Capt. John Weeden takes the power out of the twin rotors of the
Huey and shuts down the aircraft. The helicopter has exhausted nearly
all its fuel supply since taking off for a second time after lunch and
needs to be refueled once again. Weeden exits the aircraft with Lt. Bill
Hastings of New Hampshire Fish and Game and the AMC's Misha
Kirk, and the three head to the administration building where they'll
join AMC Manager Dave Warren and Forest Service Snow Ranger
Walter Winturri to debrief about the day's search.

The arrival of the helicopter prompts the parents of Hugh Herr
and Jeff Batzer and Batzer's oldest brother, Richie, to leave the
building where they are hunkering down to ask if there's any news.
They are told that Hugh and Jeff have not been located. "The families
of the youths, looking stunned with the ordeal of waiting, came out
for a few moments," wrote Janet Hounsel for *The Reporter.* "Then they
returned to what must [have been] the resigned, bitter seclusion of
their rooms."

It was getting close to dark, and the debriefing confirmed that
the air search had yielded no evidence of the missing climbers. "We
couldn't find any sign of them, so the helicopter crew said they were
going to go back to Concord," says Warren.

In his official report, Weeden will write: "AMC and the New Hampshire Fish and Game decided that continuation of the aerial search would be nonproductive." At this point, as expected, no plans are made for the Huey to resume searching the following day.

Two-mile mark
Mount Washington Auto Road
3:00 p.m.

Cam Bradshaw's heart rate is at near-maximum effort. As she reaches the intersection where Madison Gulf Trail meets the Auto Road, she ponders her two options. She can descend the Auto Road to the Glen House site near Route 16 and phone Pinkham from one of the small buildings onsite, or hope to summon a passing vehicle and hitch a ride to Pinkham. Old Jackson Road, directly across from her, would require a hike of 1.8 miles. As it turns out, a much better third option quickly appears.

"I got to the Auto Road and met a couple of skiers, Liz Lancaster and Steve Johnson, who were fellow employees at Pinkham," says Bradshaw of her unexpected good fortune. "They pointed their skis downhill to get word back to the search and rescue headquarters at Pinkham."

Lancaster and Johnson head down the Raymond Grade slope to gain momentum and speed for the two-mile descent. Using the lines and apexes of the curves between there and First Lookout, they tuck and ski past the one-mile and 2,000-feet posts, pass the Glen House Lookout, and arrive at the Auto Road Toll House. Johnson unclips from his skis, and with Lancaster following, runs up to Route 16, where he attempts to stop an approaching vehicle. Two cars drive past him, so the frantic Johnson takes the more drastic measure of stepping out into the middle of the travel lane. The third car stops.

Gratefully, Johnson and Lancaster load themselves and their skis into the back of the car, and the generous driver agrees to make the 2.8-mile drive to Pinkham Camp.

Emergency Bivouac Site
Great Gulf Wilderness
Shortly after 3:00 p.m.

It's been only 30 minutes since Cam Bradshaw left to summon help. Having dropped into a meditative state for their anticipated wait, Hugh Herr and Jeff Batzer are suddenly jolted into alertness when they hear male voices growing increasingly louder.

"The voices were yelling for us," Batzer recalls. "I tried to yell back, but my voice was almost gone. I croaked in a screeching kind of voice, "We're over here.""

Geoffrey May and Dave Boudreau are following tracks onto the snow-clogged bridge spanning the West Branch of the Peabody River. "The only thing we failed to get from Cam was what side of the river they were on," says May. "So when we got there, we actually started across the bridge, but then fortunately Jeff saw us and yelled out."

The two turn around to see the two young climbers lying beneath a boulder. "Jeff's cry was practically inaudible because it sounded like someone whose throat is frozen or starting to fill up with phlegm," Boudreau recalls.

Perched atop the snow load on the bridge, May and Boudreau gingerly turn 180 degrees—not an easy task wearing long wooden snowshoes. Once back on the correct side of the river, they turn right at the trail junction and follow Bradshaw's snowshoe tracks a short distance up Great Gulf Trail until they drop down the embankment to the river's edge.

"There was a large boulder, 20 feet high or so, leaning toward the river, which gave them a little bit of a dry, overhanging area," says Boudreau of the emergency bivy site. "They had created a floor of spruce boughs and were kind of tucked down in a little hole. Jeff was excited and started talking a mile a minute. He told us to help Hugh first. We scrambled down there and thought we should try to get Hugh up on a flatter surface."

Because Batzer is partially ambulatory but clearly feeling the effects of the cold, May and Boudreau start off by rewarming him. "Jeff was obviously wet, and the outer layers of his clothes were starting to freeze," recalls Boudreau. "It was easy to get him on top of a sleeping pad. We pulled off his wet fleece jacket, and I got my thick wool top and my down parka on to him."

May remembers that Jeff was in better shape than Herr but that his hands were severely frostbitten. "Dave had a really nice, fluffy down jacket, what I call a "pièce de résistance," he says. "In other words, when things get really bad, you always have a piece of clothing you can put on to save your ass. And that jacket was it. Dave gave him some water and a candy bar. He just couldn't stop talking."

Jeff tells their two unexpected visitors how long they've been out and how happy they are to have been found. "He was very relieved when we told him we had encountered Cam, and that she was on her way down to get help," says Boudreau.

With Batzer as stable as they can make him, May and Boudreau turn their attention to Herr. May still remembers the alarming condition in which they found him. "Hugh was inside the little boulder cave, huddled up and sitting on some branches. He wasn't saying anything. I learned that day that there's a smell that goes along with these kinds of desperate situations, the smell of frozen flesh and the necessary act of urinating on yourself. I had never smelled that before."

The 6-foot, 190-pound May, who once played defensive tackle for his high school football team, ignores the uncomfortable odor and moves to get Herr out of the pocket of the boulder and onto flatter ground where they can treat him. "I put my hands underneath his armpits and just pulled him out where we could get stuff off of him and put warm clothes on him," says May. "He was totally incapacitated. I tried to take off his outer jacket and his pile jacket, and they were frozen to his back."

Boudreau, who's 5-foot-11 and 190 pounds and played rugby and linebacker in high school, recalls their difficulty in trying to help Herr. "I had never seen someone in that advanced stage of hypothermia," he says. "His body was contracted, and his arms were across his chest. I tried to pull his arms out to put a dry shirt on him, and it felt like he was frozen solid and if I pulled his arm any harder it would break off in my hand. He wasn't wearing any boots. He was incapacitated from the knees down. His legs and feet were swollen, and they were as hard as rocks. We got a couple of moans out of him, but he was pretty much comatose the whole time. We finally got a pile jacket on him and got him into a sleeping bag, but he was in very, very rough shape."

"They were fantastic," says Herr today of May and Boudreau. "They gave us gorp to eat, and the sleeping bag was incredible."

"I recall Jeff trying to drink the water we had on hand, but not wanting any chocolate," says Boudreau. "Hugh was not fully conscious and too stiff for us to do much more than take off his wet outer layer and get him into my down jacket and fiber bag."

With Herr secure in his sleeping bag, May and Boudreau place Batzer in the remaining one. "It took a while and a lot of work on their part to get us into sleeping bags," says Batzer. "Talk about encouragement! They cheered us on, telling us, 'You're going to be OK, hang in there!' But Hugh was delirious at that point, and not saying much at all."

The two impromptu wilderness first responders stand over their two unexpected patients. Lying in winter-rated sleeping bags atop insulated sleeping pads, Herr and Batzer will begin to thwart the cold's efforts to claim them.

May and Boudreau anticipate a long night of waiting for the arrival of a ground team, and an even longer night of helping to carry Herr and Batzer out of the backcountry. They are unaware that Cam Bradshaw, with the help of Liz Lancaster and Steve Johnson, has arranged to speed things up. "As soon as we got done settling Hugh and Jeff in warm clothes and sleeping bags, the helicopter was overhead," says Boudreau, still amazed at the speed of the rescue team.

Pinkham Camp parking lot
Approximately 3:10 p.m.

Dave Warren looks on as the engine of the Huey Victor fires back up and the rotors slowly gain speed. Warren offers his thanks to Capt. John. Weeden for his crew's efforts and prepares to bring the day's search to a conclusion. Amid the loud hum of the Huey, Warren hears the sound of screeching tires and an accelerating engine nearby. He turns his attention away from the small group gathered in the parking lot.

"We had just finished the debrief," says Warren. "The pilots were going back out, and we were all saying goodbye. All of a sudden, this car comes careening around the corner, stops short, and these two people start getting out. I knew immediately it was Liz Lancaster and Steve Johnson. With tremendous force, they said something like, 'We found them, and they're alive!' They bolted from the car and came running over."

Misha Kirk, who's just concluded his second trip of the day in the Huey, is in the middle of an interview when the day's search is suddenly extended. "I was talking to a reporter and concentrating on what I was trying to say," he wrote in his journal. "When I saw Steve and Liz just run up and interrupt Dave Warren, who was obviously busy with important people, I knew something was wrong. I excused myself from the reporter and ran over. My first thought was there had been an automobile accident just down the road and they came to report it. I couldn't comprehend what they might have to say that would be so important. 'They're alive. Cam found them in the Great Gulf.' We were in shock. I just couldn't believe it. How could they have survived four days and three nights without any bivy gear or food?"

Warren immediately rejoins Lt. Bill Hastings from New Hampshire Fish and Game, Snow Ranger Walter Winturri, Capt. John Weeden, and Misha Kirk to discuss a response. "Everyone at Pinkham knew what was going on at that point. We were like, OK, let's figure this out. We all went back in to get a better understanding of where they were."

Glen House site
Route 16
3:20 p.m.

Cam Bradshaw is shaking as the adrenalin fueling her two-mile descent of the Auto Road begins to wear off. After getting inside one of the small buildings at the Glen House site, she removes her mittens, and steadies her hand as best she can to ensure she is dialing the correct number for Pinkham on the rotary dial phone. Bradshaw reaches someone at Pinkham and informs them she's located Hugh Herr and Jeff Batzer, that they are alive and bivouacked at the junction of Great Gulf and Madison Gulf Trails just up from the bridge. She goes on to explain that two backpackers with overnight gear are en route to help them. She adds that one of the climbers is ambulatory and the other badly hypothermic and incoherent. Once she returns to Pinkham, she will prepare to begin her night watch duties at 10:00 p.m.

Standing by at Glen House as Bradshaw makes her call is Phil Labbe, who will shepherd the ground team being organized by AMC crew member Jack Corbin to the two-mile mark of the Auto Road in the WMTW-TV Thiokol. If they are required to carry Herr and Batzer out, he will be waiting there at the Madison Gulf Trailhead to transport them down.

Labbe himself had disappeared in a storm on the Auto Road just over 40 days earlier. It sparked a massive response from the very same agencies and groups who've been searching for Herr and Batzer, including fallen MRS member Albert Dow.

Pinkham
3:30 p.m.

Mike Waddell, who will soon join a ground crew to respond into Great Gulf, remembers hearing the news of Bradshaw's discovery. "When the call came in, it was late afternoon. Everyone was hovering around the radio room because they'd been found, and by Cam Bradshaw. She was known as someone who'd wander off into the middle of the mountains for miles and miles all by herself, for fun."

"We quickly convened in the office," Kirk wrote. "Dave [Warren] was great at keeping things under control. We decided the pilots would fly over to the Great Gulf to see if they could see anything, while Pete [Furtado] and I were to get ready and be first responders."

The Herr and Batzer families are drawn to the unexpected commotion and informed that their sons have been found alive. They are told that a ground crew will be getting underway toward Great Gulf via the Auto Road to the two-mile mark on the Auto Road and then over the Madison Gulf Trail.

"They had basically called off the search," recalls then *Union Leader* correspondent Barbara Tetreault. "Most of the press had left. I was in the process of calling in my day's story on a pay phone. This was a time before cell phones, so I had to wait my turn. I had just called in to give *The Union Leader* an update and was packing up to go back home. I was in the Joe Dodge Lodge and people started running. It seemed like this spark. I thought, 'Something's going on here.' They told us they had found them. I remember Jeff's parents coming out, and I asked them their reaction."

A shocked Richard Batzer tells Terreault, "I couldn't believe they could survive three nights and then a fourth [day]. I have three boys, and I thought this morning that I had two. I thought I had lost a son. Now I'm going to get to know this one better."

Jim Cole, then a photographer for the Associated Press who'd spent most of the day at Pinkham shooting film, recalls being overwhelmed with emotion when he heard of the discovery. "I was at the Conway Chamber of Commerce, where I had built a temporary darkroom developing the day's film," he says. "Word came down that they'd found them. It still chokes me up to this day. They were alive. Right then and there, I started crying. For them to have survived was actually amazing. I immediately headed back up to Pinkham."

Because Herr and Batzer are located outside of the Cutler River Drainage and in Great Gulf Wilderness, jurisdiction for their rescue immediately shifts from the U.S. Forest Service to New Hampshire Fish and Game under the two agencies' Memorandum of Understanding. Misha Kirk, who is tasked with responding on foot into Great Gulf, is once again in battle mode. He has his marching orders and moves swiftly to prepare himself for his foray into the backcountry.

"I was still in shock," wrote Kirk in his journal. "I still couldn't believe it. As I ran through the Trading Post [to my room], the press tried to stop me. They knew something was up, and it was driving them crazy not to know. As I was fully dressed in my climbing clothes, and my pack was still preloaded and ready to go from yesterday, I went running back through the Trading Post in minutes. By this time, the rumor that they had been found and alive had flooded Pinkham. I came flying in asking for help. 'Get me some food, fill this thermos with hot lemonade, find me some extra batteries, and then meet me back in the office.'"

"Misha had this presence," says Patrice Mutchnick of her late partner and former Green Beret. "He was big, and so severe looking, but so compassionate. He wasn't in search and rescue for anything else but this incredible sense of compassion for others. He was generally light and happy sounding, but he was sometimes a rather serious and severe person when he was around other rescuers. He had this "Don't fuck with me" kind of attitude at times."

Kirk heads into the parking lot in search of a ride over to the Glen House site at the Auto Road. The plan is for him to be picked up by the Huey, while AMC Assistant Manager Pete Furtado is transported to the two-mile mark by snow machine. Kirk wrote, "I was ready to go, fully packed with snowshoes. I had enough bivy gear, food, liquids, and chemical hot packs to last me a week. The chopper hadn't left yet, and they wouldn't let me on until they made their primary search."

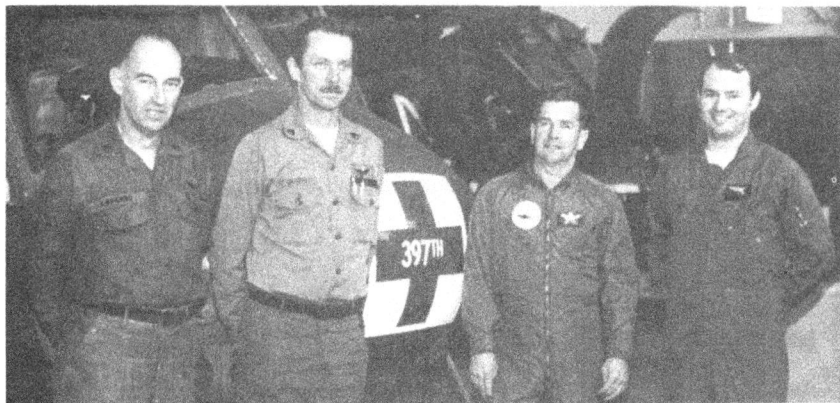

The crew of the Huey (left to right): Staff Sgt. Walter Lessard, Staff Sgt. James Halub, Chief Warrant Officer 4 Ronald Boyer, and Capt. John Weeden.

LVI
INBOUND

As we express our gratitude, we must never forget
that the highest appreciation is not to utter words, but to live by them.
—President John F. Kennedy

Great Gulf: Temperature: -5°F; visibility dusk.

Pinkham
Tuesday, Jan. 25, 1982
3:30 p.m.

Misha Kirk is task focused as he marches across the parking lot looking for a ride to the Glen House site so he can head over to Great Gulf and begin preparing Hugh Herr and Jeff Batzer for hospital transport. His impatience is making him edgy.

"I was getting frustrated," he wrote in his journal. "I could have left 10 minutes ago and with approaching darkness I was anxious to get in there. Finally, I collared a F&G cop and told him to get me out of here and down to Glen House. … As we left, the chopper lifted off. During this whole time, I kept saying to myself out loud, 'I've got to be careful about rewarming them. They're going to be borderline. I had to be careful that my excitement, joy, and anxiousness didn't impair my judgment. On the way down, in the F&G pickup truck, I heard on the radio 'Where's that paramedic?' The chopper was to pick me up at the Auto Road parking lot."

Emergency Bivouac Site
Great Gulf Wilderness
3:50 p.m.

Hidden below the canopy of tall pines, Geoffrey May and David

Boudreau try desperately to signal the Huey that's arrived in the airspace directly above them. As they jump and flail their arms, they're concerned the helicopter will fly off without spotting them.

"I'm waving this red parka and trying to get their attention, and they're just flying around," says May. "It was still a little light out and I thought, 'Oh shit, they can't see us.'"

Boudreau remembers how close the circling Huey seemed, but how far away it truly was. "We were standing there, and there was a little bit of a clearing where the trail crossed the Peabody. So there wasn't as much tree cover at the junction. It seemed to me that the helicopter was so close that I could have just hit it with a snowball. But even the trained individuals in the helicopter couldn't see us. They just kept buzzing. They'd loop around, find the brook, go right up the brook bed, and miss us. Here we were, two grown men jumping up and down waving our hands above our heads and yelling and screaming."

The two know time is running out before the Huey flies off to look for them elsewhere. May drops his jacket to the ground and immediately removes his heavy backpack. "That's when I remembered I had flares with me," he says. "I took them out of my pack and shot one off. It sent up a plume of orange smoke as the helicopter was banking away. It went above the 70-to-80-foot hardwoods, and that got them to finally focus on where we were. It made the difference."

May purchased the flares just before Christmas during a trip to L.L. Bean in Freeport, Maine. He recalls the moment he saw them behind the counter. Having just completed a wilderness first-aid course, he thought they might come in handy someday. And it turns out he was right.

Boudreau remembers the unsettling moment his companion pointed the flare toward the sky and let it rip. "I know it's all perspective, and we were all pumped up on adrenaline and nerves and all, but when he shot that flare up, it looked like the flare went through the rotor blades. It probably wasn't that close, but that was my first impression. The pilot knew what he was doing. He banked immediately and came right up over us."

Airspace over bivouac site
3:50 p.m.

Capt. John Weeden and copilot CW4 Ronald Boyer have been vainly trying to locate the stricken climbers by executing short grid patterns over the trail junction, while Crew Chiefs Staff Sgts. James Halub, Walter Lessard, and Lt. Bill Hastings have been scanning the tree-covered terrain out of the side windows of the aircraft. At last, they get a break.

Hastings will write in his official report, "As we approached the confluence of Parapet Brook and the West Branch, we were aided in pinpointing the exact location by a red flare fired by one of the two passing backpackers that Cam Bradshaw had enlisted to assist at the scene."

With fuel consumption a major concern, the crew members immediately begin to search for a place to set down. "A hasty examination of the area revealed a relatively open space nearby (100 to 150 yards) on the Madison Gulf Trail where I knew the trees to be less than 25 feet in height," wrote Hastings.

But Weeden knows he cannot possibly put the Huey down there. There is too much tree cover and not a wide enough radius to bring the aircraft in. "We couldn't land because it was a very confined area," says Weeden. "The snow was so deep that if we were able to land, we would have just stayed light on top of it and loaded patients in that way. But we just couldn't get down there."

With no time to spare, Weeden points the Huey back in the direction of Glen House where Misha Kirk awaits word on whether he'll be flying in or hiking there. The plan is to pick up Kirk, fly back to the bivouac site, and drop him down to the victims on a hoist. He can then make a medical evaluation that will help decide whether the two men can be carried out on rescue litters or if one or both must be hoisted up into the helicopter for more urgent transport to Littleton Hospital. It isn't an ideal solution, but it is the only option they have to get Herr and Batzer the help they need as quickly as possible.

LVII
BEHIND THE SCENES

Later, back in the Whites, we used to work our butts off
getting somebody down in a litter. Then everybody else would go home,
and I would go take a shower, get in the scrub suit, and fix them!
—Dr. Harry McDade, surgeon and pioneering cold-weather
physician, quoted in *Mountain Voices: Stories of Life and Adventure in*
the White Mountain and Beyond

Littleton Hospital
Littleton, N.H.
Tuesday, Jan. 26, 1982
3:30 p.m.

Because it is likely that Hugh Herr and Jeff Batzer will be transported to the hospital by helicopter, whether they are first littered out of the backcountry or immediately hoisted up into the aircraft, the Emergency Room at Littleton Hospital is notified to prepare for their potential arrival. At the time of this incident, and because of the groundbreaking work that began here years before under the direction of Dr. Harry McDade and other medical experts, Littleton Hospital has earned a national reputation for the treatment of cold-weather injuries.

The official Mount Washington Rescue Report, dated January 23-26, 1982, tells a story few are ever aware of. During any emergency, those involved are focused entirely on the victims and on their own roles in the crisis. Most give little thought to the massive preparations needed to save a life that is on the line. From the report, we learn how many people and resources must be put into play to ensure that patients suffering from critical cold-induced injuries have the best chance at survival.

In this case, in order to prepare to receive two hypothermic, frostbitten patients at Littleton Hospital, Administrator LeRoy Deabler will handle overall coordination. Dr. Campbell McLaren and the Emergency Room staff will notify all the hospital's other services.

Public Relations Director Donald Gilson will talk to the media and arrange for news releases. The Respiratory Department, X-ray Department, and lab will be alerted. Nicholas Sterling, in charge of hospital maintenance, will clear the parking lot of snow to make room for the helicopter landing. Ross Ambulance Service will be notified and have three units ready to light the landing area and mark its boundaries with red rotary emergency lights. Dick McGinnis, director of nursing, will coordinate the use of additional in-house staff. The house supervisor and the head of dietary services will prepare hot water for rewarming the two climbers and coffee for the incoming guests. Any extra Emergency Department personnel will be called in as needed.

In addition, the Hypothermia Blanket Unit will be set up and prewarmed. Stretchers will be equipped with aluminum space blankets and sheets. Hypothermia mercury thermometers and disposable rectal probes will facilitate body core temperature monitoring. Respiratory therapy will set up cascades for warming humidified air through insulated tubing. Cardiac monitors will be ready to identify arrhythmias. Blood warming coils and heaters will heat blood and fluids prior to their delivery to the patients. Intravenous bottles of low-molecular Dextran, Ringers Lactate, Normal Saline, and D5W (dextrose 5% in water) will be preheated to 104–108°F and wrapped in aluminum foil to preserve heat. A peritoneal lavage tray with catheters will be made available, as well as Foley catheters and a central venous line set up. A hydro tub will be filled and heated to 104–108°F.

It is a mind-boggling preparation plan. But for Hugh Herr and Jeff Batzer, every bit of it is essential. Given their desperate condition, it is their best—perhaps their only—chance at making it through.

LVIII
JOINING FORCES

The best way out is always through.

—Robert Frost

Great Gulf: Temperature: -4°F; visibility darkness.

Emergency Bivouac Site
Great Gulf Wilderness
Tuesday, Jan. 26, 1982
4:05 p.m.

Capt. John Weeden guides the Huey back toward Hugh Herr and Jeff Batzer's bivouac site after picking up Misha Kirk on the Auto Road. He and his crew are forced to select an area on the opposite side of the Peabody River because the bivy site poses significant challenges. The aircraft is now 100 yards from the two climbers and their caregivers, David Boudreau and Geoffrey May.

At this point, it is still unclear exactly how Herr and Batzer will be removed from the bivy site, but Weeden must choose his spot assuming he will be carrying two patients in bad shape. "The terrain over the site was steep on both sides with 80-foot trees, and it was right on the river, which was not entirely frozen, presenting an additional problem with respect to having good footing," he wrote in his official report. "We were also concerned about further aggravating the patients' injuries if they were accidently exposed to the water. The site that was selected instead necessitated a very short lift, i.e., 30 feet, and was relatively flat."

Below the Huey is a small knoll about 15 feet wide, with embankments on both sides and minimal tree cover. This will allow Weeden and copilot CW4 Ronald Boyer to hover while Staff Sgt.

James Halub and Misha Kirk are lowered to the ground on the jungle penetrator. SSG Walter Lessard will manage the rescue hoist. Lt. Bill Hastings of New Hampshire Fish and Game will coordinate communications between Kirk, the helicopter, and Pinkham.

"I had to determine whether Hugh and Jeff should be lifted out or littered out," wrote Kirk in his journal. "I was too excited to be scared as we took off."

Lessard prepares the jungle penetrator and Halub slides open the large cargo door. He will descend first. As soon as the door opens, dangerously cold air pours into the crew cabin along with the nearly intolerable noise from the Huey's shrieking engine and spinning rotors.

Although the noise and wind levels result in communications challenges and uncomfortable conditions for the crew, Weeden says such stimuli can have their advantages during a rescue mission. "The crew chiefs and medic wear safety harnesses, heavier gloves than the rest of the crew, insulated underwear, and heavier jackets, all to protect them from the extreme cold. Pilots feel the elements and the noise but not to the extent that the crew chiefs and medic do. When the door opens, it can heighten the sense of urgency and focus among the entire crew, especially during critical missions. The exposure to the elements and the increased sensory input can lead to heightened alertness and adrenaline levels."

In short order, Lessard has Halub securely fastened to the jungle penetrator and begins to lower him. Weeden holds the Huey in hover as Lessard controls the speed of the winch. Once Halub is on the knoll, the penetrator returns to the aircraft for Kirk to descend next.

Kirk's medical kit and backpack will be lowered after he safely reaches the ground. He will soon be up close and personal with the 50-mph rotor downwash that awaits him. Fortunately for Kirk, who is trained in combat rescue, he recognizes the distinctive sounds of the Huey. As he prepares to swing out beyond the landing skids of the aircraft, he reminds himself, 'You've been here before, Misha.' He understands the importance of maintaining his situational awareness as he descends.

"I got myself ready as [Crew Chief Lessard] readied the jungle penetrator," Kirk wrote. "Basically, [it's] a three-foot cylinder with pegs and a bottom that snaps down, perpendicular, to sit on. The top is attached to a cable and a winch with a movable boom that swings out. I put the peg between my legs, and the crew chief harnessed my torso to the cylinder so I didn't fall backward. ... Slowly I was picked up by the winch, still sitting inside the chopper, and was swung out. Dangling in the air, I felt the adrenaline rush as I looked 60 feet down. I love heights; then again, most climbers are adrenaline junkies."

Charles Barry, then director of New Hampshire Fish and Game, told Tom Hanley of *The Sunday News*, "When you're lowering men out of a copter onto a mountain in the dark, that's risk with a capital R." But though he has considered the risk, Kirk will write in his journal, "I really trusted those guys."

With Halub and Kirk on the ground, Weeden flies off and goes into a hover nearby to await word from Kirk on the condition of the two climbers. Halub will wait on the knoll for Kirk to complete his assessment after he reaches the bivy site.

"Once on the ground I waited for my pack to be lowered," Kirk wrote. "I noticed my snowshoes were no longer on my pack. Anxious to get to the boys, ... I left and punched through the snow and slid down the knoll toward the river. I crossed the bridge, which was tricky due to it being full of snow. Looking down at the cold river, I definitely didn't want to fall into it."

Across the river from the knoll, May and Boudreau watch as Halub and Kirk are lowered. Having fought with deep snow since arriving at the trail junction, they recognize the challenge of getting to the bivy site without snowshoes. Still wearing their own snowshoes, the two work to break trail for Kirk to ease and hasten his passage.

When he reaches Boudreau and May, Kirk identifies himself as a paramedic and follows them down the embankment to the bivy site. He first assesses Batzer, who lies prone in the borrowed sleeping bag but is alert and oriented. Herr is semi-comatose and will clearly require more time and care.

"When I told [Jeff] I was a paramedic, it was as if I was Jesus," wrote Kirk of Batzer's exuberance. "He burst into happiness and said, 'Hugh, Hugh! God, we're going to be saved!' He started talking a mile a minute."

Batzer explains to Kirk, in great detail, what has occurred since he and Herr topped out on Odell Gully four days earlier. "I found out Jeff had tolerated some water and food from Dave so I gave him several sips of warm lemonade," wrote Kirk. "I felt Jeff's foot that only had a mitten over it. It was rock hard. Jeff said, 'Hey, no problem. I'm going to lose a few things, but it's better than dying'. I was pleased with his attitude. He'll do just fine."

Kirk engages Boudreau and May to assist him with treatment. In addition to their warrior roles, Green Berets are also skilled trainers. Part of the Special Forces ethos involves boosting the capability of allies and partners. While the bivy site Kirk is now managing is not a military stronghold, he recognizes Boudreau and May as force multipliers. He gives them hot packs and tells them to pop them and stick them on Jeff, one layer from his bare skin, one in his groin, one in his armpit, explaining that these are critical areas to warm up.

Kirk learned the usefulness of hot packs from MRS team member Bill Kane during a winter rescue in 1980. He was so impressed with their effectiveness in rewarming a hypothermic patient that he added them to his medical bag from then on.

"Misha definitely stood out because he remained calm the whole time," recalls Boudreau. "He was very patient with us, explained to us what he was doing, and told us what to do. He was very professional, and we were so glad he was there."

Because Batzer is suffering from severe frostbite and is not ambulatory enough to walk, Kirk determines that he will require a rescue litter for transport over to the knoll where he will be evacuated by the jungle penetrator. He then turns his attention to Herr, already aware that Herr will require a litter carry to get him to the knoll and raised by the rescue hoist.

"I bent down close to Hugh to determine his state of hypothermia," wrote Kirk. "He was just barely conscious and kept mumbling, 'Cramps, I've got bad stomach cramps. My feet, I don't want to lose my feet.'"

Although Herr can communicate to this extent, his level of awareness is far lower than Batzer's. Kirk unzips the sleeping bag and begins his head-to-toe assessment. "I felt his abdomen: rigid and sensitive," wrote Kirk. "His feet were rock hard. Feeling them gave me a chill. I knew he was going to lose them. I kept talking to Hugh, trying to boost his spirits. I said they had come a long way. I didn't want to lose him now. I quickly radioed [Pinkham] my findings."

The Huey has been in a hover for approximately 40 minutes

while the crew awaits Kirk's medical assessment and plan for evacuation. As the aircraft burns through its fuel, the blistering cold continues to besiege the crew of three still in the aircraft. "We just stayed there hovering, realizing it was going to be a mission requiring the Stokes litter and the rescue hoist," recalls Weeden. "We had the door on the hoist slid all the way back, and there's a jump door that had to be open, too. We'd lost the sun, and everyone was very cold."

With the Fish and Game portable radio he's carrying, Kirk tries to communicate with Bill Hastings in the Huey to devise a plan for evacuation. But he is unable to relay his findings. "At about this time, we began to run into communications problems," wrote Hastings in his report. "It became next to impossible to copy any transmission from Misha on a handheld radio without a headset due to the engine and blade noise from the helicopter.

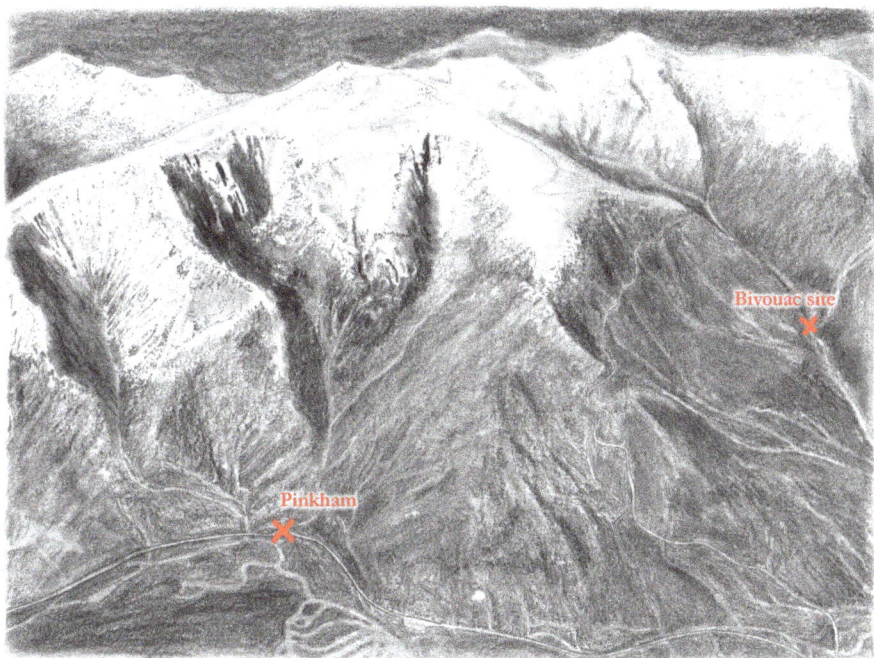

The distance from Pinkham Notch Camp to the Great Gulf/Madison Gulf Trail Junction is 3.33 miles as the crow flies. There are two high points between: Lily Ledge at 2,758 feet, and Lowe's Bald Spot at 2,868 feet.

352

Kirk silently curses at the radio as static blasts out of its speaker. "The problem was now, I couldn't talk to [Hastings]," wrote Kirk. "Feeling frustrated, but not wishing to alarm Jeff or Hugh, I made some joke about it and began to prepare Jeff for evacuation."

Low on fuel for the imminent rescue mission, Weeden leaves the scene and heads for Pinkham to refuel. There, they'll be able to communicate directly with Kirk, who has an AMC radio, and devise a plan to bring Herr and Batzer to safety.

LIX
EVACUATION

Those ravines on Mount Washington are formidable reminders
of a past and harsher climate; even to alpinists who have been often
among much more exalted peaks, they remain stark,
deadly, and challenging.
—William Lowell Putnam, *The Worst Weather on Earth*

Great Gulf: Temperature: -1°F; visibility darkness.

Emergency Bivouac/Evacuation Site
Great Gulf Wilderness
Tuesday, Jan. 26, 1982
5:00 p.m.

After refueling at Pinkham, Capt. John Weeden pilots the Huey back into the airspace over the bivy and evacuation sites. Crew Chief SSG Walter Lessard is joined in the cab by New Hampshire Fish and Game Officer David Hewitt. While at Pinkham, Hastings assigned Hewitt to take his place onboard so that he could assist Dave Warren with post-rescue coordination.

Hastings' first order of business in that role is to arrange for the families of Hugh Herr and Jeff Batzer to be escorted to Littleton Hospital by New Hampshire state troopers.

Staff Sgt. James Halub, thankful to be wearing a bulky warm jacket, remains on the knoll at the evacuation site. Once the Huey is back in hover mode, a rescue litter drops from the aircraft in anticipation of a hoist rescue of both Batzer and Herr.

In the early stages of planning, Kirk believes Batzer should be littered to the knoll above which the Huey is hovering and then hoisted into the aircraft on the jungle penetrator. But with the snow so deep and so few people to carry a litter up two slopes ranging from 30-to-60 degrees, Kirk soon ascertains that the only viable option is to get Batzer to the knoll on foot. He knows the clock is ticking rapidly for Herr, and they must hurry to get him the help he needs for survival.

"When the decision was made to get Jeff to the landing spot, I volunteered to carry him over," says Geoffrey May. "I had 50 feet of nylon cord with me, so I used it to make a one-man split that I learned in the wilderness first-aid course. You split the rope in two and put a coil on each shoulder. Jeff could put a leg into each of the coils, and I would be able to carry him on my back like a backpack."

It is pure luck that May has nylon cord with him. "I worked for an independent rental car agency in Harvard Square for a couple of weeks while on winter break," he says. "I would wash cars in the basement, and people left things in the cars all the time. Someone left quarter-inch nylon rope in the back of one of the cars, and I thought it would be good to have. I brought it on that backpacking trip on a whim."

As May and Dave Boudreau prepare to head for the knoll with Batzer, Kirk quietly tells them about the tragedy that occurred the day before. "Misha informed Geoff and me that Albert Dow had been killed," recalls Boudreau. "The ground crew was approaching the site, and I believe he wanted us to curb our excitement for the benefit of the approaching crew. He took great care to deliver that news out of Jeff and Hugh's earshot. Misha showed nothing but leadership and composure throughout the entire rescue."

Kirk and Boudreau hoist Batzer onto May's back and feed his fragile legs through the coils. With the fingers of one of his hands frozen solid, Batzer latches onto May's shoulder with the other. "Because it was dark at that point, Misha told us to take our headlamps with us," recalls May.

May and Boudreau move toward the steep embankment heading up to Great Gulf Trail. Boudreau takes the lead and makes small, driving steps up the slope. He hopes to further solidify the trough for his trailing companion and the fragile cargo he's carrying. At the footbridge spanning the West Branch of the Peabody River, Boudreau stops and moves aside so May can walk up the short snow ramp and onto the top of the narrow mound of snow clogging the bridge. Boudreau follows close behind. "I can remember the snow was so deep that it was up to the handrails on the bridge," May says of his delicate traverse. "It fortunately held, and I didn't fall. I can remember telling Jeff, 'Look, if I fall, I'm falling forward so just hang on to me.' It was a 10-to-12-foot drop to the river below."

With May and Boudreau in the process of transporting Batzer to the evacuation site, Kirk refocuses his attention on Herr, who remains woefully detached.

Meanwhile, Peter Furtado, who was transported on snow machine by Snow Rangers Brad Ray and Rene LaRoche to the Madison Gulf Trail at the two-mile mark on the Auto Road, is making his way to the scene. AMC crew members Mike Waddell and Dennis Tupick will also be snow machined to Madison Gulf Trail and hike into the site. In addition, a ground crew of a dozen AMC volunteers is being transported to the two-mile mark by Phil Labbe in the WMTW-TV Thiokol. They will all stand by there in case Herr cannot be evacuated with the rescue litter and must be carried out.

Kirk, alone now with Herr, is trying to keep hope alive. "I got down with Hugh and continued to talk to him," wrote Kirk. 'Hang on buddy, you're doing great.'"

About 10 minutes after they leave, Kirk sees May carrying Batzer across the footbridge, with Boudreau following. Shortly thereafter, he looks up to see Peter Furtado arriving. He informs Furtado of Herr's condition and then leaves for the knoll to help hoist Batzer into the Huey. "I had the utmost confidence in Pete," he wrote. "We had worked together before on accidents and he was very good."

As James Halub readies the jungle penetrator on the knoll below the helicopter, Boudreau and May traverse the bridge and soon arrive at the base of the steep slope leading up to him. Kirk joins them.

"We got to the other side, and the snow was so deep it was up to my waist," says May. "I was trying to get through the snow with Jeff on my back. Dave was hanging on to me. He had one arm on a tree, and we'd grab hands so he could pull me up the embankment through the snow. We finally got over to the opening on the knoll. The Huey was just above us, the lights were flashing, and [Holub] was there to help get Jeff on the jungle penetrator and raise him."

To this day, Batzer remains grateful to May and Boudreau for their extraordinary efforts. "He was a really strong guy,'" says Batzer of May. "Both of them were really calm, good guys. On the bridge, it was difficult. He would slip down into the snow, and I thought we would both go over the guy wire. He got me to the clearing, and I remember Misha was there, too. The whole time I was thinking, 'This is just insane.' I wasn't afraid because I said to myself, 'They've got this; we're safe.' I felt completely taken care of at that point. They had told me they were taking us to this place with all of these hypothermia and frostbite experts."

Weeden slides the Huey into position above the knoll and maintains a hover. The powerful downwash of the spinning main rotor system creates a ground blizzard on the small patch of terrain. May and Boudreau rest as Halub secures Batzer to the jungle penetrator.

"[Halub] harnessed him in as I talked to Jeff," Kirk wrote. "Jeff was great. His attitude was confident, happy, and he knew he was going to live. I gave him a hug, and up he went. Jim and I huddled to protect our stinging faces."

Batzer warmly recalls that exchange with Kirk. "When I was on the jungle penetrator, Misha said to me, 'This is nothing for you, you're a climber!' I told Misha, 'I'm fine.' The penetrator started to spin as I was going up, and it was a battle for them to get me inside. They strapped me into the seat and gave me thumbs up. They asked me, 'You, OK?' I said, 'Yes, I'm good to go.'"

LX
GOING FOR IT

Never interrupt someone doing what you said couldn't be done.
—Amelia Earhart

Great Gulf: Temperature: -1°F; visibility darkness.

Emergency Bivouac/Evacuation Site
Great Gulf Wilderness
Tuesday, Jan. 26, 1982
5:30 p.m.

With Jeff Batzer safely and securely on the aircraft, Crew Chief James Halub joins Misha Kirk, Dave Boudreau, and Geoffrey May as they move back to the bivy site with the rescue litter.

Kirk is pleased to find that he can now communicate with Pinkham. Both he and Paul Cunha, then a member of the AMC crew, have AMC and Fish and Game radios. But since Kirk and Cunha cannot communicate with the Fish and Game officer on the Huey because of the cabin noise, Kirk must communicate with Cunha, who has been ducking in and out of a second-floor window of a small building at the Glen House site for a better signal. Cunha can speak with Kirk, then relay word to someone at Pinkham. From there, Pinkham can communicate with the Huey through Staff Sgt. Ronald Bellerose, the flight operator and radio operator who is also at Pinkham. This complicated communication loop will last throughout the remainder of the mission.

As the four rescuers return to the bivy site and join Pete Furtado, the Huey hovers just east of them and awaits word on next steps. The experience of carrying Batzer to the knoll convinces the rescuers that they cannot transport Herr over the bridge safely in such deep snow.

The reality of having to litter him along the Great Gulf Trail all the way out to the Auto Road is beginning to set in.

"We had gotten Jeff out, and I was sure he'd live," wrote Kirk. "When we got back to Hugh, it was dark. I fully expected to litter Hugh out all night. I heard through my radio [that] Dave [Warren] was organizing and sending out litter teams. I decided to at least get Hugh packaged in the litter."

Boudreau hears Kirk on the radio with Pinkham, saying they won't be able to carry Herr over the bridge to the knoll. As difficult as it will be, a long carryout appears to be their only safe option. "But I didn't think Hugh had that long," Boudreau says. "It would be very hard to get him out of there."

As they finish packaging Herr into the litter, the Huey slowly moves overhead. "I heard the chopper and looked up to see a marvelous sight," Kirk wrote. "The chopper with full lights ablaze, lighting up the whole river, hovering just above the trees and downriver. I heard from [Pinkham] that 'Capt. Weeden is going for it.'" They are going to try to hoist Herr up from where he lies.

An attempt is made to lower Kirk's snowshoes on the rescue hoist to aid him in navigating the deep snow at the site. Caught in the vortex of the rotor's downwash, they swirl violently, striking the branches of the tall spruce and fir trees around them. Unable to get them down to Kirk, Staff Sgt. Walter Lessard pulls them back into the aircraft.

"The pilot was incredible maintaining his position," recalls May. "He had to move back and forth to pick up Jeff, and then he had to move forward to where Hugh was. I'm not a doctor or anything, but to me, if we had to carry Hugh out, I don't know if he would have made it."

The crew is fortunate not to be dealing with the high winds and mountain turbulence they had encountered on their earlier flights. Throughout the afternoon, winds had decreased, especially in more protected areas like Great Gulf. Were winds and turbulence a factor now, an already tenuous hoist rescue would be completely out of the question.

The airspace directly over the bivy site is congested with heavy tree cover, and there is no clear path for the rescue hoist from the Huey to the ground. "This particular hoist maneuver was significantly more difficult than other, routine evacuations because of the exactness of decisions required by all crew members necessitated by metrological conditions, darkness, blowing snow, and the extreme tightness of the evacuation site," wrote Weeden in his report.

"Misha was in radio contact with someone in the helicopter and told us to bring Hugh out to the highest point we could find in the brook bed," Boudreau says. "It was covered with dry snow and ice. The pilot did what he said he couldn't do and didn't want to do. He hovered low enough to get that tow line down onto the riverbed. From where we were standing, it appeared that the rotors were almost touching the treetops."

In his official report, Weeden describes their careful approach, "It was then dark with absolutely no lunar illumination. In order to best effect the evacuation, the helicopter had to hover at approximately 110 feet above the site. There were trees on either side and a very narrow path for the litter to pass through. It took precise coordination and aircraft control in order to maintain a constant position over the site. Darkness was an inherent inhibitor of the evacuation effort."

Because there are not enough of them to carry the litter, the five rescuers slide it across the snow-covered ground to a site out on the river, as instructed. Dark patches of open water serve as traffic cones, signaling spots to avoid. "There was a high boulder just out in the river," wrote Kirk. "A snow bridge 20 feet-by-5 feet had been blown in. We dragged the litter with Hugh in it out to the boulder. Pete [Furtado] was in front, Jim [Halub] on the right, and I was on the left. Suddenly Jim started to fall backwards into the river. I reached out and grabbed him back in by his big bulky jacket. If anybody fell in that river, we'd been in more trouble. I stacked us there, and we waited for the cable."

Even with the Huey 110 feet above them, Herr and his five rescuers are pummeled by the downwash of the aircraft's main rotor system. The five huddle around Herr's litter as the rescue hoist is lowered to them. At Kirk's direction and using a rope that was packaged in the litter, May attaches a bowline knot to the end of it. Known as a tagline, it is used to prevent a dangerous spin of the rescue litter as it is raised to the aircraft and exposed to rotor wash and wind.

"During this type of rescue, the individual is securely strapped into the Stokes litter, which is designed to immobilize him and prevent further injury," says Weeden. "This can provide a sense of safety despite the chaotic environment. There can also be a tendency for the litter to spin. The crew member operating the hoist stabilizes it from the helicopter while the crew member on the ground sometimes attaches a tether to the litter to prevent excessive spinning."

May recalls the blowing snow under the Huey and the strong downdraft. "It was really an awakening experience!" he says.

With his shield frozen to his face, James Halub attaches the rescue hoist to the litter. May hands the tagline over to Kirk, who keeps it taught and feeds it out as the litter ascends to the Huey.

"I had to shout in my radio to let [Pinkham] know we were ready," wrote Kirk. "Soon the litter began to rise. Pete and Jim let go, and I pulled to keep the litter from going sideways up into the blades. It was a battle. I had to force myself to look up as the whirling snow blinded me."

May, who is huddled directly behind Kirk and feeding him rope, remembers how impressed he was with Kirk's medevac skills. "Misha grabbed a sleeping pad, pinned himself against a rock, and peeked

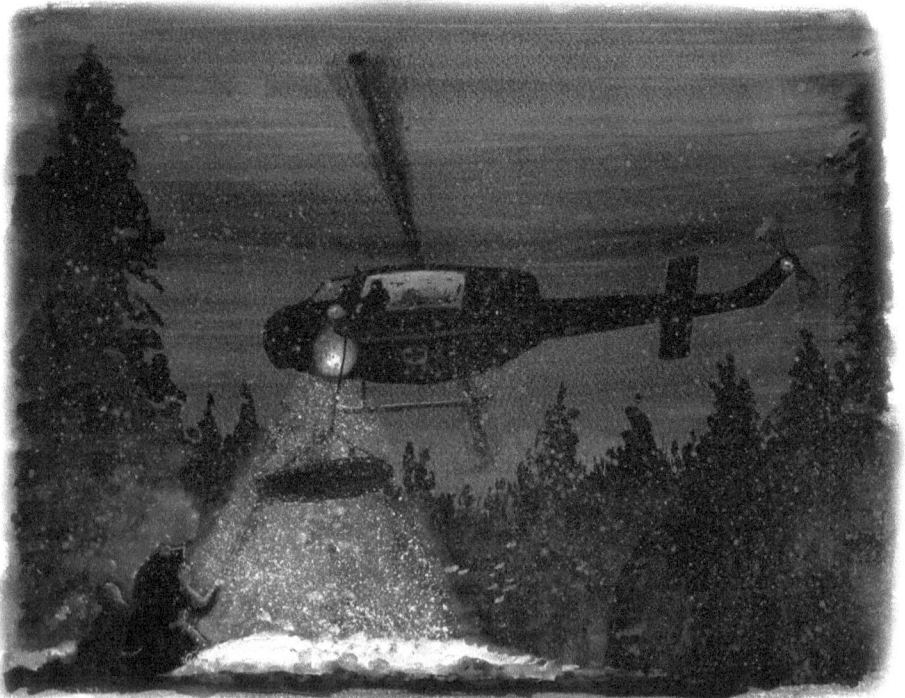

around the pad as they lifted up the basket," he says. "He had to face the helicopter as he let the tagline out. I was behind him making sure the tagline didn't knot up. I had my back to the wind."

As Weeden keeps the Huey in its stoic hover, the litter holding Herr continues toward it. Although semi-conscious and wrapped tightly in an insulated sleeping bag, Herr is aware of what's happening to him.

"Being lifted on a rescue hoist in a Stokes litter can be an intense experience," says Weeden of what Herr is likely experiencing. "The person will feel the vibrations and movements of the helicopter, which can be quite pronounced. The initial liftoff can be jarring as the hoist begins to pull upward. The downdraft from the helicopter's rotor creates strong winds and loud noise, which can be overwhelming. The patient may feel a significant amount of air pressure and loud sounds from the operating helicopter. The experience can be anxiety-inducing, especially for someone who is already injured or in distress."

As Kirk releases the slack in the rope, the litter slowly rises. "I had on a waist belay, but still my hands screamed as my grip was shutting off blood to my fingers," he wrote. "My frost nip from Albert and CPR brought tears to my eyes. My exposed nose and cheeks screamed with the biting of frost nip. What an eerie scene. Jim and Pete huddled behind me protecting their hands from the blowing snow. I could barely see them. Finally, the stretcher was in the chopper."

The ground crew believes Herr is safely on board. But that is not, in fact, the case. Because of the blowing snow and blinding search and landing lights, they cannot see that the head of the rescue litter is caught on one of the landing skids beneath the aircraft.

"That's normal," says Weeden. "People on the ground hook ropes to the litter because it inherently wants to swing, So when it gets up to the skids, you've got to work the litter outside them to continue lifting it up level to the floor of the aircraft."

Although normal for the crew, the disruption is anything but normal for the ailing Herr, whose level of consciousness has just reached its highest level in days. "Going up in the helicopter was terrifying," he says today. "I couldn't see anything. I heard the blades, and it was terrifying because I had trouble breathing. I was so packed in, and the sleeping bag was over my face. I thought I was suffocating.

I started screaming for help."

From inside the aircraft, Walter Lessard, who is wearing a safety harness attached to a ring on the Huey, removes his gloves and steps out onto the skid on which the litter has become tangled. With his hands numbed in seconds by the subzero windchill, he manages to free the litter, allowing it to be brought up into the helicopter.

"All of a sudden I saw Hugh, and he was completely encased in the sleeping bag," recalls Batzer of his reunion with Herr. "They slid the litter in and closed the door. I remember hearing, "Hey, we've got to get moving, we're running out of fuel!' I thought to myself, 'We might go down.'"

Herr, who is still screaming in fear as the litter slides into the cargo area, remembers the chilly welcome he received once inside. "When I got into the helicopter, I first felt anger, because the person who pulled the bag away from my face was gruff," he says. "At that point, I was just trying to survive, but he seemed to be angry and frustrated. His reaction is completely understandable today, though, because they had just put their lives on the line. The story is miraculous. So I would have responded to me the same way he did: 'These damn kids!'"

On the ground, amid all the noise, the blowing snow, and the general chaos, Kirk and the others are unaware of the situation with the litter and the landing skid, and the delay it's causing. "It was a little confusing for a few minutes," says Cunha, who is monitoring the scene from the Glen House site. "You know these things are always a little funky. I can remember a couple of minutes of 'What the hell is going on?' There was some confusion about whether the team at the evacuation site should let go of the tag line they'd been holding on to. But then I saw the chopper lift up and head out of Great Gulf, and that was that."

Weeden says he was eager to lift off because the Huey was very low on fuel. "It was a long mission just hovering there," he says. "The heaters didn't do much because all the doors were open, but it was just enough to blow some warm air on you. We were committed to getting both those guys onto the helicopter and to the hospital. Once we got Jim Halub back on board, we closed the doors, and we pumped the heat up as hot as it would go. We had to leave Misha behind because it was more critical to move the patients. They were in pretty dire straits."

Because the mission has lasted well over an hour, the Huey must head for Pinkham to refuel before transporting Herr and Batzer to Littleton Hospital. In reflecting on that night's evacuation, Weeden says today, "There was good crew coordination once we got a handle on what had to be done. Sergeant Lessard was on the hoist and constantly communicating with us: 'Slide left.' 'Slide right.' 'Lift.' Ron Boyer and I would split the duties. One of us would be on the controls and the other handling communications. It was a total crew effort to communicate, operate, and execute the mission."

For the remaining rescuers on the ground, it is a strange moment that brings them back abruptly from chaos to calm. "The helicopter was gone, and it was weird feeling to be all of a sudden without all that noise and light and in total darkness," says May. "We were in the mountains again."

Boudreau recalls that he and May seemed to be handling the aftermath differently from Misha Kirk. "Misha had been very, very businesslike and very, very subdued throughout the entire thing," he says. "I was thinking that this was his training, that he knew what he was doing and was trained to remain calm, but Geoff and I were getting emotional. The other members of the rescue crew who arrived divulged that they had lost one of their colleagues, which added even more emotion to the moment."

But it turns out Boudreau is not aware of what is really going on in Kirk's mind. Kirk will later capture his feelings in his journal, feelings he kept for himself: "The chopper lifts Jim up, flies off, and suddenly it's over. I realize how quiet it has become. I sit down in the snow, shut my headlamp off, and take a breather. I look up to a beautiful star-filled night and think, 'Albert would have been proud and glad we got them out alive.' For the first time since his death, I cry. First tears of sadness that he's gone, then tears of joy. I'm suddenly filled with the joy of being alive. It feels so good. I break into a smile and break out in a low 'Whoop!' We did it."

LXI
TRANSPORT

You must stand on a cliff of death to understand your purpose in life.
It's the only place you can see it.
—Mo Brings Plenty, Oglala Lakota and actor

Mount Washington Observatory Surface Weather Observations (6:00 to 7:00
p.m.): Temperature -14°F; winds out of the northwest averaging 47 mph;
visibility 0 miles; fog; clouds below summit; windchill -50.2°F; peak wind gust:
52 mph.

Airspace west of the Presidential Range
Tuesday, Jan. 26, 1982
6:40 p.m.

After a 10-minute stop at Pinkham to refuel, Capt. John Weeden
and copilot Ronald Boyer have the throttle of the Huey Victor matted.
The rotary-wing aircraft's 1,400 horsepower turboshaft engine
screams as the aircraft reaches its maximum speed of 127 mph. Even
though Hugh Herr and Jeff Batzer are way beyond the "golden hour,"
a term used for emergency or trauma victims that suggests a patient
must receive definitive medical care within 60 minutes of the onset of
injury or symptoms, the ethos of the 397th Medical Detachment is to
effect as rapid a transport as is safely possible.

"When we landed at Pinkham and refueled, they didn't take us
off because we were in such bad shape," recalls Jeff Batzer of their
brief stop. "The rotors stopped, and I could hear muffled screaming.
It was Hugh inside the sleeping bag. He was zipped up in it and felt
like he couldn't breathe, so they unzipped it enough to free his face."

Weeden and Boyer are both intimately familiar with this part of
the North Country. "We knew the area extremely well because one of
our primary training areas was the White Mountain National Forest,"

says Weeden. "We'd spent a year or more just flying mountaintop to mountaintop, picking out places that might be good extraction points that we would plot on maps working with New Hampshire Fish and Game. So we knew the area, and I knew where Littleton, New Hampshire, was from Mount Washington."

Maintaining what is called "terrain awareness" in military aviation, Weeden and Boyer monitor their airspeed, direction, and altitude while keeping a visual reference of the undulations in the terrain ahead of them. Each peak in the White Mountains has a distinctive shape, which also helps them orient themselves without the benefit of night-vision goggles, which were not available to them at the time.

"Even though there wasn't much ambient light that night, there was lunar illumination, so everything was all white," says Weeden. "With the snow cover, we did have some residual effect with the reflection. You can see the White Mountains very clearly at night, especially when there's a fresh coat of snow on the ground. From there, you look for civilization, and I knew what Littleton looked like from the air. Once I saw the lights of Littleton, it was very easy to find the hospital."

Batzer sits buckled to the bench seat in the crew and cargo area along with Staff Sgt. James Halub, Staff Sgt. Walter Lessard, and Conservation Officer David Hewitt of New Hampshire Fish and Game. Herr has quieted since the adjustment was made to his sleeping bag. He no longer feels he's suffocating. Batzer, who is also feeling calm now that the evacuation is behind him, begins to realize the scope of his cold injuries.

"My feet were solid blocks of ice," he recalls. "I can remember they were sliding across the hard floor of the helicopter. It felt like we flew for 40 minutes or so. It was complete darkness in the back, and they were trying to get Hugh stabilized. I remember feeling very upbeat during the flight."

Batzer is a man of deep religious faith. He believes that God has saved them through the selfless intervention of many. As the Huey approaches Mount Eustis, then a popular ski area in Littleton, Batzer's salvation is affirmed by an unexpected sign. "We came over this rise, and I saw the cross," he says. "I knew immediately that it was the same cross I saw the year before when Hugh and I were here to climb in Huntington. I took the moment in and thought, 'This is astounding.' I was thinking how cool and meaningful it had been when I first saw that cross on top of the mountain from our car. But seeing it from the helicopter after we were rescued, I thought, 'Oh God, I cried out to you, and you answered.' I knew without a shadow of a doubt that God rescued us. It was a profound moment."

Weeden can see the muted glow of the hospital ahead of him. As the Huey descends on a gradual angle toward the parking lot, he sees the red rotary emergency lights sitting atop the fleet of ambulances outlining the landing area. "We'd spent a lot of time before this mission setting up these landing areas not just at hospitals but at other sites, so we could use them in emergencies," he says.

At 6:45 p.m., Weeden sets the aircraft down amid a cloud of blowing snow and takes the power out of the main rotors. Boyer shuts down the engine and pauses as the jet-like whine of the engine ebbs and the main rotors slowly spin to a complete stop.

Mission accomplished.

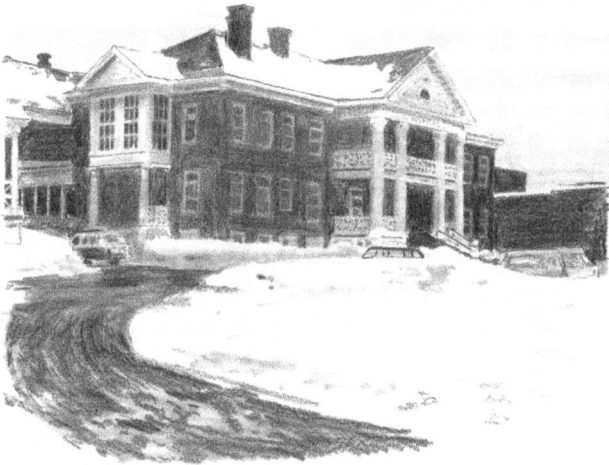

The front entrance of Littleton Hospital as it looked in 1982.

LXII
YOUTHFUL RESILIENCE

Accidents are never one event.
They're usually a combination of things that happen beforehand.
—Rick Wilcox, quoted in *Mountain Voices*

Littleton Hospital
Littleton, N.H.
Tuesday, Jan. 26, 1982
7:00 p.m.

Conservation Officer Jeff Gray does a double-take as he and other officers from New Hampshire Fish and Game move Hugh Herr and Jeff Batzer from the Huey into the Emergency Department. "I remember getting called out to meet the helicopter at Littleton Hospital," Gray says today. "I responded, as did several other COs, and I was surprised when we were carrying them in. They were small, wiry guys."

While Gray and the others wheel Herr and Batzer to their respective treatment rooms, security officers stand guard at the entrance and nearby ambulance dock. Members of the press arrive and are hastily diverted to the hospital's solarium, dining room, or front lobby, where they'll wait anxiously for updates on the condition of the rescued climbers.

Standing just inside the Emergency Department's main entrance, Dr. Campbell McLaren and Dr. Howard Pritham ready themselves for the long night ahead. Earlier, when the hospital was alerted to the discovery of the missing climbers and told that both were alive, McLaren knew he'd need every resource available to him when they arrived.

"I was working a 24-hour shift that day," recalls McLaren. "For a situation like that. I would always call in the on-call surgeon, and that night it was Howard Pritham. Back then, Howard was a companion surgeon to Dr. Harry McDade. They were both extraordinary guys."

McLaren and his family arrived in the U.S. from Scotland in 1976. An avid mountaineer and wilderness survival expert, he'd worked for a small hospital in the Scottish Highlands through the early 1970s. The cold, wet climate of the region frequently brought hypothermia and frostbite victims to his facility, so when McLaren arrived in the U.S., he was already well versed in cold injuries. After working at Androscoggin Valley Hospital in Berlin, N.H., he took a job in Littleton Hospital's Emergency Department in 1979.

"Dr. Harry McDade was the reason I came to Littleton," says McLaren. "He and I were among the first trauma life-support instructors in New Hampshire, and we taught out of Dartmouth-Hitchcock. It was a very interesting time because we were breaking down barriers with the treatment of trauma and cold injuries. We were aggressive, and we were getting treatment algorithms going. We were as data driven as possible."

At that time, McDade and McLaren were part of a small cadre of hospital and pre-hospital medical professionals who were developing innovative methods and protocols for the treatment of cold injuries. As a result of McDade and McLaren's work, Littleton Hospital quickly positioned itself as a go-to medical facility for hypothermia and frostbite treatment, and a national and international resource for hospital and wilderness medical professionals seeking guidance.

McLaren makes a quick visual assessment of his new patients and is surprised at what he observes. In the years leading up to 1982, McLaren had seen numerous victims who'd been in the cold for far less time than Herr and Batzer. He assumed their level of consciousness would be significantly altered that night. "I was amazed they were both conscious when they arrived," he says. "With Hugh and Jeff, I had two alert victims. They were not delirious. Both boys were clear, lucid, and aware."

McLaren says Herr's return to lucidity from his state of disorientation at the bivouac site can be explained by the treatment he received at the site and after the evacuation. "If a person hasn't eaten, you can have low blood sugar and be hypoglycemic," he says. "If the person is dehydrated, under stress, or has a lack of sleep, all of this can alter brain function."

Herr is wheeled into the first-aid room, where he will be under the care of McLaren. Batzer, whose condition is considered less severe, is brought into the observation room with Pritham.

Herr's room is equipped with a hypothermia blanket, known as a Blanketrol. After being removed from the sleeping bag, he will be placed on top of this warming blanket and covered with space blankets. In the event Herr requires a transfusion to increase blood volume, blood warming devices are on standby to warm the blood as it is introduced into Herr's circulatory system.

The room itself is heated with humidified air, and Herr is fitted with an oxygen mask allowing him to breathe in warm air. Boiled water arrives from the cafeteria in case Herr requires peritoneal lavage. If he is found to be severely hypothermic, a catheter will be inserted into his peritoneal cavity (the space within the abdomen that contains the stomach, intestines, and liver) and the warm water infused to aid in rewarming him from the inside.

Batzer's room also has space blankets and a whirlpool filled with hot water, and he too is fitted with an oxygen mask. "At first, I snapped it away because the air was so warm, and I just wasn't used that," he recalls. "There was this amazing sense of being in a warm building. With the lights over my head, I felt an overwhelming sense of warmth and safety. I was thinking, 'Wow, we made it.'"

Herr and Batzer's temperatures are first taken orally using standard mercury thermometers. It is no surprise to McLaren and Pritham that the readings bottom out for both patients at 94°F. "At that time, it was well known that oral mercury thermometers only read down to 94," says McLaren. "We were expecting hypothermia. We had to use something accurate, so we ordered rectal probes because I wanted to be sure. Rectal probes read core temperatures well below that measured by the oral thermometers that were available at the time. We had them brought down from the lab. For hypothermia back then, a rectal thermometer gave us ongoing, minute by minute temperature changes."

With the probes ordered, McLaren, Pritham, and their nurses attempt to remove the clothing Herr and Batzer are wearing. This will allow them to perform a thorough visual and physical assessment of their condition and start treatment. It will also allow them to apply monitors and start intravenous fluids. The process is painstaking for the staff and painful for the patients.

"They started to take the mitten off my left hand, and skin came off," recalls Batzer. "So they decided they'd leave the mitten on and remove it when I was placed in the tub. The fingers of my right hand were completely frozen and bonded to the silk gloves by the time we got to the hospital. The fingers on my left hand were frozen too, but not as bad as the right." To remove Batzer's one remaining boot, they use a blow dryer to thaw it enough to slide it off his badly frostbitten foot.

Decades later, Jeff Gray remembers the moment when the layers of clothing covering Herr's lower extremities were removed. "They allowed us to stay in the room during the initial assessment," recalls Gray. "With Hugh Herr, it was the worst case of frostbite I've ever seen to this day. His feet were just black right up through his lower legs, totally black and blue, just frozen solid."

For McLaren, a seasoned medical professional who'd seen horrific bodily trauma, the sheer magnitude of Herr's cold injuries continues to amaze him. "I'll remember this for my whole life," he says. "When I tapped Hugh's legs, it was like the thickest, densest wood. They were ice blocks, and I immediately knew he wouldn't have his legs much longer. He was totally frostbitten right up to the knee area."

Because both survivors are severely dehydrated, they are given a warm solution of Ringer's Lactate, an IV therapy used to replace fluids and electrolytes. "I was gulping ginger ale at the hospital," says Batzer. "I was never really hungry on the mountain. It was thirst that dominated the whole time."

Cardiac monitors are placed on the two patients to watch for heart arrhythmias. Hypothermia weakens the heart and slows the heart rate. A lower heart rate decreases the volume of blood the heart perfuses. A lack of blood flow reduces the oxygenation of tissue, which leads to a buildup of toxic acids. Because of these and other cold-related complications, the heart rate of a victim can become erratic. In instances of severe hypothermia, ventricular fibrillation can occur, which then ceases blood flow altogether.

At 7:06 p.m., Herr and Batzer's treatment plan takes an unexpected turn. With the rectal probes now in place, both Herr and Batzer are showing a core temperature of 94°F, the same readings obtained by the oral thermometers. Not only are their core temperatures identical, but they are much higher than anyone expected. The two are just barely hypothermic, despite their frozen limbs.

"I was surprised they didn't have a much lower core temperature," says McLaren. "We had things ready to treat them for hypothermia when they got here. As a physician, I have to cut to the chase and deal with what's going to kill them first, and that's hypothermia. But in this case, we didn't have to go into hypothermia protocol. Once we got the readings, hypothermia was not an acute concern; of concern was the frostbite."

McLaren says today that there's no clear explanation for Herr and Batzer's stunning core temperature readings. "Every case is unique. Every individual is unique. When you're at 92 to 93, some patients exhibit signs of hypothermia, some not. When you get down to 90 degrees, you're out of it. Hugh and Jeff weren't grumbling, mumbling, or confused. They were alert and aware. How astonished we all were! These were young men suffering from vasoconstriction, and boy, they had been constricted. It was pure frostbite. Ultimately, physiology had won over: these were young, healthy bodies."

When asked if the rewarming efforts at the evacuation site had a positive impact, McClaren says, "I wasn't aware of any pre-hospital warming when they first arrived, but it probably did alter their core temperature. The pre-warming by the rescue team at the scene was done well, but it wouldn't have been by much using external warming devices. It's pure conjecture on my part, but it may have brought them up two or three degrees."

By 7:30 p.m., with their core temperatures rising and life-threatening hypothermia ruled out, focus shifts to treating the climbers' severe frostbite. Preparations are made to submerge their frozen extremities into tubs of water that have been preheated to 104°F. "The tub we had was one I found at the Lancaster trash dump," says McLaren. "It was a good tub because it had lion's foot legs on it. Harry McDade had pushed for one, and I found it."

In a room nearby, the crew of the Huey sits quietly and attempts to rewarm as well. "We elected to stay at the hospital," says Capt. John Weeden. "I think we were all slightly hypothermic. We were all extremely cold and soaked."

In his two-part article in *Yankee Magazine*, Evan McLeod Wylie wrote, "Captain Weeden and his crew, looking for 'the warmest spot in the hospital,' downed large quantities of hot coffee and rested after what had turned out to be the longest, most exhausting, and most perilous rescue mission in which they had participated in the White Mountains."

Copilot Ronald Boyer still cannot forget how brutally cold he felt during and after the rescue. "We were so into that mission," says Boyer. "We had quite a crew. We were happy to save their lives. But I've never been so cold in my life. I don't think I've ever warmed up!"

When they feel just warm enough to resume flight, the four crew members head back to the New Hampshire Army National Guard base in Concord, arriving at 8:50 p.m., followed by the ground support crew, who arrive by truck at 9:30 p.m.

For their actions that day, Capt. John Weeden, CW4 Ronald Boyer, SSG Walter Lessard, and SSG James Halub will be awarded the Air Medal, a distinguished military decoration given for single acts of heroism or meritorious achievement while participating in aerial flight. It will be presented to them by the commanding general of the United States First Army. The four will also be recognized by New Hampshire Gov. Hugh Gallen, and in September 1983, they will receive the Hero Award at a dinner sponsored by *The New Hampshire Union Leader*.

Such honors are, of course, far from everyone's mind as the crew focuses on recovery and vigorous efforts continue to save Herr and Batzer. Complicating those efforts is the news that Albert Dow has died, which the two survivors are now aware of. "I can only remember bits and pieces on arriving at the hospital," says Herr. "We learned of Albert's death pretty immediately. I went from elation at being saved—because we were sure we were going to die—to seeing my parents and realizing they had believed they'd lost their son. The elation of all that and then hearing about Albert—it was just utter sadness and depression."

In a 2011 interview with National Public Radio's "Fresh Air," Herr said, "Our physical condition, to me, was the least of my concern. We were plucked from the mountain. We were told that a volunteer rescuer had died in an avalanche. The news of that was just horrible, so I really didn't care what was happening with my physical body. I was just devastated by the news that a fellow climber had perished."

Batzer has a similar response when a nurse asks him, "Did you know there was a rescuer who died trying to rescue you guys?" He recalls collapsing in the whirlpool and starting to weep. "My mom and dad and older brother came in," he recalls. "I wept so hard that I had to be held up in the tub. I was grieving and sobbing. Here we'd made it, but I said, 'We don't deserve to be here.' Hugh and I had made decisions that started this situation and pulled the rescuers into this dangerous search. We had made decisions that would end in tragedy."

Batzer's mother Joan, in an interview that night with John Hawkes of *The Intelligencer* newspaper said, "They are both conscientious kids. They really are going to have to deal with this."

Fortunately, though they are devastated by the news of Dow's death, Herr and Batzer gradually improve. Their core temperatures continue to increase and the heated, humidified air they've been breathing through oxygen masks is discontinued. At 8:30 p.m., when their core temperatures reach a normal 98°F, all heating devices are stopped.

Herr and Batzer's frostbitten feet are removed from the hot tubs. They are both able to move their feet and toes, but their skin is markedly discolored. Neither McLaren nor Pritham are able to detect pulses when they palpate their frostbitten extremities. "We do a percussion test with frostbite. You get a resonance with healthy tissue, but when I tapped Hugh's legs, they were dead. They were not getting blood flow."

The two are given morphine intravenously. "The battle would occur over the next week to try to save our hands and feet," says Batzer. "There was so much pain."

Once they are heated, the boys are transferred from the Emergency Department to the Intensive Care Unit for further monitoring. Shortly after 10:00 p.m., Batzer develops acute renal shutdown and is given a rapid infusion of mannitol. Fortunately, his body responds well to the treatment, and his renal failure is stopped within 20 minutes.

"Renal failure is usually a combination of things," says McLaren. "This was a transient failure, likely due to lack of fluids during their ordeal."

Care for Herr and Batzer now transfers to Pritham and the ICU staff. McLaren is still struck by the outcome of Herr and Batzer's harrowing, near-fatal ordeal. "How do you survive when it's impossible?" he asks, then goes on to offer some insight on how that happened. "They vasoconstricted in their limbs, but that peripheral vasoconstriction in two healthy young men protected their core, their brains, their livers, and their hearts. The blood where all the crucial functioning of the body was going on was maintaining a useful working temperature. It was amazing. The outcome was severe, no question. But it was due to their frostbite, not hypothermia. And they survived."

Note: In February 2008, 26 years after the rescue of Hugh Herr and Jeff Batzer, Dr. Campbell McLaren and Dr. Richard Merrick will treat James Osborne at Littleton Hospital after he arrived by Black Hawk helicopter. Osborne was rescued on the summit of Little Haystack Mountain in Franconia Notch at night and in full conditions by the four-person Black Hawk crew, two members of the New Hampshire Fish and Game Advanced Search and Rescue team, and five members of Mountain Rescue Service.

Osborne arrived at the hospital with a core temperature of 76.28°F. To this day, Osborne remains the coldest dryland hypothermia patient to be fully revived in the northeastern United States.

LXIII
RECOVERY AND LOSS

There is no education like adversity.
—Benjamin Disraeli

Littleton Hospital
Littleton, N.H.
Wednesday, Jan. 27, 1982
11:00 a.m.

Geoffrey May sits quietly in the passenger seat of the 1980 Jeep CJ-7 as David Boudreau pulls into the parking lot of this small regional hospital. Still reeling from their involvement in the rescue in Great Gulf, they are becoming aware of the extent to which events of the past four days have attracted widespread press and public attention.

"The next day was beautiful and crystal clear, one of those blue-sky days you remember," May recalls. "We were out in the Jeep at Pinkham letting it warm up and listening to the local radio station, and that's when we realized how big of a thing this was. They were going through the list of people who would attend Albert Dow's funeral the next day. I can remember that they mentioned he had been going to be married soon."

The previous night, when they returned to Pinkham with the rest of the rescue team, AMC Manager Dave Warren gave the two friends a room in the lodge for the night. Because he had lent his cold-weather gear to Herr and Batzer at their bivouac site, Boudreau was relieved to have a warm space to sleep. The kitchen crew reheated leftovers for them and the other returning rescuers.

Boudreau recalls the awkward moment when people in the dining room learned of their involvement in the rescue. Like May, he remains humble about their efforts. "As the Pinkham employees were reheating food for us, one of them said, 'These guys helped with the rescue.' So, we were momentary celebrities for some of the other guests. But we were trying to emphasize that we really didn't do anything much. Cam Bradshaw asked us to do something, and we did it. Then Misha Kirk showed up and told us what to do, and we did it."

After a welcome night's sleep that night, May and Boudreau head to Littleton Hospital to retrieve Boudreau's cold-weather gear. Neither wants to linger there, however. "When we got to the hospital we're going to get in and get out," says May. They know they are peripheral to the all-out effort to treat Herr and Batzer, and they don't want to be in the way. They are also a little stunned to see how many people are at the hospital, including the media. When they walk into the Emergency Department, they encounter a number of television cameras perched on tripods and reporters milling about. They make a beeline past the cluster of press to the nurse's station. "I explained who we were," says May. "The nurse said, 'Come with me.' We went into this room on the other side from where the ICU was. She handed us a garbage bag and told us, 'This is what we took off them.' We opened the bag, and all of these down feathers came flying out."

Boudreau digs through the garbage bag as errant feathers float to the floor. One at a time, he pulls his gear out of the bag to inspect it. "My sleeping bag was intact, but the parka and the shirt had been shredded," says Boudreau. "When the boys got to the ER, I figured the doctors did what they needed to do. They just took a scalpel to all their clothes to help get them off."

Boudreau places the tattered items back into the garbage bag, and he and May head straight for the exit. They are able to bypass reporters without being interviewed, but they do not go undetected by the parents of Jeff Batzer, who intercept them in the hallway. "They wanted to thank us, but we said we were just bystanders who were able to help a little. We were not the actual rescue crew," says Boudreau.

The Batzers look at the garbage bag in Boudreau's hand and know immediately what's inside.

"They heard we had lost some gear, and they wanted to get out their checkbook right there and write a check for what the gear was worth," says Boudreau, still moved by the gesture. "I said, 'No worries. The hospital administrator has already assured us the hospital insurance is going to cover the loss.'"

About two months later, Boudreau will receive a letter from the insurance company saying that they had reviewed the case and determined that the damage was not due to any fault or negligence on the part of the doctors. So they did not cover the loss. "That was not a big deal," says Boudreau. "It was only a parka and a shirt."

After expressing their good wishes to the Batzers for their son's recovery, Boudreau and May leave the hospital and arrive back at Pinkham in late afternoon. They are greeted by Cam Bradshaw, who will be filling in as caretaker for Joe Gill in Tuckerman Ravine that night and invites them to stay. "There were a couple of extra bunks there, and since their own backpacking trip had been interrupted by the rescue, I invited them up for the night," says Bradshaw. "The invitation was out of character for me, but I guess I felt some solidarity."

"That was a very nice gesture of kindness," says Boudreau. "We were able to cook indoors, and they had some nice chairs in the cabin and a little library. Cam was able to explain to us how extensive the rescue had been and where the avalanche had taken place. That was an eye opener to me, because it inspired me to read up on avalanches."

For their selfless actions in Great Gulf, Boudreau and May will be recognized in a letter from New Hampshire Gov. Hugh Gallen, who wrote: "On behalf of the people of New Hampshire, I want to thank you … for your efforts in the recent rescue operation on Mount Washington. Without your efforts, two lives would have been lost. By staying with the two climbers, you played a crucial role in the successful rescue. Congratulations for your good work … and thanks."

Intensive Care Unit
Littleton Hospital
11:00 a.m.

Hugh Herr and Jeff Batzer are stabilizing, Their kidneys are functioning properly, and no damage has been found to their vital organs. The big unknown is whether or not their frostbitten extremities can be salvaged.

A line of demarcation has developed at the point where their boot tops reached their legs. Batzer has blistering on his ankles and down toward his toes, and Herr's feet are purple and still cold to the touch. Herr has fewer blisters than Batzer, and both are able to extend and flex their feet at the ankle and move their toes.

In between visits from Dr. Howard Pritham and the nursing staff, the two are interviewed throughout the day by David Warren, Misha Kirk, Cam Bradshaw, Peter Furtado, and Lt. Bill Hastings. Though both remain on morphine to help manage the waves of excruciating pain that arrive unannounced, they are lucid enough to recount in detail what happened to them.

On Thursday, Herr's calves will swell to a point where Pritham must release the pressure. The condition is known as compartment syndrome and can lead to tissue death and even prove fatal if left untreated. Herr is taken to an operating room, where Pritham makes four incisions into the muscle compartments of his calves and feet. Following the procedure, the circulation in Herr's lower extremities shows such marked improvement that the procedure is repeated on Batzer's feet, which had swelled to the size of footballs. Because their frostbite has resulted in decreased blood volume, both receive ongoing doses of dextran to increase circulation.

That same day, members of the press are brought in to talk with Herr and Batzer. "They took us to the ICU for five minutes," says Barbara Tetreault, a correspondent for *The Union Leader*. "There were 10 or so newspaper people. I can vividly remember someone asking them, 'How did you feel when you learned someone was killed trying to find you?' I'll never forget the answer one of them gave: 'We felt horrible, and we're going to dedicate our lives to doing something good.'"

One recurring question Herr and Batzer field from reporters during their hospital stay and in the months that follow challenges their goodwill. "A common question was, 'What does it feel like to almost freeze to death?' says Herr. "We got so sick of the question that we started giving it a flippant response."

Jim Cole, a photographer for the Associated Press, returns to the hospital later that afternoon and is given access to Herr and Batzer, who remain in the ICU. "I can remember Hugh was passed out. He was in such pain that they had just sedated him. I said to Jeff, "Can I

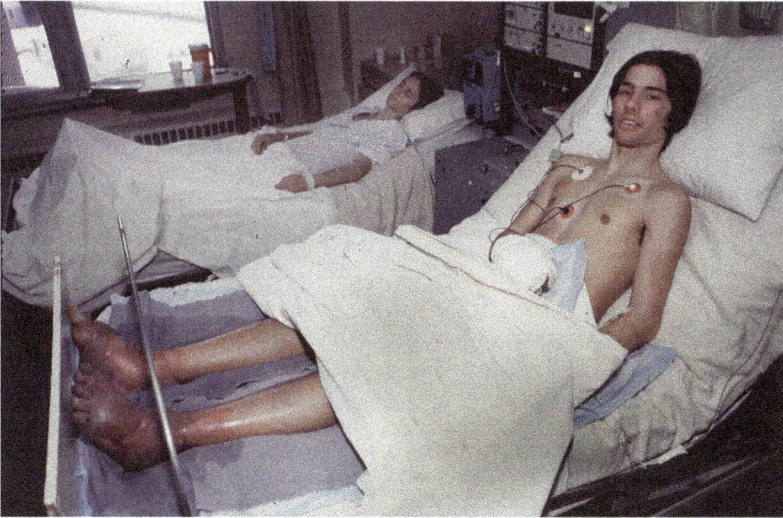

Jim Cole of the Associated Press took this widely published photo of Hugh Herr (background) and Jeff Batzer. Note the severe frostbite on Batzer's feet.

see what your feet look like, and he said, 'Yes.' I'd never seen anything like that. I took a photo, and that's the picture everybody remembers."

By their second week at Littleton Hospital, Herr and Batzer are in good physical condition, but there is still no clear prognosis for the viability of their extremities. In an interview with Steven Garfield of *The Littleton Courier* (March 24, 1982), Joan Batzer, who has been a nurse for 25 years, will tell him, "I can't say enough about the people of Littleton Hospital, or for that matter, the people of Littleton. We could never forget or repay the kindness and courtesies extended to us during our stay. ... Thank goodness for a medical facility so knowledgeable about frostbite."

On Feb. 11, Herr is transferred to Presbyterian Medical Center of the University Hospital in Pennsylvania. There, the circulation to his feet remains poor, and necrosis of tissue causes infection to develop. Batzer remains at Littleton Hospital, where his left foot and right hand show signs of deterioration.

On Feb. 20, Batzer is transferred to Lancaster General Hospital in Pennsylvania, where circulation to his right hand and left foot remains problematic. He is also showing signs of infection.

On March 2, Batzer's right thumb and all but one inch of his four other fingers are amputated, as well as the tip of the middle finger of his left hand and the toes of his right foot. His left foot is still showing no sign of improvement.

On March 5, Batzer's left leg is amputated six inches below the knee, and plans are made with physical therapy for training in the use of a prosthesis.

On March 10, both of Herr's legs are amputated six inches below the knee. Plans are made for him to undergo extensive physical therapy and training for use of prosthetic legs.

During these weeks and months of painful treatment and loss, Herr and Batzer's rescue, and the death of Albert Dow in the throes of it, will garner a good deal of public response. Elected officials will call for more oversight of the mountains, and several published opinion pieces will focus on the event, some insisting that Herr and Batzer be billed for the cost of rescuing them. Some people even suggest the mountains be shut down altogether.

The June 1993 *Appalachia* journal includes an article submitted by the AMC Search and Rescue Committee entitled "Multi-day Search on Mount Washington and Death of Rescuer." The piece contains this note: "Shortly after the events of Jan. 23-26, [1982], cries were heard throughout the North Country from many sources, demanding some sort of regulation of the mountains. Mandatory hiker's insurance, a policy of closing the mountain completely during bad weather, programs charging hikers a user's fee, and other less realistic ideas were discussed on radio programs, in newspaper columns, and in letters to the editor."

These strongly-worded opinions will begin almost immediately following the rescue. In his first few days at Littleton, Batzer will receive a phone call from MRS Team Leader Bill Kane. "Some of the opinion pieces and letters being written were rough on those kids," recalls Kane. "Jeff started crying on the phone. I said, 'Listen, you're no different than any of us. The reason we do what we do is because we're a brotherhood, and we don't leave our friends behind. You didn't do anything more than anybody else. What happened, happened, but it wasn't because of you.'"

Amid the heated debate, the voices of the climbers who went out to help— and lost a friend and teammate doing so—will advocate for a more reasoned approach to positive change, change that will become the legacy of Albert Dow.

LXIV
FAREWELL

We don't have to turn to our history books for heroes.
They're all around us.

—President Ronald Reagan, State of the Union Address,
Jan. 26, 1982

White Funeral Home
Conway, N.H.
Wednesday, Jan. 27, 1982
2:00 p.m.

Albert Dow Jr. holds open the front door of the funeral home for wife Marjorie, daughters Susan and Caryl, Susan's husband, Charlie, their 5-year-old daughter Amy, and his late son's girlfriend, Joan Wrigley. Inside, they are greeted by the director of the funeral home, who offers condolences for their unimaginable loss. Family members remain in shock over what has transpired.

"The day before, we had gone with Joannie to her and my brother's house in Brownfield, Maine, to get clothing," recalls Caryl. "We went to see Albert at the funeral home, but we couldn't see him that day. We brought the sweater that our Aunt Caryl had knitted for him. Albert went to see her once while on one of his road trips. She made him a reindeer sweater that he always wore."

Prior to leaving their home in Tuftonboro, N.H., for the funeral home, the family had received a continuous line of visitors, phone calls, and deliveries. "The phone didn't stop ringing," says Caryl. "People were calling from all over the country because they came to Lake Winnipesauke and were customers in my parents' antique shop."

"A reporter came to the door and asked me how I felt about my brother being killed on Mount Washington," recalls Susan. "I was nasty. 'How do you [expletive] think I feel?' I said. 'Leave us alone; we want our privacy.'"

"There was a neighbor who came to the house whose young son, my playmate, had been killed in a freak accident in the store they owned. She brought a bottle of whiskey and told Mom, 'It's for the day you just can't seem to get through. It will numb the pain a bit.' She knew what my mother was going through."

In addition to visits and calls, the family received copious amounts of comfort food from friends and residents of their small community. There were cards and telegrams, and flowers sent by the parents of Hugh Herr and Jeff Batzer. "I don't think any of us were angry with Hugh and Jeff," says Caryl. "We were all just in shock. It was really quite blurry."

Susan recalls the moment the family learned that Herr and Batzer had been found alive. "We all cheered. We were very excited that they'd been found alive. If they had found two corpses, it would have been a lot harder. We knew then that Albert had not died in vain. I'm very glad they survived. and the fact that both have done service for the world has really helped."

At the funeral home, there is concern among family members for Albert Jr., who is trying hard to remain a pillar of strength for his grieving family. But to his younger daughter, the loss is taking a toll on him. "I can remember my father holding his head a lot, trying to get his head around the fact that his son was gone," says Caryl. "I remember him trying to be strong for us."

The family is also concerned for Susan, who is six months pregnant. For Susan, the death of her brother in an avalanche has not only brought on debilitating grief but has also triggered memories of her own near-death experience in an avalanche on Mount Washington. In spring 1972, Susan and three classmates from Dartmouth College set out for a day of backcountry skiing in the Gulf of Slides. Susan was attending nursing school at the time and looked forward to getting out to ski amid intensive study. The gulf is the southernmost glacial cirque on Mount Washington and a popular spot for backcountry skiers and boarders.

"I was taking a run, and the snow suddenly broke away under my skis," says Susan. "My friends watched as I rode on top of the slide for a long time until it went over a drop-off and dumped me on some rocks. I can remember the snow filling in around me as I lay there. My friends told me that when I went over the drop, they thought I might have died. They were very glad to find me alive at the bottom of it. But I did suffer a skull fracture."

Albert's funeral will take place the following day in nearby Melvin Village. The major snowstorm and the aftermath of the World Airways jet's slide into Boston Harbor over the weekend are still creating complications for transportation in New England and for mourners trying to reach New Hampshire. "The storm prevented our nana from flying in from Florida," says Susan. "And our Aunt Caryl [Jorgensen] couldn't get there from California." Even some friends closer to home were unable to make it."

For now, the close-knit Dow family is cherishing their time with Albert before those who can make it will join them on Thursday. Each is able to spend time alone in the reception room where Albert lies in repose, wearing his beloved reindeer sweater. And each feels a wave of grief on remembering that he wore it last during their joyful Christmas together at the family home.

"I remember feeling fear," says Caryl. "Maybe it was because Albert was my big brother and protector, and he was now gone. I was going have to face life without him."

Susan remembers a more incongruous response. "My first reaction when I saw Albert was that they had done his hair wrong," she recalls. "I was upset about that. I focused very hard on my 5-year-old, who really loved her uncle. She insisted on going in to see him, and I wasn't about to deny her. I remember he looked peaceful."

The initial death certificate indicated that Albert had died as a result of asphyxiation, which was inaccurate. When Marjorie Dow first saw the certificate, she was devastated. "My mother was so haunted by the thought of her only son suffocating alone under the snow that my dad asked the medical examiner to change the cause of death to reflect the fact that it was immediate and that he didn't suffer," says Caryl. "It was changed to say Albert had died from multiple blunt-force trauma. We had been told that had happened when he hit the tree during his slide."

As the Dow family gathers around the coffin together and prepares to depart, their memories of Albert's impact on each of them and on so many others over his 28 years are making it impossible for them to imagine life without him. Only when their grief begins to subside will they understand that his death will help serve others in positive ways, just as he was so intent on doing throughout his life.

Note: Since Albert Dow, there has been one other avalanche death on Lion Head. On Jan. 5, 1996, Alexandre Cassan, 19, of Bécancour, Quebec, started up the old Lion Head Winter Route with three companions. This old route was closed in late 1995, and because it was no longer marked, the hikers lost the trail but continued up. While crossing an open snow slope that was fairly close to the location where Dow was killed and Michael Hartrich was injured, the four were caught in an avalanche. Cassan was buried and died of asphyxiation. He was the seventh avalanche fatality and 120th person killed on Mount Washington.

LXV
RECOMMITING

We do not learn from experience.
We learn from reflecting on experience.
—John Dewey

Eastern Slope Inn
North Conway, N.H.
Wednesday, Jan. 27, 1982
7:00 p.m.

On the eve of Albert Dow's funeral, members of Mountain Rescue Service gather for the first time since rushing to the avalanche site on Lion Head Monday afternoon. There's an understandable tension in the room brought on by the range of emotions each man is feeling. The meeting is convened by Team Leaders Bill Kane and Joe Lentini, who understand the importance of being together as a team in the aftermath of the tragedy they've experienced.

The only missing member is Michael Hartrich, who was injured in the avalanche that killed his partner in the weekend's mission. "There was nothing I could do about it," says Hartrich. "I just kind of shut down and stayed in bed for two to three days."

The rules for the meeting are informal, but the expectation is that what is said there, stays there. Counseling services for backcountry search and rescue volunteers who have suffered trauma are not available at the time. Dr. Nicole Sawyer, who works with search and rescue teams in New Hampshire, says the fact these men met to debrief about the loss of one of their own was an important step in their healing process.

"Humans are communal creatures," says Sawyer. "The concept of professional stress debriefings, which we use today, did not manifest as a result of science and research as much as it did from the natural inclination of humans to connect over impactful experiences. We celebrate together and we grieve together. Psychology just came along and put a label on something that humans have been doing naturally for millions of years. Despite western society's valuing of toughness, stoicism, and masculinity, humans feel an innate compulsion to gather over shared emotion. This is the primary reason rituals such as funerals and birthday parties evolved. It's why the water cooler in the office and the kitchen table in the firehouse are landmarks in their respective communities. They are gathering spaces for information, experiences, and belonging."

The recollections of some of those who were at the evening meeting offer insights into the tenor and tone of that gathering. It emerges from their memory as a moment when they could feel comfortable and safe airing their honest feelings and opinions, knowing they are among kindred spirits.

Getting things underway, Kane takes on the role of facilitator and opens the floor for candid discussion. "I can recall that Joe [Lentini] was openly angry at the two climbers, and some others were asking, 'Should we have been there?'"

Over the years, Lentini has been forthcoming about his early anger at Hugh Herr and Jeff Batzer. He serves as an excellent example of how one can work through such strong emotions and find understanding and forgiveness on the other side. "In those early days, I had no idea who those two were, except that I had heard they were a couple of young climbers who'd gotten themselves lost," he says. "I didn't care. I was so burnt at that point, I didn't care. The fact that it was Albert, that it was one of our team members, is what really caused me to feel rage and blame. I feel badly about that today. It actually wasn't that long before I started realizing that I was seeing all of my friends out there, and the mountains aren't safe. I now have so much respect for Jeff and Hugh, and so much empathy. I was a young climber once, just like them."

Doug Madara, who climbed Odell Gully with Steve Larson during the search, says he recalls sensing anger within the community but harbored no ill will himself. "I remember more reaction from the town than the team'" he says. "People in town were pretty pissed off. But I didn't hold Albert's death against Hugh and Jeff. They were kids, for one thing. I was curious about how the whole thing went down, how they ended up where they did. I really admire what Hugh's done since. Every time I've read anything about him, it's obvious to me that he feels some drive to pay a debt. I think that's impressive."

Larson says he also felt at the time that it was important to put the events in perspective. "We all get to be forgiven," he says. "Because you make a mistake doesn't mean you can't learn from it."

But the meeting is meant to allow free rein to everyone in the room, and those present take that to heart. "We were encouraged to vent, analyze, grieve or whatever we wanted and maybe make it a learning experience," says Dana Seavey, who carpooled to Pinkham with Albert Dow on Monday morning. "I remember being told no subject was inappropriate as long as it stayed in that room."

Seavey recalls asking how Albert's death could have happened. "I was more of a junior member, so I was nervous to speak out but just went for it," he says. "Some members agreed and supported me, while others were a little defensive." Seavey adds that some were asking where the team should go from there and even if their volunteerism was worth the risks. "We kind of had it out on a few topics," he acknowledges.

Kane, who is still taking the tragic outcome personally, talks openly with the group about the process the planning team followed. "Everyone knew we were the tip of the spear for that search," he says today. "I explained again how we had talked with the snow rangers every day about the avalanche risk and where it was highest. We all really felt the snowpack would be more consolidated that Monday, meaning less risk."

Someone questions whether it was reasonable to think Herr and Batzer could have been alive in Huntington Ravine after multiple days in subzero temperatures. Should they have even searched there that day? Others counter that the day's climbs, while in difficult conditions, were still well within their technical capabilities, and that the avalanche on Lion Head had been in terrain all thought was safe ground.

Gradually, resolutions will be made that spring from the lessons they've just learned. But before they can arrive at such decisions, they must first confront the question of their continued existence as volunteer rescuers. "The true emotional impact of Albert's death on MRS was after the fact," says Dr. Frank Hubbell, an MRS member who participated in the rescue. "It's when the reality of what happened settled in. Do we really want to do this? Should we do this? There was talk of disbanding. Why should we risk our lives to go out and help people? It was Bill Aughton who stood up at the meeting and said, 'This is not what Albert would want. He'd want us to do better.'"

With this comment, Aughton, one of the elder members of the team, turns the discussion away from second guessing and refocuses it on their belief in their purpose—and in the value of that purpose. Discussion turns to steps the team can take to improve.

All agree that the team should bolster its medical capability and undergo training. "We decided to hold a wilderness EMT course for the entire team," says Hubbell. "We had most of the team there at Pinkham two nights a week for three months." Hubbell and Kane were the primary instructors, and Misha Kirk led classes as well. "I became an EMT not long after Albert was killed," says Joe Lentini. "I felt like I had to have that knowledge."

In the following months and years, the MRS team will devote significant attention to bringing their already high level of technical competency and expertise to even higher levels.

"Up to that point, we were improvising," says Larson. "Many of us had done various walls, multi-day climbs like El Capitan in Yosemite, where we'd go up five or six days. So, we knew how to haul. But we didn't know how to raise somebody up a cliff as we do today."

Larson credits then MRS President Rick Wilcox with leading the team forward. Wilcox was guiding on Aconcagua during the search and would not learn of the tragedy that befell his team until his return home in early February. "For the next two to three years after Albert's death, Rick would bring in experts from the Tetons and elsewhere to come teach courses, which we were able to attend for free," says Larson. "People like Marc Chauvin, who was American Mountain Guide Association-certified, Kurt Winkler, Alain Comeau, and others started doing trainings for us on technical rescue skills. Today, we get to the top of the cliff, rappel down to the person, and bring them back up. In 1982, we didn't have the technique to do this. We went from scratching our heads and figuring out how to do it to being highly trained. We developed an ever-expanding bag of tricks to execute these rescues. Now we have scheduled trainings and people looking for terrain to play out potential scenarios. In 1982, we weren't there yet."

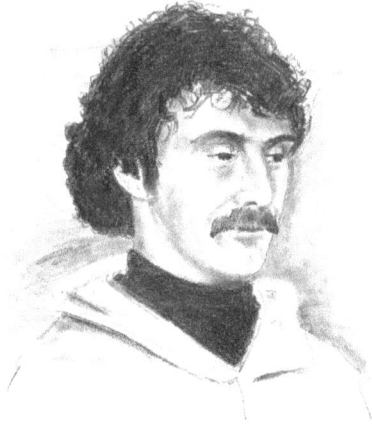

Rick Wilcox

Comeau, a member of MRS and a close friend of Albert Dow who was away during the search, says the team was mindful and methodical about how it moved beyond the tragedy. "The changes were slow to evolve. Like anything, it takes time to process, analyze, and reflect to see how and what should change."

Soon after Dow's death, MRS will participate in avalanche awareness training and acquire new equipment through donations. "I can remember that summer in 1982 we got avalanche transceivers, and we trained with them in the sand at Echo Lake below White Horse Ledge," recalls former MRS member Todd Swain. "It was the first time I had ever seen one. In retrospect, we were way behind the curve on avalanche awareness. I'm not sure why it took so long for us to figure out that avalanches were a danger in the northeast outside of Tuckerman Ravine."

"I think MRS has had a gradual and continual evolution since Albert's death," says Dow friend and teammate Alec Behr. "They've become more organized and better trained, and yet they still have that same kind of loose organization of local climbers. There are at least a half a dozen who were on the team in 1982 and are still on the team today."

One of these longtime members is Steve Larson, who along with a handful of others has served for over 40 years. "We took our role more seriously after Albert's death," he says today. "It was the catalyst and the first of many dominoes that led to the progression of MRS. We became a much better rescue organization because of him."

Note: On Jan. 29, 1982, New Hampshire Gov. Hugh J. Gallen issued a commendation that read: "I do hereby posthumously commend ALBERT DOW for his courageous efforts to save the lives of two others, and for which he gave the ultimate human sacrifice of his own life."

On Feb. 3, 1982, the New Hampshire State House of Representatives passed a resolution to "pay tribute to the memory of Albert Dow and to the example of courage and unselfishness which he set and … express deep sympathy to his family and friends."

On March 25, 1982, the New Hampshire State Senate passed a resolution "honoring the volunteers of Mountain Rescue Service for their dedication, skill and courage in times of emergency in the mountains of New Hampshire."

On Sept. 23, 1983, Albert Dow and Michael Hartrich were recognized with the Hero Award by *The Union Leader.* Hartrich, resistant to any form of recognition, elected not to attend the awards dinner.

Mountain Rescue Service also received the 1983 Outstanding Volunteer Award from the U.S. Department of Health and Human Services.

LXVI
OUTPOURING

Do not stand at my grave and weep.
I am not there. I do not sleep.
I am a thousand winds that blow.
I am the diamond glints on snow.
　　　　　　—Mary Elizabeth Frye

Melvin Village Community Church
Tuftonboro, N.H.
Thursday, Jan. 28, 1982
2:00 p.m.

Weather Observations (2:00 to 3:00 p.m.): Temperature 29°F; winds south/southwest averaging 13 mph; cloudy. Peak wind gust: 18 mph.

For some, the walk into church feels colder than what the thermometer reads. Others, already numbed by grief, are oblivious to winter's unforgiving chill. Within the four walls of this small, white, wood-shingled church scores of mourners will honor the life of Albert Dow. He and his sisters Susan and Caryl attended Sunday School here as children.

Standing prominently near the iced-over waters of Lake Winnipesauke and lying in the shadow of the deep blue Ossipee Mountain Range, the 115-year-old church seats only 150 people, according to fire regulations. But no one is keeping count on this day. More than 500 people are here. Some occupy the wooden pews; others stand shoulder to shoulder in the basement as they listen to the services on the loudspeaker. Those who could not squeeze into either space, including Albert's friend and MRS teammate Alec Behr and his girlfriend, huddle just outside the large front doors of the church or stand on top of snowbanks.

Everyone is here to celebrate the life of the young boy who brought lemonade to highway workers on hot days, frolicked on stone walls and in the forests and fields of Tuftonboro, and gracefully climbed railroad trestles in nearby Ossipee. They are honoring the man who was devoted to his family, paid kind attention to others, and went out to help those who were lost.

To make room for all the vehicles, the town's front-end loader moved heavy amounts of snow from the parking lot and front lawn, creating a wall of five-foot-high snowbanks surrounding the building. The Governor Wentworth Highway out front is lined on both sides with the overflow for as far as the eye can see. The Tuftonboro police chief shares with a reporter that it's by far the most people he has seen in the church in his decade of service.

Bea Lewis, a correspondent for *The Union Leader* will write, "Many members of the Mountain Rescue Service, with whom Dow was working at the time of his death, attended the service. Some were distinguished by the addition of a heavy woolen sweater under a sport coat or worn leather hiking boots beneath dress slacks."

Lewis, who grew up knowing the Dow family, remembers her experience as a new journalist covering the funeral. "It was the largest group of people I had ever seen, all just ruined and abject. A 28-year-old kid in the prime of his life, and such a nice kid. And his parents salt of the earth. That he was a volunteer going out in sub-arctic conditions trying his best to find fellow climbers just made it all the more awful."

Not all from MRS are there. Some avoid the services altogether, not out of a lack of respect for their fallen teammate, but because they are wrestling with a grief they have never before felt at their young ages. But there is one teammate present who could have chosen to stay away, a decision all would have understood. "Someone took me to the funeral," says Michael Hartrich, acknowledging that his memory is a bit blurry. "I remember the state police were all lined up as we got there."

The church is filled with a wide variety of mourners, reflecting the many kinds of people who were touched by Albert's life. Wearing the department's signature bright red jackets, with their green felt hats resting on their laps, are members of New Hampshire Fish and Game, offering a strong show of support. They are joined by friends, community members, fellow climbers, members of the AMC, local and state elected officials, and others who just felt the need to be there.

One of these is Marti Shoemaker, who has driven from Lexington, Mass. Her son David, along with Paul Flanagan, was killed in Odell Gully in 1979. "A closeness drew me there," says Shoemaker today. "I knew how it felt when someone came to tell me that David had died. There's no describing those feelings. So that's why I went. I was still fresh from David's wounds."

The service has drawn a heavy media presence as well. Reporters mingle with mourners and they, too, are feeling the weight of Albert's loss. John Howe, a correspondent for *The Lakes Region Trader*, will write that he watched as a member of the media offered apologies to the church's deacon for their intrusion, but the deacon would not accept it. "This is good," the deacon said. "It recognizes Albert's contribution to life, almost as a hero."

Two hours away, at Littleton Hospital, Richard Batzer stands at his son's bedside. When asked by correspondent Margery Eagan of *The Boston Herald American* about the services for Albert, he says, "Our hearts and deepest feelings are with the Dows today. Their son tried to save mine, and my son is alive today."

At the funeral, Albert Jr. tells Richard Mertens of *The Concord Monitor* how much he admires his son and his sacrifice. "I'm proud of my boy going up there. Anybody would be. You can't leave somebody up there. You just can't. He would go up there again tomorrow, and so would every other boy. ... They were all just as brave."

Orrin Welch, a childhood friend and neighbor of Albert's, sits quietly beside the Dow family. He's never forgotten the love and support he received from them. At only 5 years old, Albert insured that Orrin always had food, clothing, and companionship. "I drove all night from Cincinnati to get to the funeral," says Welch today. "I walked in, and I must have looked like a bum. The ushers jumped up and said, 'Family only.' But Mr. Dow got up and said, 'He's part of our family.' When I went to hug him, I could feel every bone in his body trembling. Albert's death tore him apart. Mr. Dow was a quiet and gentle man. He was extremely kind and intelligent, and when he spoke you listened to him."

Rev. Dr. Robert Thurston opens the service citing scripture from the Old Testament and offers these words: "We live in deeds, not years; in thoughts, not breaths; in feelings, not figures on a dial. We should count time by heart throbs. He most lives who thinks most, feels the noblest, acts the best. How one lives is more important than how long one lives.

Rev. Greta Dow, Albert's aunt, has traveled from Cavendish, Vt., to participate in the service. She reads from several pieces of scripture, intermingling them with poetry, choosing passages that evoke stories of Albert. "Little Al had a way of making us all feel individually special," she says in part. "I'm sure most of you here can recall a time when, by some simple deed or expression, he made you feel like royalty, too." She adds that Albert's happiness "was the contagious type," and that it was important to realize "how much he crowded into 28 short years—sports, education, helping, giving, loving, just plain being the best self he could be."

Albert's sister Susan says, "There were all of these accolades that Albert wouldn't have been comfortable with. He would not have liked being put on a pedestal."

The congregation is told that Albert was to have announced on Valentine's Day that he was engaged to marry Joan Wrigley, who is seated with his family. This heartbreaking news causes many who have thus far held it together to weep.

At the conclusion of the service, friends and relatives file out of the pews, and Albert's casket is brought outside where it is placed in the waiting hearse. With arms interlocked, members of the Dow family steady one another as the heavy door closes.

Over the course of several hours, hundreds of mourners will file through the receiving line at the Willing Workers Hall near the church. It is an opportunity for the Dow family to thank those who have come to honor Albert and show support. "We were there for a couple of hours," recalls Susan. "I met Misha Kirk in the receiving line. I stepped out to talk with him and to thank him because I knew he had tried to resuscitate Albert."

The funeral marks the moment when the Dow family must move on with their lives in the absence of a beloved member. Though difficult for everyone, it is especially hard for Albert and Marjorie Dow. "To lose an only son who was such a good man, it absolutely tore my father right down to shreds," says Caryl. "Daddy was a very humble man. He knew his son was out there serving the public, and that's what he'd raised his son to do. But he had a hard time coming to terms with the price Albert paid. There was always that "But... .""

Caryl adds that her mother coped at first by writing hundreds of thank-you letters. "This went on for years," she recalls. "It was one of the ways my mother worked through her grief. My father did what a lot of men do, really digging into something he could get his teeth into and focusing on it as a distraction. For him that something was flying lessons, which they both decided to take. My dad got his visual and instrument rating, and my mother got her visual-only rating. It turns out he had always wanted to learn to fly. He told me he did it then because he wanted to fly over Albert's mountains."

LXVII
LEGACY

I think it's because of Albert that we are where we are today.
—Lt. Mark Ober, New Hampshire Fish and Game

Nearly 1,000 man-hours by five organizations were devoted to finding and rescuing Hugh Herr and Jeff Batzer in 1982. Rescuer Albert Dow's tragic death on Lion Head during that mission became a watershed moment for search and rescue in New Hampshire. Important changes at the volunteer, state, and federal levels were a direct result of his sacrifice.

The most profound change occurred within weeks of the tragedy. In the years leading up to it, there were discussions within the legislative and executive branches of state government about whether volunteer search and rescue personnel should be covered by workers' compensation. But the proposal never advanced because up to that point no volunteer had required medical attention. Dow's death in the line of duty placed the issue front and center, resulting in the formation of a 15-member special senate committee called the Search and Rescue Study Group. Comprising three state senators and representatives from a variety of organizations involved in search and rescue, the committee initially focused on two critical issues: workers' compensation coverage and communications capability during missions.

Less than two months after Dow's death, Senate Bill 22, sponsored by State Senate Majority Leader Raymond Conley of Center Sandwich, passed by a vote of 22-0 and was signed into law by Gov. Hugh J. Gallen on March 18, 1982. The law provides workers' compensation coverage to those "voluntarily assisting in search and rescue missions' who are injured or killed while working under the oversight of New Hampshire Fish and Game. The law was made retroactive to January 1, 1982, to offset burial costs for Albert Dow and to cover Michael Hartrich's medical bills. Because Dow had no dependents, his parents received $1,200 from the State of New Hampshire for burial expenses.

Federal workers' compensation benefits soon followed under the Federal Employees' Compensation Act for those assisting in search and rescue missions in the Cutler River Drainage while under the oversight of the U.S. Forest Service. Today, volunteer search and rescue personnel are also covered by a first-responder death benefit at both the state and federal levels.

Responding to the challenges search teams faced on Mount Washington during the Herr/Batzer mission, the New Hampshire State Legislature approved a $77,000 appropriation to New Hampshire Fish and Game for the purchase of emergency equipment, most of which was earmarked for radios. It was the first step in what remains a continuous effort to improve interoperability between agencies and organizations conducting search and rescue operations.

Jeff Gray was a conservation officer with Fish and Game at the time of the 1982 search. Now retired, he remembers the lasting impact Dow's death had on his agency. "Albert's death was the impetus for us to improve our training," he says. "We did a lot of avalanche training and attended specialized courses that dealt with understanding snow conditions. As a department, we purchased better equipment and trained more with MRS, SOLO, and the Forest Service."

In 1986, the all-volunteer/nonprofit New Hampshire Outdoor Council (NHOC) was founded to support search and rescue teams and other organizations involved in backcountry safety. "The NHOC was formed as a result of Albert," says founding board member and former MRS team member Bill Aughton. "We needed an organization for the rescuers and a mechanism with which to interact with the public and the legislature on backcountry safety and responsibility."

In addition to providing funding support for search and rescue teams and other organizations involved with backcountry safety, NHOC has recently turned its attention to the mental health of the search and rescue community, whose members must sometimes face the lingering aftereffects of traumatic circumstances they face during dangerous, sometimes heartbreaking missions.

"I think volunteer search and rescue in New Hampshire is gradually becoming part of what I call the trickle effect," says Dr. Nicole Sawyer, who provides training for the state's SAR community.

"As service members were returning from Iraq and Afghanistan, the military began to focus on their mental health. From the military, that attention made its way into the public safety environment and is now starting to trickle down into the volunteer community that supports Fish and Game and the Forest Service. Critical Incident Stress Debriefing services are now available to these volunteers."

Though not a direct result of Dow's death, but in keeping with the effort to continually improve, the White Mountain Search and Rescue Working Group was formed in the mid-1990s. The group of 15 agencies and organizations meets monthly to discuss pertinent issues related to search and rescue operations. "Discussion in the working group is intended to promote safety, professionalism, and communication, and to serve common interests among all the SAR teams, such as education, training, and search management skills," says Lt. Jim Kneeland, a 30-year veteran of New Hampshire Fish and Game and team leader for the department's Advanced Search and Rescue Team. "The group also helps promote backcountry safety among the public."

Since the 1982 avalanche that claimed Albert Dow, the danger of such events has increased. This is due in part to a sharp increase in the number of backcountry skiers, winter hikers and climbers on Mount Washington who benefit from advanced equipment that was unavailable four decades ago, and in part by the effects of climate change.

"The change with backcountry skiing here is that it's no longer a springtime event," explains Nick Aiello-Popeo, an MRS member since 2014 who is American Institute for Avalanche Research and Education Level 3-certified and an avalanche course leader. "The equipment and the trends have changed, and everyone wants to ski powder in the cold snow months. All things being equal, there's a greater risk of triggering avalanches in those months versus the springtime. It's a more dynamic environment in the cold snow months because there are many distinct layers in the snowpack."

Charlie Peachey, a weather observer and research and IT specialist for the Mount Washington Observatory, says that a recent study conducted by the Observatory shows rain-on-snow events—the kind that contributed to the snowpack instability that led to Dow's death and injured Hartrich on Lion Head—are increasing on the mountain. "Temperatures at the summit in recent decades have warmed dramatically in the winter," he wrote. "Rain-on-snow events can lead to high avalanche danger due to the freeze/thaw cycle weakening the snowpack."

The Observatory study recorded weather data obtained over four decades, broken down into two 20-year periods—1981 to 2010 and 1991 to 2020. One of the most telling findings for today's outdoor community is that a 27 percent increase in the number of rain-on-snow days was noted from 2011 to 2020, especially in early winter. It is not surprising, then, that avalanche awareness and prevention have become high priorities for outdoor educators. Jeff Fongemie, the lead snow ranger for Cutler River Drainage and director of the Mount Washington Avalanche Center, says that "the biggest challenge for the center is getting the word to people who are going into the terrain. They just don't know avalanches are there, so they don't look for an avalanche forecast. We see this a lot with the new backcountry skiers."

The increased danger is also a major concern for rescuers. MRS President and Team Leader Michael Wejercht says that avalanche hazard is a big part of the team's calculus when they are out on a winter mission. "We're often in avalanche terrain, and it's something we don't necessarily know we're going to be in at the outset. Just like with Albert and Michael, you have no idea where you're going to be on the mountain at any given time or what your backup plan is going to have to be. So these days—and especially informed by that particular accident, which still resonates with all of us—we always take avalanche hazard into consideration. The thing in winter is that a mission can turn technical very quickly, especially on Mount Washington."

An exceptional climber himself, Wejercht is aware that he and others in New Hampshire's search and rescue community owe a great deal to their predecessors, including Albert Dow, who helped bring about today's advances and improvements. "The utter unknown of what those folks were going into is unimaginable," he says. "Today we have the knowledge of avalanche hazards that they didn't. They were doing the absolute best with what they had. The snow science and our understanding of it has come such a long way since then. The White Mountains are a fickle and unpredictable range that can become extremely dangerous extremely quickly. In a tragic way, we're lucky to have the knowledge of what happened back in 1982. We benefit from it, we use it, and we take it quite seriously."

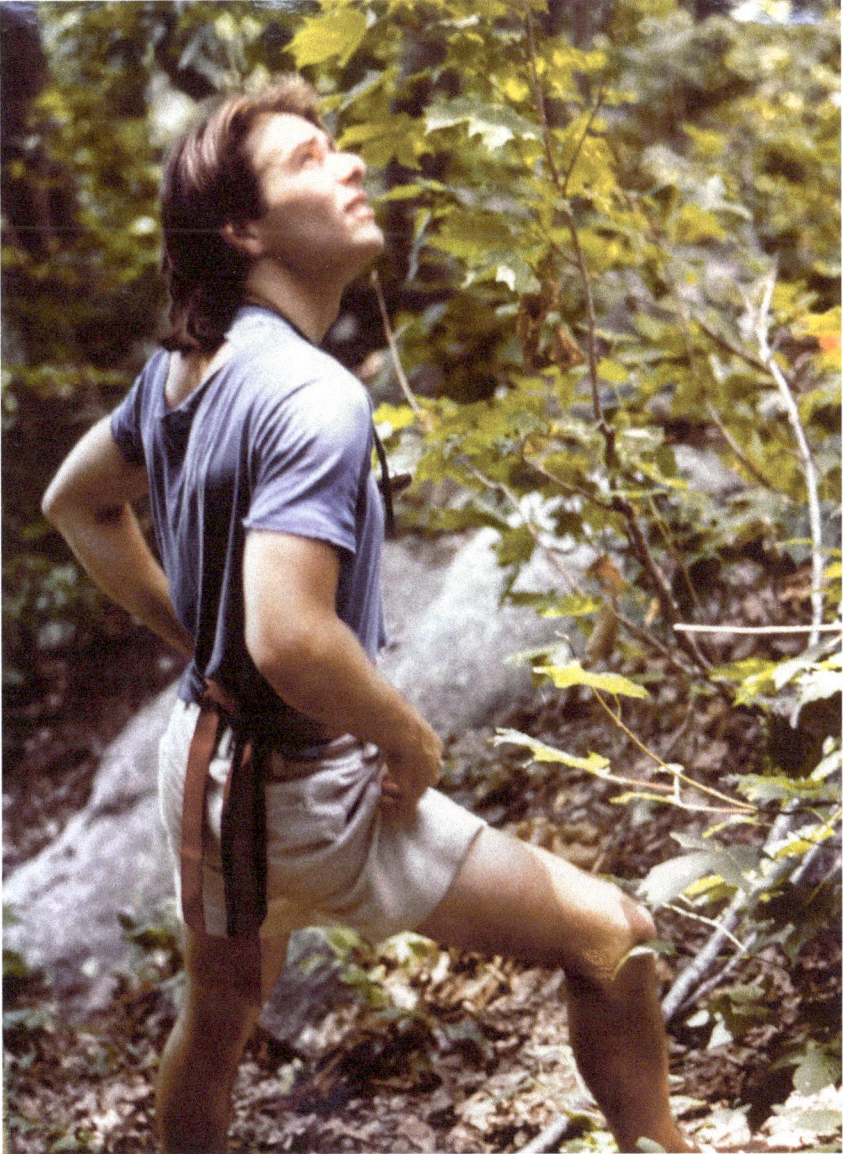

Albert Dow, 1953-1982.

EPILOGUE

Albert put forth tremendous service in his life, tremendous love, and I
thought it would be a disgrace to his memory to give up the fight.
—Hugh Herr

On the morning of Aug. 17, 2018, eighteen members of the Dow family are making their way up the Mount Washington Auto Road. It is a mild, cloudy day, with fog below the summit. They are here to participate in a ceremony that will dedicate the Mount Washington Observatory's Extreme Weather Exhibit in the name of Albert Dow, a fitting tribute to a man who, along with other rescuers, braved extreme conditions on this mountain in 1982 in a desperate search for Hugh Herr and Jeff Batzer.

Albert's sisters, Susan Dow-Johnson and Caryl Dow, along with their children and grandchildren and Albert's fiancée, Joan Wrigley, have boarded the Auto Road's stagecoach van to take the 7.6-mile ride to the Sherman Adams Building, part of Mount Washington State Park, where the ceremony will be held. On the way, just beyond the five-mile post, the van takes a sharp right turn at Cragway Corner. The family traveled there in August 1982, the month of Albert's birth, to spread his ashes. "We chose a spot on the road where we could get as close as we could to Huntington Ravine," recalls Susan. "It was Caryl and I, our mother and father, my husband and two children, and Joan Wrigley. We walked out onto Nelson Crag as far as we could and spread his ashes. We set him free in the mountains."

Because of the low cloud cover and fog, the rim of Huntington Ravine is barely discernible out of the large left windows of the van, but Susan and Caryl know the ravine is the site of their brother's last climb. Today, it is the location of the Dow Emergency First-Aid Cache. The cache was unofficially dedicated to Albert when his friend and MRS teammate Matt Peer asked a woodworker to make a sign for the structure that read: ALBERT DOW KILLED BY AVALANCHE JANUARY 25, 1982.

In March 2001, after a large avalanche in Huntington Ravine significantly damaged the cache, the Forest Service repaired it and placed it lower down in the ravine. It was officially rededicated on Jan.

26, 2004, and a new bronze memorial mounted in its place.

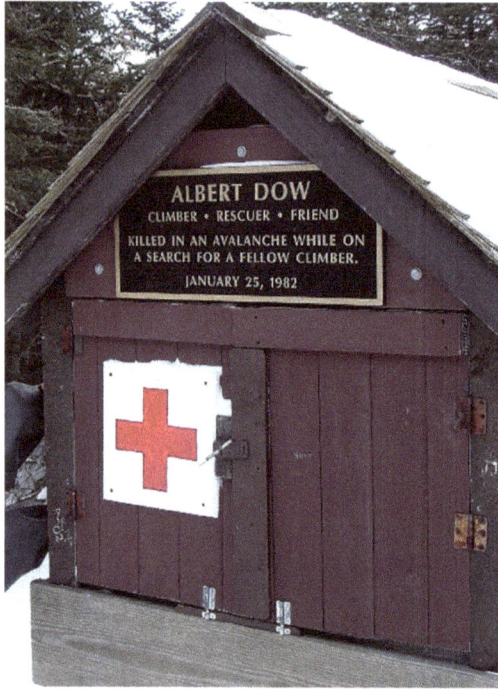

Once they arrive at the summit, the Dow family and Joan Wrigley are warmly greeted by members of the Observatory board and staff, current and former members of Mountain Rescue Service, members of the New Hampshire Fish and Game Advanced Search and Rescue Team, snow rangers, AMC personnel, and many others who knew Albert or are friends of the family.

Amy Brown takes a deep breath and marvels at the vast number of people who've gathered in to honor her late Uncle Albert. At 41, she is the only one of Albert's nieces and nephews who was born early enough to have known him. She was too young to remember when he called her 36 years ago in his classic Kermit the Frog voice to wish her a happy fifth birthday three days before his death. But she does remember how much she loved him "It was nice to meet some people at the dedication who I hadn't met before, like Uncle Albert's climbing buddy, Michael Hartrich," she says today.

Fourteen months after he survived the avalanche that claimed Albert, in March 1983, Hartrich left Mountain Rescue Service. He and members of the team had responded to Mount Washington for a hiker who was killed after falling into Raymond Cataract. "The mountain was a sheet of ice, and it was really pretty treacherous," he says. "We put the body in the litter and started heading back over to the Auto Road. I was giving commands, and they became brusque commands. After a teammate commented on my behavior, I started to think about it and realized I was really under stress. I thought maybe I shouldn't be involved in these situations anymore. I might be putting other people in danger."

Hugh Herr, who has established a warm relationship with Albert's two sisters over the years, is present at the summit and will offer remarks during the ceremony. "The Dow family is just remarkable," he says today. "They have been deeply kind toward me from day one."

Jeff Batzer is not among the attendees, but Susan has begun corresponding with him. For Batzer, Albert's death and his own rescue have played a decisive role in how he's chosen to live his life. "At the time, I made climbing a form of idolatry," he says. "I pushed off other things in my life—God, family, friends. I knew I needed to follow God more closely and serve him. Albert's death had a profound impact on me. I learned that my actions could have a lasting effect on others. My family and I have felt a deep sense of sorrow for the Dow family's loss and for a life short lived. I'm incredibly grateful to Albert for giving everything in order to try to get to Hugh and me. Both Hugh and I carry a deep sense of humility for our part in what happened. While I realized from the beginning that God had forgiven me, I am grateful to the Dow family for their kindness and forgiveness through the years."

A year after his rescue, Batzer was asked to speak at the Milton-Hershey School in Pennsylvania. "I was terrified of public speaking at first. From there I got one call after another to speak. Over the course of the next 10 years, I spoke almost 300 times along the eastern seaboard and shared the story of how God saved my life. I received a seminary degree and started pastoral work, spending 17 years with my congregation. I also did leadership work with international missions for 26 years."

Hugh Herr says that while he and Batzer have taken different paths in the aftermath of their rescue, they have both lived their lives with a sense of purpose in an effort to give back to others for the price Albert paid in searching for them. "I was so inspired by all these humans that selflessly acted to help a stranger: Albert giving the ultimate cost, all the rescuers, all the medical personnel, the helicopter crew, the nurses," he says. "I became this incredible fan of humanity. That was my response to what happened, to the extraordinary level of love and empathy we received."

Almost two years after he was rescued, Herr returned to North Conway to live until he attended college in Pennsylvania in 1985. With the assistance of prosthetics, he had started climbing again. Although his presence in town generated a lot of interest and some controversy, he quickly integrated into the climbing scene. Many of those with whom he climbed and socialized were some of the very people who had searched for him.

After earning a degree in physics from Millersville University, Herr went on to attend the Massachusetts Institute of Technology, where he was awarded a degree in mechanical engineering. From there, he earned a PhD in biophysics from Harvard University. Today he is a professor of media arts and sciences at MIT and the director of the Biomechatronics Group at the MIT Media Lab, where he is helping create bionic limbs that emulate the function of natural limbs.

"Everybody has written about what Hugh has become and how the rescue transformed him into the person he is today," says Michael Hartrich. "I've always said they're really doing an injustice to Hugh because he was an extraordinarily intelligent and driven person at age 17, when it all happened. The avalanche and their getting lost didn't make him what he is. It might have directed where he went, but he was an extraordinary person to begin with."

A small camera crew is following Herr from a distance. They are here to film *Augmented*, a documentary about Herr and his groundbreaking work in the field of prosthetics. But he and the crew are doing their best to stay on the sidelines in order to give the family the place they deserve at this event.

Sharon Schilling, executive director of the Mount Washington Observatory, welcomes the gathering and introduces Caryl Dow. With sister Susan standing beside her, Caryl offers opening remarks about their brother and his impact on others:

Recently, I hiked just outside Denver at the Garden of the Gods, a place where Albert had been to climb. I walked with intention and a sense of wonder at the beautiful things I might see: birds, trees, animals, clouds, heart rocks, I saw them all! I saw them all because Albert taught me to see beautiful things by doing the simplest thing of all; slow down, breathe, smell the roses. My sense is he learned this from the simple life our parents gave us, simple but full of love and acts of kindness toward others at every turn.

Albert was a humanitarian. This is why he was a member of MRS. We are all part of Albert's legacy when we slow down and smell the roses.

Caryl then turns to Herr and addresses these words to him:

No one is more Albert's living legacy than Hugh Herr. Yes, Albert gave his life searching for Hugh and Jeffrey, and Hugh has given his life back to science by changing the world's view of disability by changing the lives of amputees. Without Albert, we might not be slowing down to smell the roses. Without Albert, we would not have Hugh's work.

Herr is visibly moved by her words as he steps up to offer his own remarks. Saying that he has dedicated his life to service in honor of Albert's sacrifice, he adds in part:

I am certain wherever Albert is in the universe, he continues to rescue people. He continues to make souls smile and laugh and continues to emulate love. I know here on Earth, he continues to make us smile in his memory and provide us with inspiration and hope. So thank you, Albert, for all your inspiration to me and to so many other people. And thank you so much for venturing out in the young winter of 1982 in search of two lost boys.

Rick Wilcox, who is here on behalf of Mountain Rescue Service, recalls the response to Caryl's and Hugh's words. "Albert's sisters stood side by side with Hugh and told us that Albert's life was given so that Hugh would have his career to help so many people. It was a tear-jerker."

MRS members Joe Lentini, Steve Larson, Rob Walker, and Bill Kane, who all took part in the rescue, are also present at the event with several other current and former team members. Lentini, who is next to speak, offers these reflections:

There are days in your life that change everything forever. The day Albert died on Mount Washington, that cold and windy day, was one of those days. Each of us must decide, when we're dealing with a life-changing experience, whether it's going to lock us into that time or become something that helps us grow. I feel it would be a disservice to Albert if I carried bitterness in my heart over his death. That's not the person he was. Over time, he's helped me strive to be a more forgiving person, to try to be someone who doesn't judge others.

People often ask me why we do it, why we go out in dangerous conditions. I know Albert would answer the same way I'm answering now: Climbers take care of climbers. It's not for us to judge when we're called out. We go out for those in need. I believe it is the best of human nature that we strive to help people in need.

Susan and Caryl then approach the exhibit and remove the cloth covering the memorial plaque.

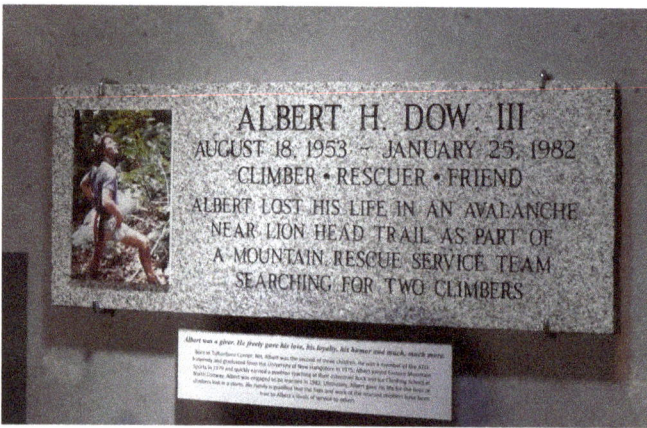

Though this ceremony is happening almost four decades after Albert Dow's death, family members say that he remains a prominent presence within the Dow family. "Albert is not somebody we never talk about," niece Amy says. "Every time something comes up or somebody does something that is honorable, someone in our family will say, 'That's something Albert would have done!' The core value in our family is "Love your neighbor as yourself."

As if to confirm Amy's words about her uncle's lasting impact, the Dow family has another Albert-inspired event to attend the following day, when they will be helping out at the Granite Man Triathlon in Wolfeboro, N.H. The triathlon was founded in 1982 to support the Albert Dow III scholarship, first awarded in June of that year and given annually to a Kingswood High School graduate who "exemplifies unselfish devotion to the service of mankind." Since its inception, it has offered approximately $200,000 to 60 deserving students from Albert's alma mater.

Abigail Morrissey, a 2016 recipient, recently explained that for her the scholarship was not so much about the money as it was about the meaning she has drawn from receiving the award. "I am acutely aware of the privilege and honor that comes with receiving the Albert Dow III scholarship," she said. "It not only supported my academic pursuits but also serves as a wealth of inspiration and motivation to continue embodying the principles of service that Albert Dow exemplified. I'm committed to honoring his legacy by upholding these values and striving to contribute meaningfully to society."

In the mountains as well, Albert's legacy will continue to be reflected in the selfless service of kindred spirits. Joe Lentini spoke for many when he said at the Observatory event: "As winter approaches, I know I'll be high on Mount Washington. I'll think of Albert and see the smile on his face, and I'll know he'll always be there with me."

RESOURCES

White Mountains Avalanche and Weather Forecasts

Mount Washington Avalanche Center: A partnership between the Mount Washington Avalanche Center Foundation and the U.S. Forest Service. Provides avalanche forecasts for the Presidential Range. (mountwashingtonavalanchecenter.org)

Mount Washington Observatory: Home of the Higher Summits Forecast and Forecast Discussion for the White Mountains of New Hampshire. (mountwashington.org)

Outdoor Education and Safety

Hike Safe: A joint program between the White Mountain National Forest and New Hampshire Fish and Game to create and develop a Mountain Safety Education Program. Learn more about the Hiker's Code and the Ten Essentials for backcountry travel and purchase a Hike Safe card, which supports search and rescue in New Hampshire. (hikesafe.com)

New Hampshire Outdoor Council: Learn more about search and rescue teams and backcountry safety in New Hampshire. This all-volunteer nonprofit organization is worthy of support. (nhoutdoorcouncil.org)

International Mountain Climbing School: Offers rock and ice climbing, mountaineering, and avalanche and outdoor training courses in North Conway, N.H. (climbimcs.com)

Eastern Mountain Sports Climbing School: The oldest climbing school in the East. Offers rock and ice climbing, mountaineering, skiing, and other outdoor courses.

Appalachian Mountain Club: Offers several four-season outdoor courses and workshops. (outdoors.org)

Professional mountain guide services: These can be found throughout the Mount Washington Valley.

Avalanche Education and Training

Eastern Snow and Avalanche Workshop: A nonprofit venture of the Mount Washington Avalanche Center that offers an annual professional development seminar for backcountry enthusiasts and avalanche safety professionals. (esaw.org)

The American Institute for Avalanche Research and Education: A nonprofit educational organization founded to create an evidence-based avalanche education model for backcountry users. Offers training at both recreational and professional levels. (avtraining. org)

East Coast Avalanche Education: Provides avalanche training to students within the Green and White Mountains of northern New England. (eastcoastavalancheeducation.com)

American Avalanche Institute: Provides applicable information for use in the field. Focuses on hands-on learning and coaching. (americanavalancheinstitute.com)

The Albert H. Dow III Scholarship Award

Donations to the scholarship fund may be made c/o New Hampshire Charitable Foundation, 37 Pleasant St., Concord, NH 03301.

HIKER RESPONSIBILITY CODE

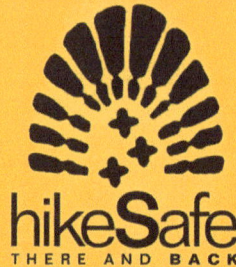

hikeSafe
THERE AND **BACK**

You are responsible for yourself, so be prepared:

1. **With knowledge and gear.** Become self reliant by learning about the terrain, conditions, local weather and your equipment before you start.

2. **To leave your plans.** Tell someone where you are going, the trails you are hiking, when you'll return and your emergency plans.

3. **To stay together.** When you start as a group, hike as a group, end as a group. Pace your hike to the slowest person.

4. **To turn back.** Weather changes quickly in the mountains. Fatigue and unexpected conditions can also affect your hike. Know your limitations and when to postpone your hike. The mountains will be there another day.

5. **For emergencies,** even if you are headed out for just an hour. An injury, severe weather or a wrong turn could become life-threatening. Don't assume you will be rescued; know how to rescue yourself.

6. **To share the hiker code with others.**

hikeSafe: It's Your Responsibility.

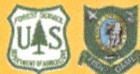

The Hiker Responsibility Code was developed and is endorsed by the White Mountain National Forest and New Hampshire Fish and Game.

Hike Safe, a mountain safety education program, was developed jointly by the White Mountain National Forest and New Hampshire Fish and Game.

Recommended Clothing and Equipment for Hikers

For Summer Day Hikes:
The Ten Essentials
  Map & Compass
  Warm Clothing
    Sweater or Pile Jacket
    Long Pants (wool or synthetic)
    Extra Socks
  Extra Food and Water
  Flashlight or Headlamp
  Matches/Firestarters
  First-aid kit/Repair kit
  Whistle
  Rain/Wind Jacket and Pants
  Pocket Knife
  Sturdy Footwear and Socks

Add for Overnight Trips and Groups:
Sleeping Bag
Foam Pad
Tent or other shelter
Extra Clothing
Pots, Cup, Bowl, Spoon
Food
Water Purification
Toothbrush, Towel, etc.
Stove, Fuel

Watch
Hat (wool)
Trash Bag (for trash or rain protection)
Light Plastic Tarp or "Space" Blanket
Guidebook
Insect Repellent
Sunglasses
Sun Lotion
Gloves or Mittens
Personal Medications
Cord/Rope
Gaiters
Extra Batteries

Add for Winter:
Extra Warm Clothing
  Insulated Parka
  Extra Mittens
  Balaclava
  Insulated Boots
  Overmitts
  Snowshoes

Add for Above Treeline:
Crampons
Face Mask
Ice Axe
Goggles

Add for Avalanche Terrain:
Avalanche Transceiver
Avalanche Probe
Snow Shovel

IN CASE OF ACCIDENT OR EMERGENCY CALL:
New Hampshire State Police 1-800-525-5555 or 911

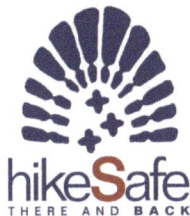

hikeSafe
THERE AND BACK

https://hikesafe.com

Acknowledgments

The support I've received throughout this project has been humbling, and I am incredibly grateful to everyone I talked with for their help and trust. I could not have shared this story, which is so broad in scope, without them.

Susan Dow-Johnson and Caryl Dow: Thank you for your time, support, and trust throughout this project. Your devotion to your brother's memory, and the love and kindness you put out in the world, have had a profound impact on me.

Hugh Herr and Jeff Batzer: Thank you for the trust you placed in me to recount your ordeal. I believe your vulnerability, transparency, and insights will save lives in the backcountry. Thank you also for pursuing a life of service to others.

Michael Hartrich: Thank you for your willingness to share your experiences over the course of your days of searching on Mount Washington and the aftermath of the avalanche that befell you. I am deeply grateful for your time and trust, and I will never forget the weight of our conversations at Pope Memorial Library. With admiration and respect for your resiliency and sacrifice.

Mountain Rescue Service (past and present): Thank you to everyone who welcomed me into your homes, shared a cup of coffee, or took the time to answer any question I posed. You and your organization are a shining example of resiliency, humility, and service to others. Nick Aiello-Popeo, Bill Aughton, Alec Behr, Peter Cole, Alain Comeau, Paul Cormier, Ryan Driscoll, Frank Hubbell, Bill Kane, Steve Larson, Joe Lentini, Doug Madara, Chris Noonan, Matt Peer, Paul Ross, Dana Seavey, Rob Walker, Michael Wejchert, and Rick Wilcox.

The Law Enforcement Division of the New Hampshire Fish and Game Department: Col. Jeff Gray (ret.), Col. Kevin Jordan, Lt. Jim Kneeland, Lt. Bob Mancini, and Lt. Mark Ober.

The U. S. Forest Service: Chris Joosen, Rene LaRoche (ret.), Marianne Leberman, Charlotte MacDonald, Jessica Marunowski, Justin Preisendorfer, Pat Scanlon, and Daniel Sperduto.

The New Hampshire Army National Guard: Chief Warrant Officer 4 Ronald Boyer (ret.), 1st Sgt. Earl Foss (ret.), Lt. Col. Greg Heilshorn, Gen. David Mikolaities, and Brig. Gen. John Weeden (ret.).

The Appalachian Mountain Club (past and present): Melissa "Cam" Bradshaw, Bill Corbin, Jack Corbin, Abigail Coyle, Paul Cunha, Alan Kamman, Bill Meduski, Gary Newfield, Chris Thayer, Jeff Tirey, Mike Waddell, Dave Warren, Chris Woodside, and James Wrigley.

Mount Washington Observatory: Jay Broccolo, Drew Bush, Charlie Buterbaugh, Donna Dunn, Brian and Stephanie Fitzgerald, Rob Kirsch,

Ryan Knapp, Gary MacDonald, Charlie Peachey, Ken Rancourt, Myha Rather, Bruce Soper, and Brenda Sullivan.

Jeff Fongemie of the U.S. Forest Service and Mountain Rescue Service, Joe Gill, formerly of U.S. Forest Service and Appalachian Mountain Club, and Dale Atkins: Thank you for your insights and expertise on avalanche hazard and analysis of the 1982 tragedy on Lion Head.

Dr. Nicole Sawyer: Thank you for your insights and expertise on critical incident stress in the first-responder community.

Dr. Gordon Giesbrecht and Dr. Campbell McLaren: Thank you for your insights and expertise on hypothermia and frostbite.

Archivists Becky Fullerton at the Appalachian Mountain Club and Dr. Peter Crane at Mount Washington Observatory for your efforts during my research. I'm so thankful to you and your organizations for preserving the history of our White Mountains.

My editor, Lucille Stott: Thank you for everything you have done to help me through our years of working together. I am so fortunate to have your expertise and perspective during the writing process. Your patience and support as I worked through some of life's inevitable challenges is something I'll always be grateful for. Thank you for your friendship.

My publisher and illustrator, Ted Walsh: It all started with a single illustration almost a decade ago. I'm so grateful for your willingness to publish these stories, and for your creativity and vision in bringing them visual context. I also appreciate your allowing me to stay close to the process from start to finish. Thank you for your friendship.

Early readers Bob Champlin, Doug Nelson, Chris Noonan, Jeff Fongemie, Paul Fitzgerald, Heather Cummings, and Laura Waterman: Thank you for your time, and for your candid and helpful feedback.

My sincere thanks to the following people who helped me during the project: Danold Ampagoomian, Henry Barber, Jaime "Stomp" Bernard Don Bolduc, David Boudreau, Amy Brown, Hank Butler, Joe Butler, Rob Buxton, Taylor Caswell, Steven Chase, Allan Clark, Gail Clark, Jim Cole, Seth Cooper, Rick Gross, Justin Cutting, Mike Dickermann, Sam Danais, Mark Doyle, Andrew Drummond, Jimmie Dunn, Tiffany Eddy, Dan Egan, Julie Fetzner, Jim Frati, Patrik Frisk, Paul Geissler, Sandy Geisler, Govenor Wentworth School District staff, Rick Gross, Les Hinson, Kingswood High School staff; Mark Kirk, Ken Krause, Laura Knoy, Jack Lawlor, Bea Lewis, Karen Libby, Spencer Logan, Lynn Lyons, Bill MacGregor, Nick Martini, Geoffrey May, Maggie McGovern, Mike McLaughlin, Fletcher Missud, Brenda Monihan, Tom Morse, Abigail Morrissey, Tom Morse, Kerry Muricchio, Patrice Mutchnick, Rebecca Oreskes, Matthew Orr, Chris Patridge, Mike Pelchat, Dr. Kristen Pierce, Matt Pierce, John Porter, Ron Reynolds, Primex Board & Staff, Ed Rolfe, Teresa Rosenberger, Gen. Richard Safreed, Linda Shoemaker, Kacy Terrell St. Clair, Steve Smith, John Stevens, Sarah Stewart, Matt Stohrer, Lin Stone, Layne Terrell, Barbara

Tetreault, Bruce Twyon, Denise Valley, Orrin and Linda Welch, Paul Woyda, Jim Wheeler, Jed Williamson, Tom Wilson, and Joan Wrigley.

My wife, Debbie: I am absolutely certain I could not have taken on this story without your love, support, and presence. You were always there for me as I struggled with writing *Lions* amid life, work, and a deeply personal loss. Thank you for your patience and encouragement. You sacrificed a lot to help me bring this to completion. And my three children, Matthew, Megan, and Tyler, and their families for their love and support.

I assume full responsibility for any errors. During my research I spoke with several technical and subject matter experts, and those who were asked to recall events from decades ago. I have done my best to present this story as accurately as possible. If I got any of the details wrong, the mistakes are mine alone.

Selected Bibliography and Further Reading

American Alpine Club (various editors): Since 1948, the American Alpine Club has issued an annual publication entitled *Accidents in North American Mountaineering*. Current and past postings are available online at http://publications.americanalpineclub.org.

Appalachian Mountain Club (White Mountain Guide Book Committee). *White Mountain Guide, 22nd Edition*. Boston, MA: AMC Books, 1979.

Billings, Marland P., et al. *The Geology of the Mount Washington Quadrangle New Hampshire*. State of New Hampshire Department of Resources and Economic Development, (Second reprinting) 1972.

Bliss, L.C., *Alpine Zone of the Presidential Range*. Edmonton, Canada: L.C. Bliss, 1963.

Giesbrecht, Gordon G., and Wilkerson, James A. *Hypthermia, Frostbite, and Other Cold Injuries: Prevention, Survival, Rescue, and Treatment*. Seattle, WA: The Mountaineers Books, 2006.

Goldthwait, Richard P., *Geology of the Presidential Range*. Hanover, NH: The New Hampshire Academy of Science, 1940.

Herr, Patricia Ellis. *Up: A Mother and Daughter's Peakbagging Adventure*. New York, NY: Crown Publishing, 2012.

Howe, Nicholas, *Not Without Peril: 150 Years of Misadventure on the Presidential Range of New Hampshire*. Boston, MA: AMC Books, 2010.

Hubbell, D.O., Franklin R., *Wildcare: Working in Less Than Desirable Conditions and Remote Environments*. Conway, NH: TMC Books LLC/Stonehearth Open Learning Opportunities, 2014.

LeBlanc, John-Paul. *Mount Washington Rescue Report*: January 23-26, 1982. Concord, NH: Department of Health and Welfare; Division of Public Health, 1982.

Lewis, Peter S., and Wilcox, Rick. *An Ice Climber's Guide to Northern New England*, 3rd Edition. Conway, NH: TMC Books, 2002.

Logan, Nick, and Atkins, Dale. *The Snowy Torrents: Avalanche Accidents in the United States 1980–86*. Denver, CO: Colorado Geological Survey, 1996.

Mayer, Doug, and Orsekes, Rebecca. *Mountain Voices: Stories of Life and Adventure in the White Mountains and Beyond*. Boston, MA: Appalachian Mountain Club Books, 2012.

Orr, Matthew. *Augmented*, Arlington, VA: PBS, 2019.

Peachey, Charlie. "Mount Washington Observatory Rain-On-Snow Research Study": Provides detailed data findings, graphics, and explanations from the Observatory's climate change research project. (https://mountwashington.org/research/current-research-projects/rain-on-snow/), 2024.

Osius, Alison. *Second Ascent: The History of Hugh Herr.* New York, NY: Stackpole Books, 1991.

Putnam, William Lowell. *The Worst Weather on Earth.* Gorham, NH: The Mount Washington Observatory and The American Alpine Club, 1991.

Roberts, David. "The Mechanical Boy Comes Back." *Outside Magazine*, Chicago, IL: Mariah Publications Corporation, 1983.

STEPT Studios for Arc'Teryx Films. *109 Below.* New York, NY, 2023.

Stott, Sandy. *Critical Hours: Search and Rescue in the White Mountains.* Dartmouth, NH: University Press of New England, 2018.

Washburn, Bradford (maps). "Tuckerman Ravine: Boot Spur and Lion Head." Boston, MA: Grand Circle Foundation for Boston's Museum of Science and the Appalachian Mountain Club, 1993.

—"Mount Washington and the Heart of The Presidential Range." Boston, MA: Boston's Museum of Science for the Appalachian Mountain Club and the Mount Washington Observatory, 1989.

Waterman, Laura and Guy. *Yankee Rock and Ice: A History of Climbing in the Northeastern United States.* Mechanicsburg, PA: Stackpole Books, 1993.

Waterman, Laura and Guy. *Forest and Crag: A History of Hiking, Trail Blazing, and Adventure in the Northeast Mountains.* Boston, MA: AMC Books, 2003.

Wejchert, Michael, *Hidden Mountains: Survival and Reckoning After a Climb Gone Wrong.* New York, NY: Ecco Press, 2023.

Wilcox, Rick, and Dogarf. *New Hampshire Ice: A Select Guide.* Littleton, NH: Sherwin Dodge Printers, 2021.

Wylie, Evan McLeod. "The Rescue That's Still Being Debated." Dublin, NH: *Yankee Magazine*, Part I: January 1983; Part 2: February 1983.

Photo and Illustration Credits

My heartfelt thanks to those organizations and individuals who provided me with images for the book. Many of these photos are over 40 years old, and I'm grateful to those who located and provided slides to me, or had them digitally converted.

Bill Hemmel, Lakes Region Aerial Photos
• Front cover

David C. D. Stone with permission of Lin Stone
• Title page, pages 141, 148, back cover

Joan Wrigley
• Dedication page

Mount Washington Observatory
• Page viii (Ken Rancourt), pages 238, 410

Ted Walsh, TMC Books
• Pages xi, 8, 10, 27, 28, 45, 56, 76, 96, 104, 123, 127, 133, 135, 158, 180, 184, 190, 202, 209, 236, 248, 257, 271, 281, 283, 286, 288, 297, 298, 300, 313, 320, 323, 330, 351, 360, 367, 391

Jeff Batzer
• Pages 2, 6, 192

Hugh Herr
• Pages 4, 7

Susan Dow-Johnson and Caryl Dow
• Pages 14, 16

Joe Lentini, Mountain Rescue Service
• Pages 19, 22, 110, 124, 200

Appalachian Mountain Club
• Page 26

State of New Hampshire Bureau of EMS
• Page 306

The Brad Washburn Gallery/Mount Washington Observatory
• Pages 30, 86, 246

Kacy St. Clair
• Page 36

Todd Swain and the Harvard Mountaineering Club
• Pages 37, 46

David Lottmann, Northeast Alpine Start
• Page 52

Jim Frati
• Page 54

United States Forest Service/Mount Washington Avalanche Center
• Pages 100, 164, 206, 258, 278, 406

Joe Gill
• Pages 119, 264, 277

Col. Jeff Gray, New Hampshire Fish and Game
• Page 145

Geoffrey May
• Pages 176, 263

Misha Kirk with permission of Patrice Mutchnick and Mark Kirk
• Pages 210, 212, 252, 314, 318, 324

Paul Ross
• Pages 216, 222

S. Peter Lewis
• Pages 234, 240

David Warren
• Page 308

New Hampshire Army National Guard
• Page 339

Jim Cole
• Page 381

Alain Comeau
• Page 403

• Author photo: Kimberly Davis, Photography by Kimberly

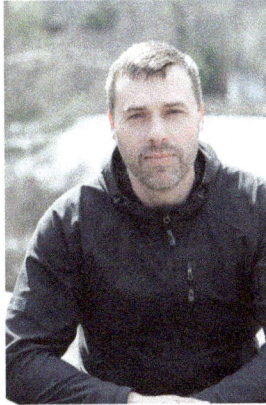

About the Author

Ty Gagne is chief executive officer of New Hampshire Public Risk Management Exchange (Primex³), a public entity risk pool serving local governments in New Hampshire. He is the author of the books *Where You'll Find Me: Risk, Decisions, and the Last Climb of Kate Matrosova* (2017) and *The Last Traverse: Tragedy and Resilience in the Winter Whites* (2020). Two of his essays, "Emotional Rescue: A hiker becomes a benefactor as she follows a set of sneaker prints" and "Weakness in Numbers: How a Hiking Partner can be Dangerous," were published in *Appalachia* journal.

www.ingramcontent.com/pod-product-compliance
Lightning Source LLC
Chambersburg PA
CBHW050806270326
41926CB00026B/4562